THE SCIENCE OF

BEAUTY THERAPY

By the same author
The Science of Hairdressing

Ruth
Bennett

THE SCIENCE OF

Beauty Therapy

Hodder & Stoughton
LONDON SYDNEY AUCKLAND TORONTO

To Martin and Frances

British Library Cataloguing in Publication Data
Bennett, Ruth
  The science of beauty therapy.
  1. Beauty care services. Scientific aspects
  I. Title
  646.7' 2' 015

ISBN 0 340 48684 8

First published 1990
Third impression 1992
© 1990 Ruth Bennett

Typeset by Taurus Graphics, Abingdon, Oxon.
Printed in Hong Kong for Hodder and Stoughton Educational, a
division of Hodder and Stoughton Ltd, Mill Road, Dunton Green,
Sevenoaks, Kent by Wing King Tong Co. Ltd.

Contents

Acknowledgments

I wish to thank Miss Della Bingley of Coventry Technical College and Ms Lyn Goldberg and Mr Alan Warren of the London College of Fashion for generous help and advice during the preparation of this book. I am also grateful for specialist advice on Chapter 15 from Dr Alan Bedford of the Open University.

I am greatly indebted to Mrs Mary Robinson of Coventry Technical College and to Mr Dick Welsh, Assistant Secretary, Northern Council for Further Education and Chief Examiner for CGLI Hairdressing and Beauty Therapy Science, for their careful reading of the manuscript and most valuable comments.

The publishers would like to thank the following for permission to reproduce photographs in this book:

Cover: Camera Press, London and The Sanctuary (see below)

Black and white photographs: Dr J Almeida, p 35; Bel-art Products 1989, p 40; Dalesauna, p 201; Empire Stores Limited, p 42; Walter Gardiner Photography, p 37; John Lawrence Photography Limited, p 31; Dr D W R MacKenzie, p 34; The Sanctuary, p 214; Tony Brain/Science Photo Library, p 62; NIBSC/Science Photo Library, p 205; George Solly Organisation Limited, pp 1, 37, 100, 136, 181, 232, 240, 254, 267, 287; Taylor Reeson Laboratories, pp 56, 77, 155, 194; Unilever, p 59

Colour photographs: pp 295–302, The Sanctuary, 11 Floral Street, London, WC2E 9DH; Beauty Therapists: Kate Jackson, Andrea Lomas; Models: Dawn Little, Mary Phillips

Every effort has been made to trace copyright holders of material reproduced in this book. Any rights not acknowledged here will be acknowledged in subsequent printings if notice is given to the publishers.

Foreword

In this book Ruth Bennett gives a full and comprehensive account of the applied science required by students studying for beauty therapy examinations. Students will find Chapter 1 particularly useful as it gives a good insight into the basic scientific principles necessary for the understanding of the materials which follow in Chapters 15 and 16.

As well as embracing all the scientific information necessary for the examinations, the science covered also concentrates on the anatomy and physiology, physical and electrical sciences and cosmetic chemistry behind the activities and treatments taking place in the beauty salon.

I congratulate Ruth on her book which has been written with great care and the wealth of detail, coupled with her illustrations, reflect her very extensive experience. It should succeed in its aims.

Richard S Welsh
Chief Examiner for CGLI:
Hairdressing and Beauty Therapy Science

Preface

This book is intended for students taking courses in Beauty Therapy who are preparing for the examinations of the City and Guilds of London Institute Certificates in Beauty Therapy (304), Manicure (302), Cosmetic Make-up (303) and Electrical Epilation (305), the International Health and Beauty Council Diplomas, those of the British Association of Beauty Therapists and Cosmetologists, and of the BTEC National Diploma in Beauty Therapy. Much of the material also has relevance to courses such as the City and Guilds Science Foundation Course, CPVE modules in Beauty Care, TVEI courses and GCSE, A/S Level Human Biology.

The material in this book aims to provide a scientific explanation of the procedures carried out in a beauty salon. Chapter 1 is intended to explain briefly those basic scientific concepts required for an understanding of the material in later chapters.

A number of self-assessment questions are included at the end of each chapter to which the answers will be found in the relevant chapter by careful reading of the text. Most of these questions resemble the shorter type of question which occurs in the examination papers set by the City and Guilds and the International Health and Beauty Council. Some longer questions placed at the back of the book resemble those in Section B of the examination papers mentioned above.

CHAPTER I

Foundation science

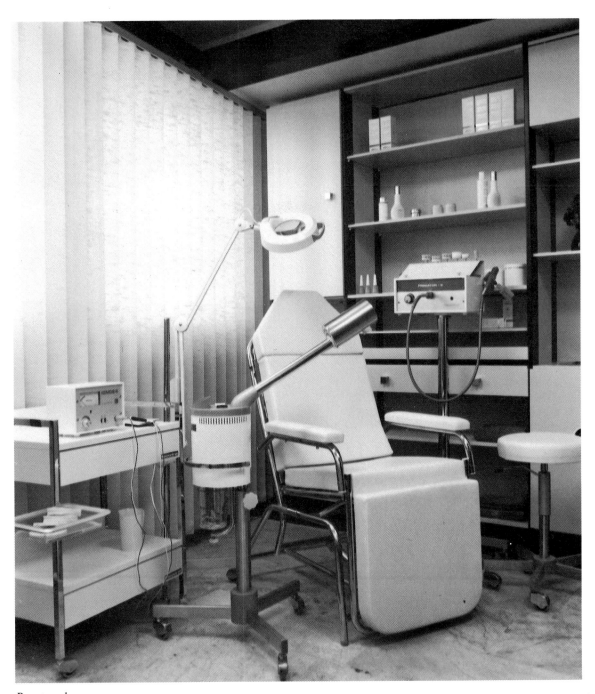

Beauty salon

Physical science

Measurement

Both a number and a unit are needed to give a value to a particular quantity such as weight or energy. The number is obtained by measurement using a specific unit. Scientists use the *metric* system of measurement, and *SI* (international system) units. Larger or smaller quantities are derived by multiplying or dividing these units by multiples of ten.

Table 1.1
Units

Name of unit	Dimension	Conversion	Subdivisions & multiples
Metre (m)	Length (distance between two points in space)	1 m = 39.37 inches	1 m = 100 centimetres (cm) 1 m = 1000 millimetres (mm) 10^{-6} m = 1 micrometre (μm) 10^{-9} m = 1 nanometre (nm)
Cubic metre (m^3)	Volume (amount of space)	16.38 cm^3 = 1 cubic inch	10^{-3} m^3 = 1 litre (l) 10^{-6} m^3 = 1 cubic centimetre (cm^3) = 1 millilitre (ml)
Kilogram (kg)	Mass (amount of matter) Weight $\left(\begin{array}{l}\text{pull of gravity on a}\\\text{mass}\end{array}\right)$	1 kg = 2.2 lbs 28.34 g = 1 oz	1 kg = 1000 grams (g) 1 g = 1000 milligrams (mg)
Kilograms per cubic metre (kgm^{-3})	Density (mass per unit volume)		
Newton (N)	Force (a push or a pull)	4.45 N = 1 lb force	
Joule (J)	Energy (makes things happen)	4.2 J = 1 calorie 4200 J = 1 kilocalorie	1000 J = 1 kilojoule (kJ)
Degree Celsius (°C)	Temperature (hotness)	1 °C = $\frac{9}{5}$° Fahrenheit t °F = $\frac{5}{9}$ (t − 32) °C	

Nature of matter

All substances are composed of matter, and are divided into two large groups called **elements** and **compounds**. If a substance can be split up into two or more simpler substances by a chemical change, it is a compound. If it cannot be split up by these means it is an element. *Chemical changes* are those which are permanent and result in the formation of new substances.

Changes which are easily reversed, such as ice melting or salt dissolving in water, are *physical changes*. New substances are not formed by physical changes. Chemical changes are often called chemical *reactions*, and many of them are *exothermic*, giving out heat.

Matter is composed of very small particles called **atoms**. An element is made up of only one kind of atom, and there are as many different kinds of atom as there are elements. As the atoms of different elements have different masses, it is useful to compare these masses to obtain the *relative atomic mass*. The carbon atom is chosen as the standard at 12. A hydrogen atom has only one-twelfth of the mass of a carbon atom, so its relative atomic mass is 1. Chemical changes do not destroy or create atoms, but during them atoms will combine together to form **molecules.**

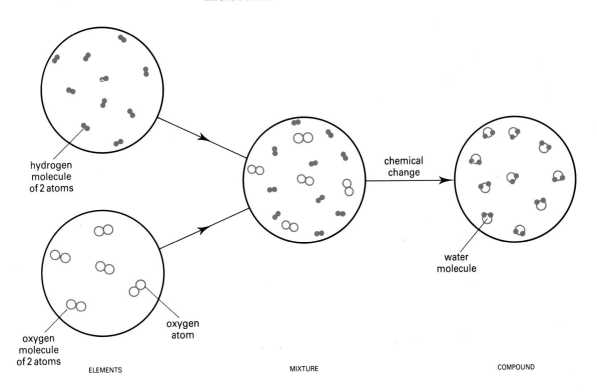

hydrogen
molecule
of 2 atoms

oxygen
atom

oxygen
molecule
of 2 atoms

ELEMENTS

chemical
change

MIXTURE

water
molecule

COMPOUND

Figure 1.1
Elements, mixtures and compounds

An *atom* is the smallest part of an element that can be involved in a chemical change. A *molecule* is the smallest part of an element or compound that can exist alone. Although both **mixtures** and compounds contain at least two substances, a mixture differs from a compound in that a chemical change is not involved in its formation. *Air* is a mixture of several elements (oxygen, nitrogen, neon) and compounds (water, carbon dioxide).

Table 1.2
Mixtures and compounds compared

Mixtures	Compounds
Are formed by a physical change (mixing)	A chemical change is involved in their formation, eg combustion or neutralization
Their properties are the sum of the properties of their components	Their properties are quite different from the properties of their components
They may vary widely in their composition	Their composition is fixed, ie the weight of each component does not vary
Their components can be separated by physical means, eg filtration, evaporation or distillation	Their components cannot be separated by physical means
The atoms or molecules they contain are arranged randomly	The atoms they contain have a regular arrangement

Atoms are made up of three smaller kinds of particle called **protons, electrons** and **neutrons**. Protons and neutrons cluster in the centre of the atom forming its nucleus. Electrons are much lighter in weight, and move round the nucleus at a fixed distance from it in a particular orbit called an *electron shell*. The number of each of these three subatomic particles varies in the atoms of different elements.

Figure 1.2
Hydrogen and copper atoms

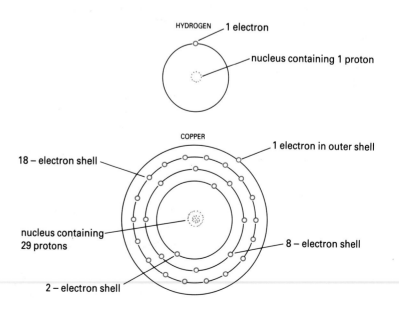

Protons have a positive, and electrons a negative electric charge. As a result of these unlike charges, protons and electrons attract one another. Neutrons have no electric charge. In each atom the positive and negative charges are balanced because it contains the same number of protons and electrons. All atoms are therefore *electrically neutral*. If an atom (or molecule) loses or gains electrons, it acquires an electric charge, positive or negative respectively, and becomes an *ion*. Ions which have a positive electric charge are *cations*, and those with a negative charge are *anions*. Both hydrogen and copper ions are cations.

Matter may occur in three forms, or *states*, known as solid, liquid or gas (vapour). If a solid becomes a liquid or a liquid becomes a gas, or vice versa, this is a *change of state*. Melting, solidifying, evaporating, condensing, boiling and freezing are all changes of state. When they occur, *latent* heat is either given out or absorbed. This explains why sweat cools the body when it evaporates; it takes latent heat from the skin when changing from the liquid to the gaseous state.

Table 1.3
States of matter

Gases	Liquids	Solids
Molecules move at high speeds	Molecules stick together (cohere) but can slide over one another	Molecules can move only very slightly
Exert a pressure which increases with increasing temperature	Exert a pressure which increases with temperature, but which is less than gas pressure	Molecules are often arranged in regular patterns so the solid is crystalline
Can be compressed to occupy a much smaller volume	Can be compressed very much less than gases	Cannot be compressed
As the temperature drops, a liquid is formed	As the temperature drops, a solid forms at freezing point. As the temperature increases a gas forms by evaporation, and the liquid finally boils	As the temperature increases a liquid forms at the melting point

Solubility

When some substances are added to a liquid they dissolve and form a **solution**. The substance which dissolves is the *solute*, and may be a solid, liquid or gas. Some solutes ionize (ie split up into ions) in solution, and are called *electrolytes*. If all the solute molecules ionize, the substance is a *strong* electrolyte. If only a few of the molecules ionize, the substance is a *weak* electrolyte.

If none of the molecules ionize, the substance is a *non-electrolyte*. The liquid in which the solute dissolves is the *solvent*.

Solid solutes will be left behind if the solution *evaporates*, eg when the water (solvent) in sweat (solution) evaporates, the salt (solute) is left behind on the skin. Liquid or gaseous solutes are separated from the solution by *distillation*. The solute molecules are evenly distributed throughout the solution, which is therefore a *homogeneous* mixture. A solution looks *transparent* (clear) as the dissolved particles are too small to be visible. The solute molecules cannot be removed from the solution by *filtering* it through a filter paper.

A *concentrated* solution contains a large amount of solute, while one which is *dilute* contains very little. A *saturated* solution contains as much solute as it can hold at that temperature. *Concentration* is usually expressed in terms of the number of *moles* of solute in one litre of solution (mol l^{-1}). A mole is the unit used to describe the amount of chemical substance and is calculated from the relative atomic masses of each element in the substance. The relative atomic mass (in grams) of every element contains the same number of atoms (6×10^{23}) and equals one mole of the element. Thus, since a mole of sodium chloride (salt) contains this fixed number of sodium atoms (relative atomic mass 23) and the same number of chlorine atoms (relative atomic mass 35.5), one mole of sodium chloride has a mass of:

$$23 \text{ g} + 35.5 \text{ g} = 58.5 \text{ g}$$

A solution of sodium chloride with a concentration of 1 mol l^{-1} contains 58.5 g dissolved in 1 litre of solution.

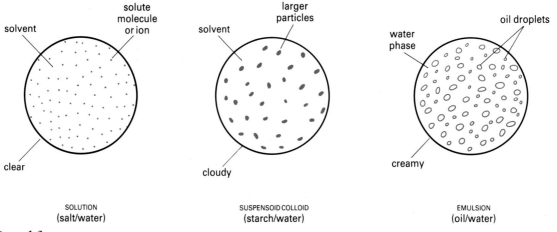

Figure 1.3
Solutions and colloids

Suspensions may form from insoluble solids which remain homogeneously mixed with a liquid. The solid particles in a suspension are usually large enough to be removed by filtering, and to be visible so that the suspension looks cloudy. On standing, the solid particles slowly separate out of the liquid as a visible layer. A clay-based face pack is an example of a suspension.

In a **colloid** the suspended particles are smaller than those in a suspension, but larger than the individual molecules in a solution. On standing, the particles do not settle out but are kept in suspension by continuous collisions with solvent molecules. This jostling effect is known as *Brownian movement*. The particles in a colloid are small enough to pass through a filter paper, and can be split into two classes: *suspensoids* where the particles are solid, and *emulsoids* where the particles are tiny liquid droplets. Soap and starch form suspensoids, mixing with water to form a colloid which is cloudy in appearance. If the colloid is very concentrated, a semi-solid *gel* is produced. Emulsoid colloids are usually called *emulsions*.

An **emulsion** is thus a suspension of droplets of one liquid in another liquid, where the two liquids are immiscible (one liquid does not dissolve in the other). An emulsion is known as a *cream* when the two liquids are oil and water, and many cosmetics are formulated as creams. The tiny droplets of the suspended liquid form the *disperse phase* of the emulsion, while the other liquid forms the *continuous phase*. Where oil droplets form the disperse phase an *oil-in-water* (o/w) emulsion is produced. When water droplets form the disperse phase the emulsion is of the *water-in-oil* (w/o) type.

Figure 1.4
Structure of an emulsion

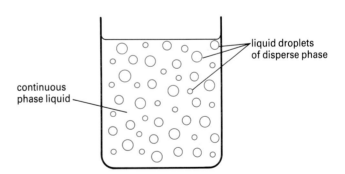

continuous phase liquid

liquid droplets of disperse phase

The two types of emulsion have different properties. An o/w emulsion is less greasy and can be rinsed off the skin with water. A w/o emulsion is very greasy and cannot be rinsed away. It must either be wiped off the skin using a paper tissue, washed off by a detergent solution, or removed by another oil which is miscible with the continuous phase of the emulsion.

When preparing an emulsion, the oil and water phases must be heated separately, and an *emulsifying agent* (emulsifier) added before stirring the two phases together.

Classification of chemical substances

The elements are divided into **metals** and **non-metals**, and each element is represented by a chemical symbol which may also represent one atom of that element, eg Cu represents copper and one atom of copper.

Table 1.4
Metals and non-metals compared

Metals	Non-metals
Solids, with the exception of mercury	May be gases, liquids or solids
Have lustre (shiny)	Solid non-metals are dull except carbon in the form of diamond
Dense (heavy)	Have a low density (light in weight)
Good conductors of heat and electricity	Poor conductors of heat and all except carbon are poor electrical conductors
Can be hammered into sheets and drawn out into wire	Solid non-metals are brittle
Form basic oxides	Form acidic oxides
Form positive ions (cations)	Form negative ions (anions), except hydrogen

Table 1.5
Characteristics of some important elements

Element	State	Metal or non-metal	Protons	Symbol
Hydrogen	Gas	Non-metal	1	H
Boron	Solid	Non-metal	5	B
Carbon	Solid	Non-metal	6	C
Nitrogen	Gas	Non-metal	7	N
Oxygen	Gas	Non-metal	8	O
Fluorine	Gas	Non-metal	9	F
Neon	Gas	Non-metal	10	Ne
Sodium	Solid	Metal	11	Na

Table 1.5 (cont)

Element	State	Metal or non-metal	Protons	Symbol
Magnesium	Solid	Metal	12	Mg
Aluminium	Solid	Metal	13	Al
Silicon	Solid	Non-metal	14	Si
Phosphorus	Solid	Non-metal	15	P
Sulphur	Solid	Non-metal	16	S
Chlorine	Gas	Non-metal	17	Cl
Potassium	Solid	Metal	19	K
Calcium	Solid	Metal	20	Ca
Chromium	Solid	Metal	24	Cr
Manganese	Solid	Metal	25	Mn
Iron	Solid	Metal	26	Fe
Cobalt	Solid	Metal	27	Co
Nickel	Solid	Metal	28	Ni
Copper	Solid	Metal	29	Cu
Zinc	Solid	Metal	30	Zn
Silver	Solid	Metal	47	Ag
Tin	Solid	Metal	50	Sn
Iodine	Solid	Non-metal	53	I
Tungsten	Solid	Metal	74	W
Gold	Solid	Metal	79	Au
Mercury	Liquid	Metal	80	Hg
Lead	Solid	Metal	82	Pb

Compounds form the majority of chemical substances and are divided into two groups:

- *Organic* compounds are those containing the element *carbon* and are usually found in, or made by, living organisms. Many have large complex molecules due to the ability of carbon atoms to link up in chains. Proteins and starches are organic compounds;

● *Inorganic* compounds are the rest of the compounds. They may contain any of the elements, and the majority have small molecules, eg sodium chloride (salt) and water.

Figure 1.5
Organic and inorganic molecules

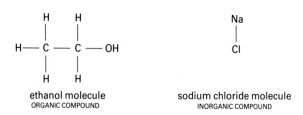

Compounds are arranged in a number of *classes* based on a study of their structure and properties:

● **Oxides** are the compounds formed when elements combine with oxygen. This occurs during the chemical change of burning (combustion). The oxides of non-metals, eg carbon dioxide (CO_2), are *acidic,* turning litmus solution red. The oxides of metals, eg calcium oxide (CaO) are *basic,* turning litmus solution blue. *Litmus* and other dyes which change colour in acidic and basic chemicals are called *indicators.*

The degree of acidity or basicity (alkalinity) is measured on the *pH scale.* This scale goes from 0 to 14. In the range 0 to 6.9 the lower the pH value, the greater the acidity. Above 7 the greater the pH value, the more basic (alkaline) the chemical becomes. A substance which is neither acidic nor basic has a pH of 7 and is said to be neutral.

Acidity is closely related to the concentration of hydrogen ions in a solution. The pH corresponding to a hydrogen ion

Figure 1.6
The pH scale

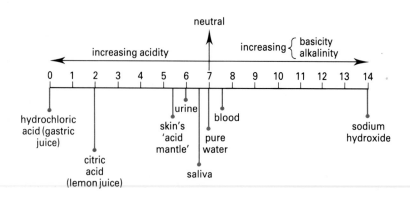

concentration of 1.0×10^{-3} mol l^{-1} is 3, ie the index figure 3 is used as the pH value. An increase in pH indicates a decrease in hydrogen ion concentration. A neutral solution contains 1.0×10^{-7} mol l^{-1} of hydrogen ions, so the index 7 becomes the neutral pH value. A basic solution has less than 1.0×10^{-7} mol l^{-1} of hydrogen ions, so its pH is greater than 7;

- **Acids** are formed when acidic oxides react with water. They ionize in aqueous solution to give hydrogen ions.

$$CO_2 + H_2O \rightarrow H_2CO_3 \rightarrow H^+ + HCO_3^-$$

acidic   water   carbonic   hydrogen   hydrogen
oxide   acid   ion   carbonate ion

   Inorganic (mineral) acids in solution usually contain a high concentration of hydrogen ions as they are *strong electrolytes*, and thus have a low pH. They are known as strong acids, examples being sulphuric acid (H_2SO_4) and hydrochloric acid (HCl). Some inorganic acids, eg carbonic and phosphoric acids, are *weak electrolytes* so they have a slightly higher pH, and are known as weak acids. *Organic* acids are also weak electrolytes and weak acids. Examples are citric acid (in lemon juice) and fatty acids. Organic acids contain a *carboxyl* group (–COOH) from which hydrogen ions are produced.
   Diluting an acid by dissolving it in a large volume of water increases its pH by reducing the concentration of hydrogen ions. (NB *It is very dangerous to add water to concentrated acid. Always add small volumes of acid to a large volume of water)*;

- **Basic oxides** may react with water to form metal *hydroxides*. A few metal hydroxides are soluble in water, ionizing to produce *hydroxyl* ions (OH$^-$), and are called **alkalis**. Examples of alkalis are sodium, potassium and calcium hydroxides. Although it is not a metallic hydroxide, *ammonium hydroxide* (NH_4OH) resembles other alkalis in its properties and is included with them.

   A solution of an acid contains *hydrogen* ions and *acid radicle* ions. A solution of an alkali contains *hydroxyl* ions and *metal* ions. When these two solutions are mixed many of the hydrogen and hydroxyl ions disappear as they combine together to form *water* molecules. The acid radicle and metal ions remain as an ionized *salt*. This chemical reaction is called *neutralization* as the product, water, is neutral. It is expressed by the following equation:

$$acid + base = salt + water$$

- **Organic bases** include the *alcohols* which contain a hydroxyl group (–OH), and the *amines* which contain an

Table 1.6
Properties of acids and alkalis

Acids	Alkalis
Turn litmus red	Turn litmus blue
Dilute solutions have a sour taste	Dilute solutions have a bitter taste and feel soapy
Many are dangerous corrosive compounds causing chemical burns	Are dangerous caustic compounds causing chemical burns
Have a pH below 7	Have a pH above 7
React with alkalis to form a salt and water by the chemical change of neutralization	React with acids to form a salt and water by the chemical change of neutralization

amine group ($-NH_2$). Examples of alcohols are methanol, ethanol, propanol and glycerol. Triethanolamine is an example of an amine. Organic bases will combine with acids to form *esters* and water:

organic acid + organic base = ester + water

- **Salts** are produced when the hydrogen of an acid is replaced by a metal or an ammonium group. They are also produced by the neutralization of an acid by a base or an alkali. Salts form metal ions which are positively charged (cations) and acid radicle ions which are negatively charged (anions). Soluble salts are highly ionized in water and are therefore strong electrolytes.

  If a salt is formed from a strong acid and a strong base (eg sodium chloride) it will form a *neutral* solution with a pH of 7. A salt formed from a weak acid and a strong base (eg sodium phosphate) will form an *alkaline* solution with a pH above 7. This is due to a small proportion of the acid radicle (eg phosphate) ions reacting with water to form acid molecules (eg phosphoric acid) and hydroxyl ions. This reduces the number of hydrogen ions present, and increases the pH.

  phosphate ions + water molecules =
  phosphoric acid + hydroxyl ions

  Where it is important to keep the *pH* of a mixture *stable*, as in acid creams and chemical depilatories, a *buffer* is

Table 1.7
Salts

Metal	Acid radicle	Common name
Calcium	carbonate	Chalk
Magnesium	silicate	Talc
Potassium	palmitate	Soft soap
Sodium	chloride	Common salt
Sodium	stearate	Hard soap
Zinc	carbonate	Calamine

required. A buffer can be made from a weak acid and the sodium salt of that acid, commonly phosphoric acid and sodium phosphate. As phosphoric acid is only slightly ionized but sodium phosphate is highly ionized, a mixture of the two compounds in water contains few hydrogen ions but many phosphate ions. If a small amount of *acid* is added to the buffer, the hydrogen ions from the acid will combine with phosphate ions to form molecules of phosphoric acid. There is thus no increase in the concentration of hydrogen ions, so the pH does not fall. Similarly, if a small amount of *alkali* is added to the buffer, the hydroxyl ions from the alkali combine with hydrogen ions to form water. Further ionization of phosphoric acid molecules then occurs to replace the lost hydrogen ions and lower the pH again;

- **Esters** are produced when alcohols react with organic acids. Ethyl, butyl and amyl acetates used as nail lacquer solvents are esters. Esters of *glycerol* combined with three molecules of long chain *fatty acids* are called *triglycerides*. They occur in plant and animal fats and oils. *Phospholipids* are more complex esters containing phosphate groups. *True waxes* are usually esters formed from long chain fatty acids and from alcohols such as cetyl alcohol or cholesterol;

- **Hydrocarbons** (alkanes) consist of molecules containing long chains of carbon atoms to which hydrogen atoms are attached. As their name suggests, they contain the elements hydrogen and carbon only. They are present in natural gas and petroleum which are *fossil fuels* derived from once-living organisms. Methane (CH_4) is present in natural gas. Alkane gases, petrol, mineral oil, petroleum jelly and paraffin wax are all obtained from petroleum.

Salon water supply

Water authorities are required to supply tap water which is free from visible suspended particles, disease-producing organisms (pathogens), and chemical substances injurious to health (pollutants). The original source of all water supplies is rainfall, which is part of the *natural water cycle* on the earth.

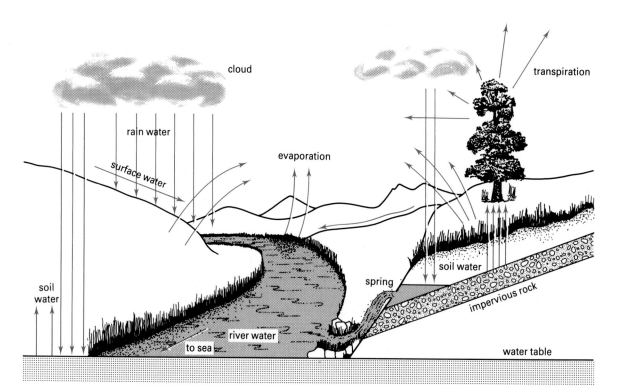

Figure 1.7
The water cycle

Water is taken from lakes and rivers, and stored in reservoirs placed at a higher level than the buildings they supply. A *head of water*, ie the distance between the water level in the reservoir and the level of the service pipes to the buildings, produces a water *pressure*. Where there is no head of water available, tap water must be *pumped* into water towers or directly into the service pipes to achieve a water pressure.

The water must be *treated* in various ways to remove suspended particles (by filters), pathogens (by chlorine) and pollutants (by suitable chemical treatments) before entering the service pipes. In some areas *fluoride* is added as a protection against tooth decay. The service pipe must supply at least one cold tap, which should be used for *drinking water*, before the

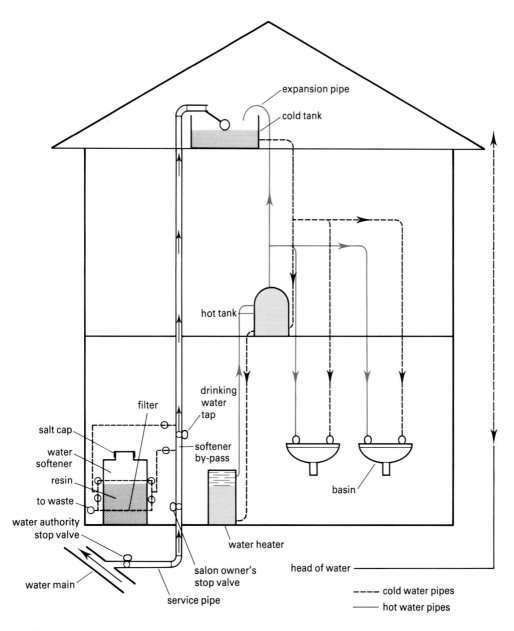

Figure 1.8
Salon water supply

water enters a cold tank for storage and circulation through the salon water system.

Distilled water and *rainwater* from clean air districts contain no dissolved solid impurities and are *soft*. Most tap water, however, does contain dissolved salts, and is *hard*. Hard water forms a *scum* with soap, which prevents it from lathering readily. It also deposits *scale* when heated. Soft water, on the other hand, forms neither scale nor scum, and lathers readily with soap.

The *impurities* which make water hard have come from the rocks over which the water source flows. They consist of the four ionized *salts*: calcium sulphate, calcium hydrogen carbonate (bicarbonate), magnesium sulphate and magnesium hydrogen carbonate (bicarbonate). The calcium and magnesium ions react with soap to form an insoluble *calcium* or *magnesium soap* called a scum. Thus, soapless detergents, such as sodium lauryl sulphate, have a great advantage over soap in that they do not form a scum with hard water.

Hardness due to *hydrogen carbonates* will be removed by boiling the water and is said to be *temporary*. Boiling converts the hydrogen carbonate into insoluble metal carbonate salts and carbon dioxide is released.

$$\text{calcium ions} + \text{hydrogen carbonate ions} \xrightarrow{\text{heat}} \text{calcium carbonate molecules} + \text{carbon dioxide}$$

Hardness due to *sulphates* cannot be removed by boiling and is said to be *permanent*. All types of hardness can be removed from tap water on a small scale by the addition of a *chemical water softener* such as sodium hexametaphosphate (Calgon), sodium carbonate (washing soda) or sodium borate (borax). Sodium carbonate and borate form insoluble particles by reacting with the calcium and magnesium ions in the hard water, and increase its alkalinity. This method of water softening does not prevent the scaling of pipes in a hot water system.

For softening the entire salon water supply an *ion-exchange* method is used. The hard water flows through a cylinder containing a column of synthetic *resin* (derived from polystyrene) which contains negatively charged *acidic groups* at the surface. These are neutralized by *sodium ions* to form a sodium salt of the resin. As hard water flows through the cylinder, its calcium or magnesium ions are *exchanged* for sodium ions from the resin. After a certain volume of hard water has passed over the resin column all its sodium ions will have been exchanged, so water softening ceases. The resin column is *regenerated* by passing a concentrated solution of sodium chloride through it. This washes out the calcium and magnesium ions and replaces them with sodium ions.

Fundamentals of heating

Heat is a form of energy. It is produced by burning fuels, by human bodies, and by friction when two surfaces are rubbed together, eg during massage. In a beauty salon heat is produced by different types of *appliances* which convert other forms of energy into heat.

A beauty salon requires a supply of *hot water* for washing and laundry all the year round. The usual temperature of a hot water supply is 60 ° Celsius. This temperature will not cause much scaling of hot water pipes where tap water is hard, but is hot enough for normal salon purposes.

A suitable *air temperature* must be maintained for the comfort of clients undergoing beauty treatments. The air temperature needs to be at least 20 ° Celsius, with an optimum temperature two or three degrees higher for maximum comfort.

Temperature is measured by a **thermometer**, an instrument which compares the *hotness* of a substance (eg water or air) with that of melting ice or boiling water. A thermometer contains a liquid (mercury or coloured alcohol) in a narrow tube with a basal bulb. The liquid *expands* as the temperature increases, giving a reading on a scale marked in degrees Celsius (°C). The *fixed points* on this scale are the temperature of melting ice at 0 °C, and that of boiling water at 100 °C. Body temperature is around 37 °C.

A special type of thermometer, called a clinical thermometer, should be used to take body temperatures. It has a strong bulb containing the mercury, and a narrow temperature range from 35 °C to 45 °C. Temperatures higher than this will cause the thermometer to break due to increased expansion of the mercury, so it must always be washed in cold water. The narrow tube containing the mercury has a *constriction* to prevent the mercury level from falling after body temperature has been registered. The thermometer must, therefore, be shaken after use to bring the mercury level down to below 35 °C.

Figure 1.9
Clinical thermometer

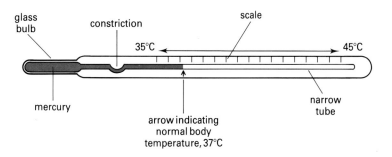

Temperature is regulated by a **thermostat**. It acts by cutting off the fuel supply to a heater once it reaches a selected temperature. When the temperature falls, the fuel reaches the heater again to bring the temperature up to its required value. Thermostats are fitted to most electrical appliances used in a beauty salon that produce heat.

The simplest type of *electrical* thermostat contains a *bimetal strip*. The scientific principle on which its action is based is that different metals *expand* by different amounts for the same temperature rise. Most metals, including *brass*, expand on heating and contract on cooling. The alloy *invar* (a mixture of steel and nickel), however, hardly expands at all on heating. Thus, if a strip of brass and a strip of invar are joined together to form a bimetal strip which is then heated, the brass expands more than the invar, causing the bimetal strip to *bend*. As the strip cools it will *straighten* again because the brass contracts to its original length.

In a thermostat, the electricity flows through a bimetal strip to reach a *heater*. The heater warms the bimetal strip which bends, breaking the electrical contact and preventing electricity from reaching the heating element of the appliance.

Figure 1.10
Electric thermostat

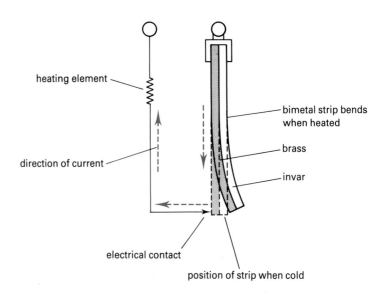

Heat produced by an appliance, or by the body, can be *transferred* in three possible ways, ie by conduction, convection or radiation.

Water heating appliances include a central heating system, immersion heaters and instantaneous water heaters. The fuel converted is either gas or electricity. *Salon space heating* appliances include a central heating system, but also an air-conditioning system, electrical floor or ceiling heating systems, balanced flue heaters and infra-red wall heaters.

Table 1.8
Methods of heat transfer

	Conduction	Convection	Radiation
How heat is transferred	Heat passes from one molecule to the next	Heat passes by the movement of heated molecules	Heat travels in straight lines as heat rays. All hot objects give out heat rays
Where the method occurs	Occurs most rapidly in solids. Metals are good thermal conductors	Occurs in liquids and gases	Occurs in gases and space
Properties of the method	Does not pass through thermal insulators such as glass, wool, plastic etc	Expansion of the heated gas or liquid increases its volume and reduces its density. The hot gas or liquid therefore rises. A stream of heated molecules forms a convection current	Dull, dark surfaces in the path of heat rays absorb them and become hotter. Shiny and light surfaces reflect heat rays and remain cool
Examples	Heat produced by friction passes by conduction through the skin to underlying muscle during massage	The movement of hot water in a hot water system and movement of warm air in a sauna are due to convection	Nichrome heating elements and infra-red heaters give out radiant heat

Fundamentals of lighting

Light is a form of **energy** which travels as waves. Light travels in straight lines, transferring energy from one place to another. A light *ray* is the direction of the path taken by light and is usually represented by an arrowed line. A light *beam* is a stream of light energy, in which the light rays may be parallel, diverging or converging.

Objects become *visible* when light rays are reflected from them and reach the eye of the observer. When all the light rays falling on an object are either reflected or absorbed, the material is said to be *opaque*. If all the light rays pass through an object, the material is *transparent*. However, if some of the light rays pass through the object while the rest are reflected, the material is *translucent*. Thus, metal objects are opaque, clean air and clear glass are transparent, and frosted glass is translucent.

When light passes from one transparent substance into another, the light rays are bent or *refracted*. When light rays are *reflected* from a shiny surface (a mirror) the angle at which the light rays strike the mirror (*angle of incidence*) is equal to the angle at which they bounce off (*angle of reflection*). These two angles are measured from a line at right angles to the mirror surface called a *normal*. A salon mirror usually has a flat surface and is therefore a *plane* mirror. The *image* produced in the mirror by reflection is the same size as the object, and appears to be as far behind the mirror as the object is in front of it.

Figure 1.11
Refraction and reflection of light rays
(a) Refraction of light
(b) Reflection in a mirror

(a)

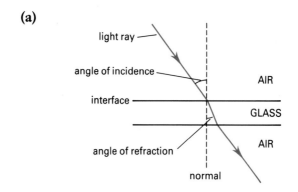

(b)

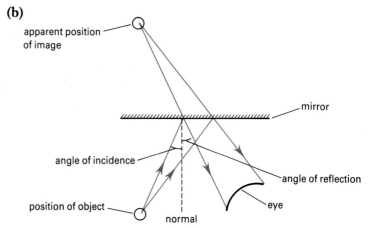

The *intensity* of light is an important factor in salon lighting since clear vision depends on adequate light intensity. This is governed by the *inverse square law*, which states light intensity decreases with the square of the distance from the light source. If you double the distance between yourself and a window allowing daylight to enter, only one quarter of the original light intensity will now reach your eyes.

Light of low intensity causes *eye-strain*. High light intensity without *glare* or deep *shadows* is required from a salon lighting system. Some form of *artificial* lighting to increase light intensity is almost always required in a salon. Electrical energy is converted by *lighting appliances* into light and heat energy. The

Figure 1.12
Inverse square law

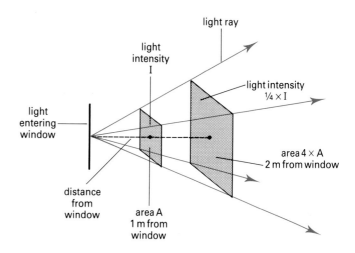

tungsten filament lamp (light bulb) converts electrical energy into 10% light and 90% heat. A *fluorescent tube* containing low pressure mercury vapour converts around 30% of the electrical energy into light so it is a more efficient lighting appliance.

Colour

The impression of colour is due to the nature of **white light**, and the way that certain molecules called **pigments** or *dyes* absorb and reflect light rays. White light can be split up into a number of component coloured light rays by passing it through a *prism*. This process is called *dispersion*, and the component colours of the light are a spectrum.

Figure 1.13
Dispersion of light

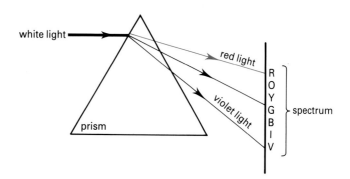

Light rays of different colours have different *wavelengths*. Red light, at one end of the visible spectrum, has the longest wavelength. Violet light, at the other end of the spectrum, has the shortest wavelength. The wavelength is the distance between the crest of a wave in the light ray and the crest of the following wave.

Figure 1.14
Wavelength differences

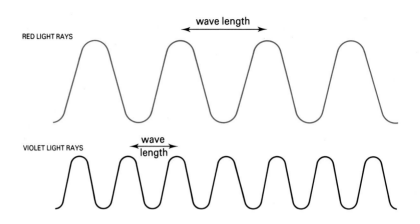

If *red, green,* and *blue* light of equal intensity are combined, white light is obtained. Red, green and blue are therefore known as the *primary* colours of light. Mixing any two primary colours of light produces the *secondary* colours, ie *yellow* (red + green), *magenta* (red + blue) and *cyan* (green + blue). A secondary colour together with the missing primary colour will produce white light. This is illustrated by the colour triangle.

Figure 1.15
Colour triangle

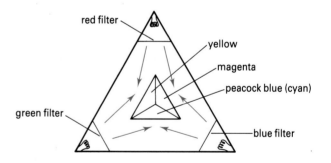

Pigments and *dyes* reflect light of the colour they appear to be, and absorb other colours. Viewed in white light, red pigments and dyes reflect the red light rays but absorb the green and blue rays. The colour of a pigment or dye will be affected by the colour of the light falling upon it. A pigment that looks red in white light will look more vivid in red light, but in blue light it will look black as there is no red light for it to reflect.

Artificial light has a spectrum which is slightly different from that of natural daylight so pigments and dyes look a slightly different colour in the two types of light. *Tungsten filament lamps* give out light containing more red and less blue light than daylight. Under this form of artificial lighting red and orange pigments and dyes will look brighter than in daylight, magenta will look redder, and blue will look duller. *Fluorescent tubes* are available to produce a range of white lights, ie with slightly different spectra. The light produced may resemble daylight, or may contain more red light (warm white) or more blue light (cold white).

This has applications in *colour matching* and in choosing coloured cosmetics suitable for day or evening make-up. Day make-up should always be applied in a salon area illuminated by natural daylight or daylight fluorescent tubes, so that the make-up will colour match day-time clothes. Evening make-up, however, should be applied in a salon area illuminated by tungsten filament lamps or warm white fluorescent tubes to obtain good colour matching of make-up with evening wear.

Fundamentals of ventilation

Humidity

During the working day the salon air will alter in composition. As a result of evaporation the air will hold more water vapour so its *humidity* will increase. If air saturated with water vapour is cooled, water droplets will condense out of it at a temperature known as the *dew point*. Air is not usually saturated with water vapour, and its humidity is expressed as % *relative humidity* (% RH).

$$\% \text{ RH} = \frac{\text{Actual amount of water vapour in the air}}{\text{Amount of water vapour saturating the air at the same temperature}} \times 100$$

For comfort, salon air should have a % RH between 40 and 50. If it reaches 70, sweat will not evaporate to cool the body adequately, and *heat fatigue* will cause headache, tiredness and irritability.

Ventilation

Stale air contains an increased amount of *carbon dioxide* and a reduced amount of *oxygen* due to human breathing. The number of *micro-organisms* is increased, and these survive well in the warm, humid, stale air, becoming a health hazard.

Ventilation is the process by which stale air is replaced by fresh air. It is needed to keep the composition of the salon air stable, and to prevent too great a rise in temperature. *Over-ventilation* causes draughts which reduce comfort and rapid loss of heat which is uneconomic. A *balance* between space heating and ventilation must be maintained for comfort.

Ventilation occurs by the physical processes of *diffusion* and *convection*, assuming that suitable entrances for fresh air and exits for stale air are provided. Diffusion is the movement of molecules to distribute themselves evenly throughout the space they occupy. Convection currents consist of the upward movement of heated molecules and the downward movement of cooling ones.

Natural and artificial ventilation

Natural ventilation occurs through open windows and doors, louvres, ventilating bricks and Cooper's discs placed in windows. Open windows and doors usually cause *draughts*, but the other three devices provide draught-free natural ventilation.

Figure 1.16
Methods of natural ventilation
(a) Louvred window
(b) Cooper's disc

(a)

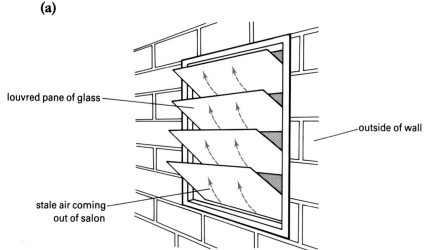

louvred pane of glass

outside of wall

stale air coming out of salon

(b)

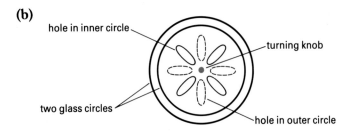

hole in inner circle

turning knob

two glass circles

hole in outer circle

Extractor fans and air conditioning are methods of ventilation by *artificial* means. They provide controlled ventilation free from draughts.

Basic electricity

Conductors and insulators

Materials such as plastic, glass, hair, nylon and ebonite produce *frictional* (static) electricity or **electric charge** when they are rubbed together. The electric charge is due to the internal structure of the *atoms* forming the material. *Electrons* from the surface atoms of one of the materials are transferred to the surface of the material rubbing against it. The surface *losing* the electrons becomes *positively* charged, while the one *gaining* the electrons becomes *negatively* charged. This happens when a plastic comb is energetically pulled through the hair. The comb gains electrons and acquires a negative charge, leaving the hair positively charged. The oppositely charged surfaces *attract* one another and, when they are close enough, the electrons jump back again. *Energy* is released as small flashes of light and crackling sounds as the electric charge is lost.

Substances which develop a *static* electric charge are electrical **insulators** so an electric charge (electricity) is unable to travel through them. Metals and water, however, will allow a flow of electric charge, called an *electric current*, through them, and are therefore electrical **conductors**. If the outside of an electrical appliance is made entirely of insulating material (eg plastic) it is said to be *all-insulated*. *Double-insulated* equipment may have some exposed metal, but extra insulation is fitted inside to prevent wires carrying an electric current from touching the exposed metal. The symbol

indicates that an appliance is double-insulated. All-insulated and double-insulated appliances do not need the safety device called an *earth wire* to prevent electric shock.

Figure 1.17
Movement of electrons in copper wire

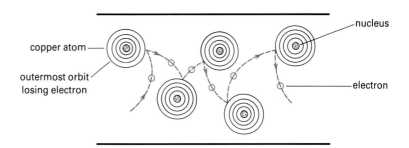

In electrical conductors the outer electrons of the atoms are able to move in a *random* way from atom to atom. The electric current passes when the free electrons move in the *same direction*. In some conductors the free electrons move less readily so there is some *resistance* to the flow of electric current. The energy used in overcoming this resistance produces heat and light, and the material is known as a *high resistance* conductor. *Nichrome* (an alloy of nickel and chromium) used in heating elements and *tungsten* used in light bulb filaments are both high resistance conductors. *Copper* has a very low electrical resistance so it will conduct an electric current without becoming hot and is used in the conductor wires of an electric circuit.

Electrical units

A *force* is needed to drive electrons round an electric circuit, which is provided by the mains supply or a battery. This electrical force, or *pressure*, is called *voltage,* and is measured in units called **volts** (V).

The number of electrons passing any point in the circuit in each second determines the *strength* or *intensity* of the electric current. The unit of rate of flow of electric current is the **ampere** (amp).

The ability of a conductor to *resist* the flow of electric current is measured in units called **ohms**. One volt of electrical pressure keeps a current of 1 amp flowing through a circuit with a resistance of 1 ohm.

$$\text{current in amps} = \frac{\text{pressure in volts}}{\text{resistance in ohms}}$$

Figure 1.18
Relationship between electric current, pressure and resistance

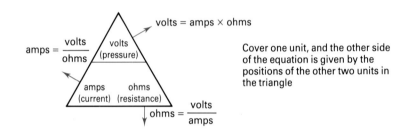

Sources of electricity

The flow of electric current from one place to another requires a *potential difference* between the two places. The size of the potential difference determines the electrical pressure and is measured in *volts.* As electrons are negatively charged, they flow through a circuit from the negative region towards a positive region where there is an electron deficit. As the direction of flow of current is usually described as being from positive to negative, this is actually in the *opposite direction* to the electron flow in a circuit.

Figure 1.19
Electron flow and direction of electric current

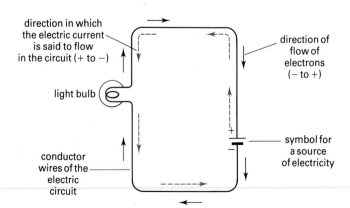

An **electric cell** makes use of chemicals to produce a potential difference which will drive an electric current round a circuit by exerting an electrical pressure. A *dry battery* is one type of electric cell in which there is an internal transfer of electrons from one of its *terminals* to the other. One terminal has a surplus of electrons, while at the other terminal there is an electron deficit. When the two terminals of a dry battery are linked by a conductor, electrons flow in *one direction* through the circuit to produce a **direct current** (DC). As electrons continue to be transferred inside the electric cell, the flow of current is maintained until the chemicals are used up. The chemicals used in a dry battery are known as the *electrolyte,* and the terminals are attached to *electrodes* made of conducting materials (a carbon rod and the zinc battery casing).

Figure 1.20
Structure of a dry battery

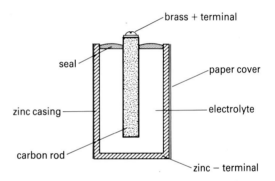

The *mains supply* is provided by large scale electric generators. The electric current they produce is usually an **alternating current** (AC) in which the direction of flow of electrons in a circuit *reverses* many times a second. A complete *cycle* is said to have occurred when the current which is flowing one way changes and flows in the opposite direction in the circuit, and then changes again to flow in the original direction. The current therefore changes direction *twice* in every cycle. The number of cycles in each second is the *frequency* of the current which is measured in units called *hertz* (Hz).

The electricity produced in power stations has a high voltage (11 000 V). This is further increased to 132 000 V when it passes into the power lines of the *National Grid.* It is then reduced to 240 V for the *mains supply* to the salon. In the UK the mains supply is usually AC with a frequency of 50 Hz and a pressure of 240 V. The mains supply may be different in other countries, so foreign appliances may not be suitable for UK mains. Continental mains usually provide AC of 50 Hz but 220 V, while in the USA AC of 60 Hz and 110 V is standard.

Effects of an electric current

In addition to heat and light, an electric current is able to produce mechanical movement (kinetic effects), magnetic fields, sound and chemical changes. On the body it causes muscle and nerve stimulation and electric shock. These effects are due to the conversion of one form of energy into a different one.

Table 1.9
Energy conversions in appliances

Appliance	Energy conversion
Fan	Electrical to kinetic
Light bulb	Electrical to heat and light
Audiosonic vibrator	Electrical to sound
Galvanic machine	Electrical to chemical effects
Faradic machine	Electrical to muscle stimulation

The amount of heat, movement or other effect that the electric current can produce in 1 second is the *electric power* or **wattage** of the appliance, measured in units called *watts*:

$$1 \text{ watt} = 1 \text{ amp} \times 1 \text{ volt}$$

$$1000 \text{ watts} = 1 \text{ kilowatt}.$$

The **heating effect** of an electric current is produced when it passes through *high resistance* wires. A nichrome heating element becomes red hot, and a thin tungsten filament in a light bulb becomes white hot producing light as well as heat. Both AC and DC produce heating effects.

The **chemical effects** of an electric current are produced when DC flows through solutions of *electrolytes*, including those in the body tissues, to cause chemical changes. Water containing dissolved substances which *ionize* (eg acids, alkalis, salts) will conduct an electric current due to the movement of the electrically charged *ions*. Pure water contains some ionized molecules, but, being a weak electrolyte, it conducts electricity less well. The process during which the chemical effects occur is called *electrolysis*. Two conductors called *electrodes* which are connected by wires to the source of the current are placed some distance apart in the electrolyte. The electrodes are called the *anode* (+) to which negatively charged anions are attracted, and the *cathode* (−) to which positively charged cations are attracted.

Chemical change occur in the region of the electrodes. In human tissues, which contain salt (sodium chloride) ionized in

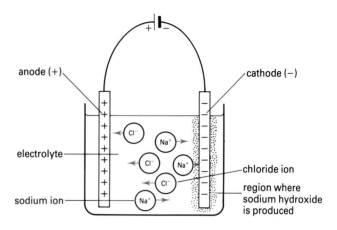

Figure 1.21
Electrolysis of sodium chloride
solution

anode (+)

cathode (−)

electrolyte

chloride ion

region where
sodium hydroxide
is produced

sodium ion

solution, electrolysis produces *sodium hydroxide* at the cathode to which the sodium cations travel, so this region becomes more *alkaline*. Acids are produced at the anode to which the chloride anions travel.

Electric circuits

Electric *circuits* link electrical appliances to the mains supply, providing a path for the flow of electrons. If a number of appliances are included in the same circuit, they may be connected in *series* or in *parallel*. When connected **in series** the current goes through each appliance in the circuit in turn. Any break in the circuit will stop the flow of current so all the appliances will stop working. Each additional appliance present in the circuit reduces the electric current as it increases the resistance.

Figure 1.22
Light bulbs connected in series

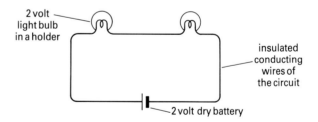

2 volt
light bulb
in a holder

insulated
conducting
wires of
the circuit

2 volt dry battery

Where the connections are **in parallel**, each appliance is connected directly to the source of electricity, and is independent of all other appliances in the circuit. In a salon *lighting circuit* each light bulb is connected in parallel so that one or several lights may be on at any one time. Provided the bulbs are of the same wattage they will all glow equally brightly however many are in use.

The individual sockets of a *ring-main circuit* are connected in parallel, and any appliance may be plugged into any socket. In

this type of circuit, one length of cable travels round the salon
and back to the mains supply, reducing the length of cable
required for power points. Extra sockets can usually be added to
a ring-main relatively cheaply. The cable carries two insulated
wires known as the *live* and *neutral* conductors which connect to
each power socket. A third wire, called the *earth*, is also
connected to each socket, and leads into the ground providing a
path of low resistance for electric current. The earth acts as a
safety device to prevent an *electric shock* occurring to a person
using electrical equipment which has become faulty.

Figure 1.23
Ring-main circuit

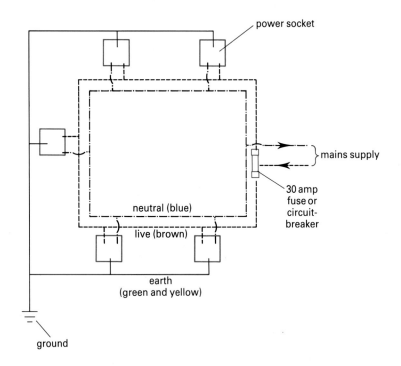

Fuses

The live conductor of a circuit passes through a *fuse* or a *circuit
breaker*. These are devices to protect the *wiring* of a circuit from
the effects of *overloading*, which can cause a fire as the wires
become very hot. A fuse is the *weakest* part of a circuit as the wire
it contains melts if too large a current passes through it, thus
breaking the circuit. A circuit breaker *switch* moves to the off
position when the circuit is overloaded. A ring-main carries a 30
amp fuse or circuit breaker while a lighting circuit is protected
by one of 5 amps.

Plugs

The appliances used in a beauty salon are connected to the
sockets by means of a *plug* attached to a *flex* from the appliance.
The plug should normally have three pins which enter the

Figure 1.24
Circuit breaker

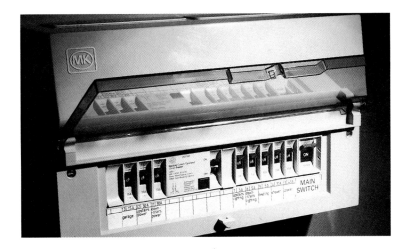

socket holes unless the appliance is all- or double-insulated, when a two-pin plug is adequate. One pin connects with the *live* wire of the ring-main, one with the *neutral* wire and the third longer pin connects with the *earth* wire. The flex must be connected to the plug so that the three wires of the flex are attached to the correct *terminals* inside the plug:

> The **brown** covered wire of the flex must be connected to the terminal marked **Live** or L;

> The **blue** covered wire must be connected to the terminal marked **Neutral** or N;

> The **green and yellow** covered wire must be connected to the terminal marked **Earth** or E.

All flex must conform to the international *colour code* described above, and all plugs to the British Standard BS/1363.

Figure 1.25
Connections between plug and flex

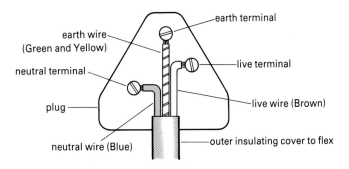

The plug contains a *cartridge fuse* which lies over the live terminal. A 3 amp fuse should be placed in the plug of an appliance with a power of less than 720 watts. More powerful appliances require a 13 amp fuse. The current normally flowing through an appliance is given by the formula:-

$$\frac{amps}{(current)} = \frac{watts}{volts} \frac{\text{(power of appliance)}}{\text{(pressure of mains supply)}}$$

For an appliance with a wattage of 720 on a mains supply of 240 volts:-

$$\frac{current}{flowing} = \frac{720 \text{ watts}}{240 \text{ volts}} = 3 \text{ amps}$$

For a wattage of 720 or more, a 3 amp fuse would not allow current to flow through it as the fuse wire would become so hot that it would burn through.

Figure 1.26
Structure of cartridge fuse

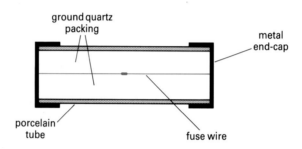

ground quartz packing

metal end-cap

porcelain tube

fuse wire

Switches

A switch allows an *air gap* to be introduced into an electric circuit to stop the current when the switch is in the off position. Some switches have a *variable* control so that different amounts of current pass through the switch to the appliance at the different numbered positions. A switch is placed in the live conductor and is a safety device. A *thermal cut-out* will automatically switch off the current to a heating element when an appliance begins to overheat.

Cost of electricity

The amount of electricity used by an appliance depends on its *power* (wattage) and the length of *time* it is operating. The unit of electrical energy is the **kilowatt-hour,** ie the electricity consumed when an appliance with a power of 1 kilowatt operates for 1 hour.

The number of units of electrical energy used in a salon is measured by the Electricity Board's *meter.* Recently installed meters display the number of units used. Older meters record the units used on a series of four large *dials.* Where the pointer on the dial lies between two numbers the lower number should be read, except between 9 and 0 where 9 is the correct reading because 0 represents 10.

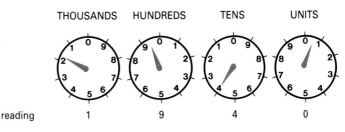

Figure 1.27
Electricity meter dials

units used 1940

The *difference* between present and previous readings represents the number of units used in that time interval. The cost is obtained by multiplying the number of units by the cost per unit.

$$\text{cost} = \underbrace{\text{kilowatts} \times \text{hours}}_{\text{units}} \times \text{cost per unit}$$

Microbiology

Micro-organisms are minute living organisms which are too small to be visible with the naked eye. Some micro-organisms become visible by using an optical microscope, but others can only be seen by using an electron microscope which has a much higher magnification. Micro-organsims are mostly either **fungi** (yeasts and moulds), **bacteria** or **viruses**. A few are single-celled animals called *protozoans*, eg Entamoeba. Micro-organisms are universally present in the natural environment and on the person. Some are responsible for infectious diseases which can be passed from one individual to another. Such disease-causing micro-organisms are **pathogens.** Many other micro-organisms are **saprophytes** feeding on dead organic material, and are non-pathogenic. Other micro-organisms are *symbiotic* living in or on a human or animal carrier. Both the symbiont and the carrier profit by the association.

Fungi

Fungi are either *unicellular* (eg yeast) or *multicellular* filamentous (eg moulds) organisms. In the moulds the filaments are called *hyphae*, and are $5-10$ μm wide and of varying length. They branch to form a flat tangled mat called a *mycelium.*
Although mycelia are visible to the naked eye, fungal spores and unicellular yeasts are too small to be visible. Fungi secrete *enzymes* which diffuse out through the cell or hyphal walls to *digest* surrounding organic material, which is then absorbed in liquid form as food. Most fungi are *saprophytic*, but a few are *pathogenic*, feeding on the living tissues of their host (eg on human skin and mucous membranes).
Structurally, fungi are *eukaryotes* as they have well-defined nuclei and other cell organelles. Fungal cells and hyphae are

Figure 1.28
Fungal hyphae

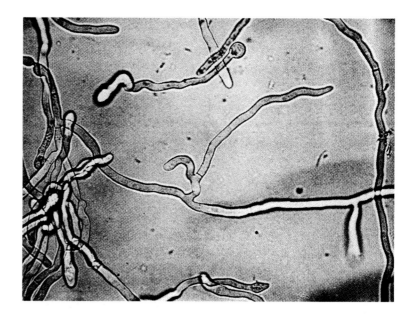

surrounded by a rigid *wall*. They never contain the green pigment *chlorophyll* which is characteristic of plants. They reproduce by tiny *spores*, or from fragments of *hyphae* which become detached from the mycelium.

Conditions which favour fungal growth and reproduction are warmth (15–30 °C), a plentiful food supply, water and oxygen, although a few fungi (eg yeasts) can respire anaerobically (without oxygen) for a short time.

Bacteria

Bacteria are *unicellular* organisms with no distinct nucleus or cell organelles. Their size varies from between 0.5 μm and 2 μm. They belong to the simplest group of living organisms, the *prokaryotes*. Each bacterium is bounded by a cell wall and has a characteristic *shape*. It is either spherical (*a coccus*), rod-shaped (*a bacillus*), spirally coiled (*a spirochaete*) or comma-shaped (*a vibrio*). Some bacteria are surrounded by a *slime capsule,* and some have one or more projecting hair-like processes called *flagellae*. Some bacteria (eg spirochaetes) are able to move around. Bacteria may form bunches or chains.

Bacteria reproduce by dividing into two (*fission*). A few form thick resistant *spores*. Bacteria produce waste products called *toxins* which, in pathogenic forms, may produce the symptoms of the disease they cause. Large numbers of bacteria live on human skin and in body cavities.

Conditions which favour bacterial growth and reproduction are warmth (37 °C for pathogenic and symbiotic bacteria), a plentiful food supply, water, and the removal of waste products. A supply of oxygenated air is needed by those bacteria which respire *aerobically*.

Figure 1.29
Characteristic shapes of bacteria

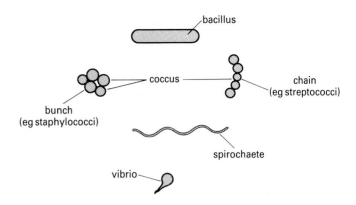

Viruses

A virus is smaller than a bacterium, eg the herpes virus is 0.1 μm in size. Viruses can grow only within the living cells of a suitable host, therefore all viruses are *pathogenic* and infect a *specific* host. A virus must pass, usually fairly directly, from an infected living cell to another cell of the same kind. Once inside the host cell, the virus takes over from the cell nucleus and programmes the cell to produce new virus material instead of the substances it would normally synthesise.

Figure 1.30
Wart virus

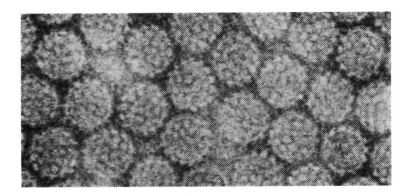

Transmission of micro-organisms

Pathogenic micro-organisms can enter the body through breaks in the skin, by being breathed in, or via the mouth, anus, urinary and vaginal openings. These pathogens are transmitted from various sources:

- the *air* which contains suspended infected *droplets* produced by the coughing, sneezing or talking of infected persons;
- equipment and towels which have become contaminated by contact with the skin of infected persons. Micro-organisms are thus transferred by *indirect* means from one person to another;
- *contaminated* food and water containing pathogens originating from sewage or insects' bodies;

- personal contacts such as shaking hands, kissing and other skin contacts such as manual massage – *contagious* diseases are transferred in this way;
- sexual intercourse can result in the transmission of *venereal* diseases;
- blood – two serious and often fatal diseases, *AIDS* and *Hepatitis B*, can be transmitted when small amounts of blood released from an infected person (the carrier) enter a small break in the skin or mucous membrane of a healthy contact. Equipment used for ear-piercing, or electrolysis needles, can transmit these viruses unless they have not been used before, or have been sterilized before re-use.

Controlling micro-organisms

Personal hygiene and disinfection provide the external methods of controlling micro-organisms. The body's natural defence mechanisms (*immune system*), due mainly to the white blood cells, provides internal resistance to attack by pathogenic micro-organisms.

Personal hygiene involves the cleanliness of skin, hair and clothing. Washing frequently with soap and water removes the layer of sweat, sebum, stale make-up and dead skin cells on which skin micro-organisms feed. It is particularly important to wash the hands after using the lavatory, and before preparing or eating food.

Disinfection is the process by which micro-organisms on salon surfaces or equipment are *inactivated* or *destroyed*. This is achieved using either *physical* processes or chemicals, some methods being more effective than others.

(a)   **Physical** methods of disinfection involve the use of heat or ultra-violet radiation:

- *Burning* will destroy all micro-organisms and is the method used to dispose of contaminated waste such as infected dressings and paper tissues;
- *Glass bead sterilizers* employ dry heat to destroy all micro-organisms on metal and plastic equipment such as applicators. These sterilizers take up to 30 minutes to reach the required temperature. The equipment is then put in to sterilize and immersed for around ten minutes in the case of a single piece of equipment;
- An *autoclave* producing steam under pressure is a very effective means of sterilizing metal and some plastic equipment, as the temperature reached is well above 100 °C and destroys all micro-organisms present;
- *Boilers* and *steamers* which reach a temperature of 100 °C are less effective than an autoclave, destroying most, but not all, micro-organisms and their spores. Natural earths used in face masks are steam sterilized to destroy bacteria. Boilers

Figure 1.31
Glass bead sterilizer

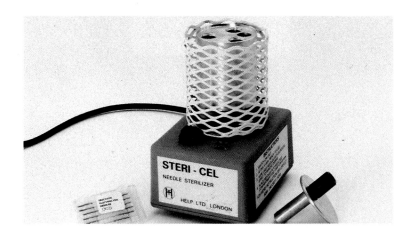

designed for use on instruments will disinfect metal and plastic equipment reasonably well during a ten minute treatment. Infected towels and linen should also be boiled;

● *Ultra-violet cabinets* contain a quartz mercury vapour lamp which emits ultra-violet rays. These rays destroy micro-organisms on the surfaces they reach, but do not sterilize the equipment placed in the cabinet, they only disinfect it;

Figure 1.32
UV Germicidal Cabinet

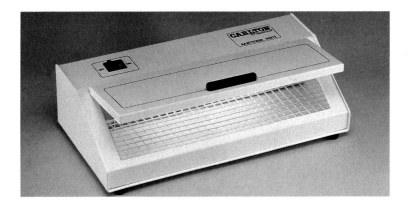

(b)   **Chemical** methods of disinfection also vary in their effectiveness. The chemicals must be used at the recommended concentration and for a sufficient time. Even when used correctly, the degree of disinfection varies with the chemical involved:

● An *antiseptic* will prevent micro-organisms from multiplying, but does not necessarily kill them. The simplest antiseptic is *soap* or *detergent* and *hot* water and is adequate for reducing the activity of micro-organisms on salon surfaces and textiles. A 1% solution of *Cetrimide* (a quaternary ammonium compound) is a useful antiseptic for human skin. Antiseptics such as *Nipagin* are added to cosmetic preparations as preservatives to prevent the growth of micro-organisms;

- A *disinfectant* kills most pathogenic micro-organisms when used correctly. A 70% solution of *ethanol* (alcohol) or *chlorhexidine* in 70% ethanol are the best disinfectants for salon use. Both disinfectants are available in liquid form or as commercially prepared wipes, and may be used on metal or plastic applicators, electrodes etc. At least 15 minutes immersion in the liquid disinfectant is necessary. Ethanol is an *inflammable* liquid, and care must be taken to keep it away from flames or heat. Other chemical disinfectants are less suitable for salon use as they may be corrosive to the equipment, damaging to the user's health, or may deteriorate on keeping;

- *Sterilizing agents* will destroy all micro-organisms and their spores. Neat *chlorine bleach* should be used as the sterilizing agent on *blood spills* following a cut or a nose bleed. This treatment will destroy the viruses which cause the diseases AIDS and Hepatitis B. Bleach should be poured on the spilt blood and left for one minute before washing the blood away with hot water and detergent. Rubber gloves should always be worn when dealing with blood spills.

Disposal of waste

Waste water from wash basins, and *lavatory waste* pass into pipes connecting to the drains where micro-organisms from sewage and dirty water flourish. Each wash basin and lavatory bowl has a *trap* below it containing a *water seal* to prevent air-borne pathogens and unpleasant smelling gases from the drains

Figure 1.33
Waste traps
(a) S-trap

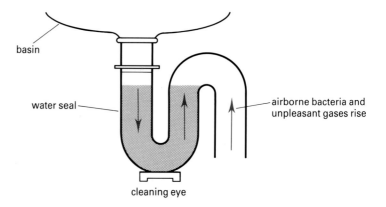

basin

water seal

airborne bacteria and unpleasant gases rise

cleaning eye

(b) Bottle trap

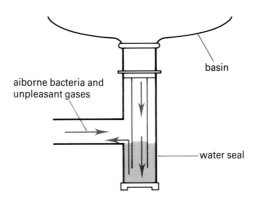

basin

aiborne bacteria and
unpleasant gases

water seal

entering the salon. Below the lavatory bowl and some older wash basins the trap is S-shaped. Modern wash basins usually have a *bottle* trap.

Below the trap the basin waste pipe runs into a waste water pipe which empties outside the building into a *gulley trap* (drain) just below the ground. The gulley trap also contains an S-shaped trap and water seal. From here the waste water enters a large underground *inspection chamber* covered by an air-tight drain cover. The lavatory waste passes from the trap into a *soil pipe* which runs down the outside of the building and opens at the bottom into the inspection chamber. The top of the soil pipe is open to allow the escape of unpleasant smelling gases at roof level, and is covered by a wire *guard* to prevent birds nesting in the opening. From the inspection chamber the waste water and sewage passes into the *main drain* which empties into the *sewer* in the road.

Micro-organisms in the traps of wash basins and lavatories can be destroyed by adding a small quantity of chlorine bleach, which is left in the trap for a short time before flushing it away. *Chlorine bleach* is a *hazardous* chemical as it is both acidic and an oxidizing agent. It should be handled with care, kept off the skin, and disposed of with large volumes of cold water. It should not be mixed with other chemicals in case violent chemical reactions take place.

Bleaches, acids, alkalis and flammable solvents must all be disposed of with great care after use, and stored and handled safely. Such chemicals bear warning signs on their containers known as *hazard symbols*.

Used electrolysis needles and other *sharp* objects should be placed in a 'sharps' box or bag for disposal. This will prevent objects which could be contaminated with blood or micro-organisms wounding the skin of a person handling the sharp object, and transmitting infection.

EXPLOSIVE
OXIDISING
CORROSIVE
HIGHLY FLAMMABLE
HARMFUL or IRRITANT
TOXIC
BIOHAZARD

Figure 1.34
Hazard symbols for chemicals

BIOHAZARD
SHARP OBJECTS
DISPOSAL POUCH

Figure 1.35
Sharps safety pouch

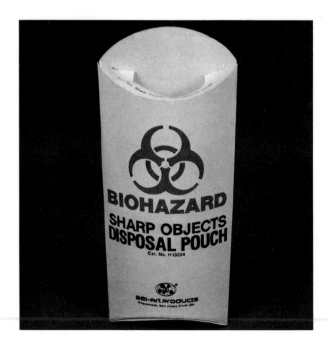

Self-assessment questions

1 When an organic acid reacts with an alcohol the products are water and:

(a) an alkali;   (b) an amine;
(c) an ester;   (d) an alkane.

2 The smallest part of a compound that can exist alone is:

(a) an electron;   (b) an ion;
(c) an atom;   (d) a molecule.

3 A suspension of tiny droplets of one liquid in another liquid is:

(a) an emulsion;
(b) a suspensoid;
(c) a filtrate;
(d) a solution.

4 When dissolved in tap water the sulphates of calcium and magnesium produce the type of hardness called:

(a) temporary;   (b) partial;
(c) permanent;   (d) anionic.

5 The physical processes on which natural ventilation depends are:

(a) humidity and condensation;
(b) diffusion and convection;
(c) conduction and radiation;
(d) evaporation and condensation.

6 A bimetal strip is part of the structure of a:

(a) thermostat;
(b) heating element;
(c) fuse;
(d) three-pin plug.

7 A device which prevents an electric shock occurring to a person using faulty beauty therapy equipment is:

(a) an appliance;
(b) a ring main;
(c) a neutral conductor;
(d) an earth wire.

8 The unit of electric power is the:

(a) amp;   (b) volt;
(c) hertz;   (c) watt.

9 Micro-organisms which cause disease are described as:

(a) pathogenic;
(b) symbiotic;
(c) saprophytic;
(d) anaerobic.

10 A sterilizing agent that will destroy the viruses causing AIDS and Hepatitis B if they are present in spilt blood is:

(a) nipagin;
(b) 1% Cetrimide solution;
(c) chlorine bleach;
(d) distilled water.

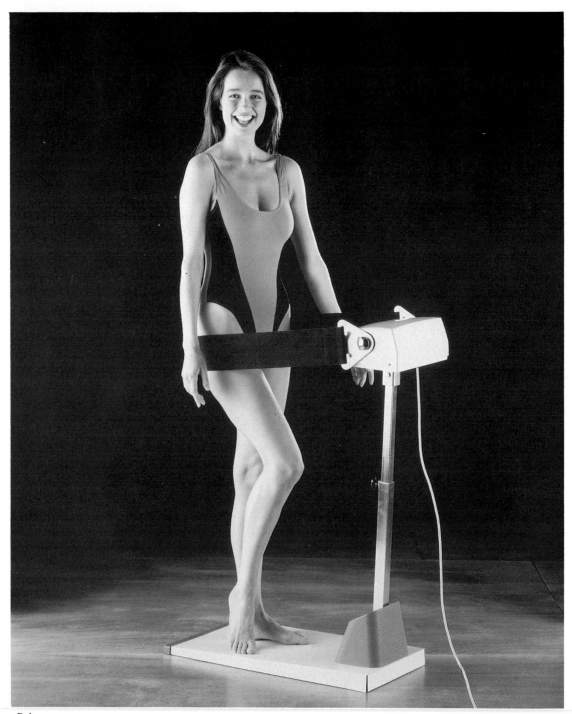

Belt massager

Cells

A human body is composed of millions of microscopic living units called *cells*.

Cell structure

Cells nearly always have the same basic structure. They are bounded by a very thin living plasma membrane which encloses the cell contents, or **protoplasm**. This consists of a number of small structures called *organelles* surrounded by a jelly-like **cytoplasm**. The central organelle, called the **nucleus**, is round or oval, and is bounded by a *nuclear membrane* pierced by pores which allow exchange of materials between the nucleus and the cytoplasm. The nucleus may contain one or two small *nucleoli*, and carries the heritable material (genes) in the form of a chemical substance called *DNA*.

Examining a cell under an electron microscope shows a system of membranes which divide up the cytoplasm into a network of channels. This membrane system is called the **endoplasmic reticulum.** Some of the membranes have small granules known as *ribosomes* on their outer surface. In one area, smooth membranes and associated vesicles form an organelle called the *Golgi body.*

Throughout the cytoplasm are rod-shaped organelles called **mitochondria** which are particularly numerous in very active cells. Other small membrane-surrounded bodies called *lysosomes* also occur in the cytoplasm. Some cells have numerous short hair-like projections from the surface called *cilia* which are able to move. Sperm cells have a single longer movable projection called a *flagellum.* Cell cytoplasm often contains *inclusions* such as granules of chemicals being temporarily stored in the cell.

A plasma membrane is a highly elastic structure composed of a central layer of fatty *phospholipid* molecules sandwiched between two layers of *protein.* Some of the protein molecules penetrate the phospholipid layer, and some completely span the plasma membrane. Within the plasma membrane the protein and phospholipid molecules can move around, giving the membrane some of its special properties, allowing substances to pass into and out of cells.

A plasma membrane must be able to respond to hormones, and must carry 'marker molecules' so that it is recognized as belonging to the individual.

Cell function

Cells carry out a series of chemical reactions resulting in the activities which keep them alive. The chemical substances involved must move into and out of the cell through the plasma membrane. Some of these substances pass, by the physical process of *diffusion*, from a region of high concentration to one

Figure 2.1
Basic structure of a cell

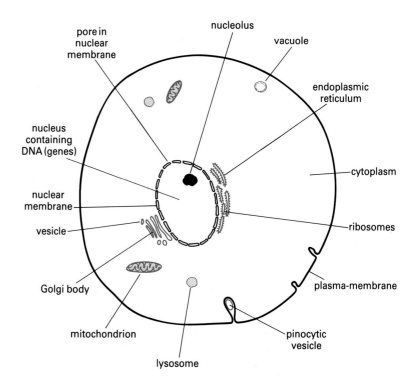

Figure 2.2
Portion of plasma membrane in section

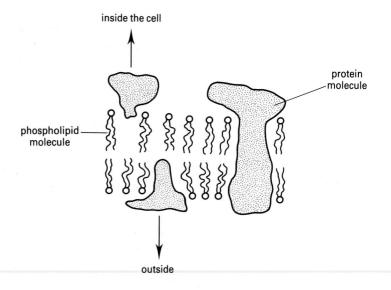

Table 2.1
Functions of cell organelles

Organelle	Functions
Plasma membrane	Protects the cell; allows substances to enter and leave the cell
Nucleus	Contains genes for inheritance; controls the cell's activities
Endoplasmic reticulum	Provides channels for moving substances round the cell; provides a large surface area for chemical reactions in the cell
Ribosomes	Provide the sites for protein synthesis
Golgi body	Region of synthesis of materials which will be secreted by the cell, eg mucus
Mitochondria	Involved in energy production within the cell; known as the 'power houses' of the cell
Lysosomes	Destroy worn out organelles and/or whole cells and foreign materials; known as 'suicide bags'
Cilia	Cause the movement of particles and fluid across a cell surface
Flagellae	Enable cells to move about

of lower concentration. Oxygen is one of the substances which diffuses through the plasma membrane, which is thus *permeable* to oxygen.

Water will pass in and out of cells by the physical process of *osmosis* from an area of high water concentration (dilute solution) to an area of lower water concentration (concentrated solution). Since osmosis occurs, plasma membranes are said to be *semi-permeable*.

Some of the substances required by a cell will only pass through its plasma membrane by active processes requiring the cell to use *energy* for their transport. Such substances, which are already present in higher concentration inside the cell than outside, can still enter the cell by *active transport*. Glucose molecules enter cells by active transport, but glycogen (animal starch) molecules stored in cells are unable to pass out through the plasma membrane, which is therefore described as *selectively permeable*. *Carrier proteins* present in the plasma membrane aid active transport of some materials across the membrane.

Another form of active transport is known as *pinocytosis*. Droplets of liquid collect on the surface of the cell membrane which folds inwards surrounding the liquid droplet and forming a vesicle by separating from the rest of the membrane. Fat droplets are taken up by the cells of the intestine lining by pinocytosis. *Phagocytosis* is a form of active transport where projections of the plasma membrane and cytoplasm surround and engulf solid particles outside the cell. The membrane closes above the particle to form a vacuole inside the cell. White blood cells engulf harmful bacteria by phagocytosis.

Cell division

As cells become damaged by disease or ageing they eventually die and must be replaced. Growth in size of the body organs also requires the production of extra cells. The process by which most cells reproduce is called **mitosis**, and results in a cell dividing into two daughter cells, each *identical* with the parent cell except in size. Each daughter cell then grows to the size of the parent cell, and contains a *complete set* of the parental genes.

Eggs and sperms are produced from cells undergoing a different type of cell division called **meiosis**. Eggs and sperms contain only *half* the genes of the parent cells.

Tissues

Some cells have special functions in the body and their structure may be modified or *differentiated*, as a result. Such differentiated cells usually occur in groups forming a *tissue*, which carries out particular activities. The body tissues are of four main types:- *epithelial, connective, muscular,* and *nervous*.

Epithelial tissue

Epithelial tissue covers the outer *surface* of the body and the *internal organs*. It also lines body cavities and forms *glands*. The cells making up the tissues have a simple shape and fit closely together. They occur as a single, continuous layer in a **simple epithelium**, or as several layers in a **compound** or **stratified epithelium**. The bottom layer of cells always rests on a non-living *basement membrane* containing a fine meshwork of collagen protein fibres.

Epithelial tissues are further classified according to the *shape* of the cells:

- **Squamous** epithelium consists of flat scale-like cells. It may be *simple* like that forming the wall of the blood capillaries and air sacs of the lung, or it may be *stratified* like that of the skin epidermis and lining of the mouth cavity where it must survive considerable friction;
- **Cubical** (cuboidal) epithelium with cube-shaped cells which have a central nucleus, may be *simple*, as in the thyroid gland and kidney tubules, or *stratified*, when lining the ducts of sweat glands;

- **Columnar** epithelium consists of tall cells with an elongated nucleus near the base of the cell. A *simple* columnar epithelium lines the stomach and intestines, and a *stratified* columnar epithelium lines the larger urinary ducts;
- **Ciliated columnar** epithelium covers wet surfaces and is often interspersed with mucus-secreting *goblet* cells. The hair-like cilia covering the free surface of the cell move a

Figure 2.3
Types of simple epithelia
(a) Simple squamous
(b) Simple cubical
(c) Simple columnar
(d) Simple ciliated columnar

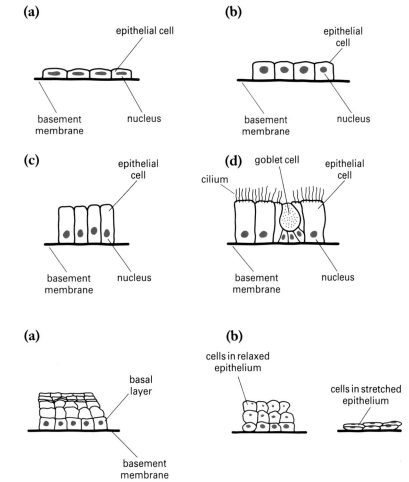

Figure 2.4
Types of compound epithelia
(a) Stratified squamous
(b) Transitional

stream of mucus and particles along. This type of epithelium lines the air passages, where it has a filtering effect on the air breathed in;
- **Compound transitional** epithelium is composed of several layers of cells when relaxed, but when stretched is reduced to one or two layers. In the bladder this type of epithelium is waterproof, and allows the large changes in volume that occur;

- **Glandular** epithelium consists of cells which secrete wanted chemicals, a process requiring the use of energy. The cells may occur singly, like the goblet cells which secrete mucus, or they may be grouped to form a *gland*. The substance secreted is passed into *ducts* in the case of *exocrine* glands, but into the blood from *endocrine* glands. The sweat and sebaceous glands of the skin are exocrine, while the hormone-producing glands are endocrine. *Multicellular exocrine* glands have an inner secretory part and an outer non-secretory duct. They are divided into a number of types, as shown in Fig 2.5. Where the duct is unbranched the gland is *simple*, while *compound* glands have branched ducts.

Figure 2.5
Types of exocrine glands
(a) Simple tubular (eg in small intestine)
(b) Simple branched tubular (eg in stomach)
(c) Simple coiled tubular (eg sweat glands)
(d) Simple acinar (eg glands storing sperms)
(e) Simple branched acinar (eg sebaceous glands in skin)
(f) Compound tubular (eg glands of liver which form bile)
(g) Compound acinar (eg salivary glands)
(h) Compound tubuloacinar (eg mammary glands of the breast)

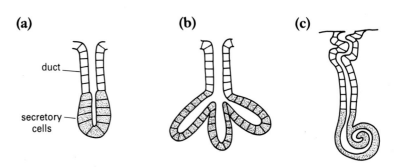

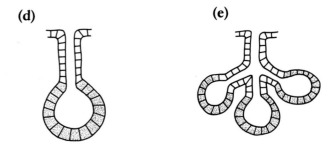

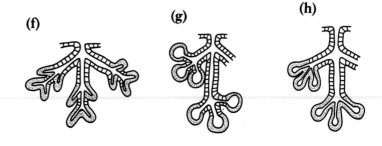

The exocrine glands release their secretions in one of three different ways:

(a) The *holocrine* type accumulates the secreted material and when the cells die each is discharged containing its secretion. Each cell is replaced by a new cell of the glandular epithelium, which becomes secretory. The sebaceous glands of the skin are holocrine;

(b) *Merocrine* glands, such as those producing saliva, discharge their secretions from the cells as they are produced;

(c) In *apocrine* glands, the secreted material accumulates near the free surface of the cell, and that part is pinched off from the rest of the cell and discharged. The large sweat glands in the armpits and the milk-producing mammary glands are examples of the apocrine type.

Figure 2.6
Secretion release methods in
exocrine glands
(a) Holocrine
(b) Merocrine
(c) Apocrine

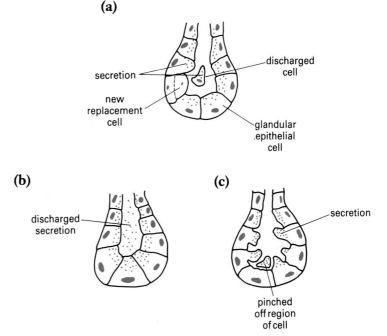

Connective tissue

The cells in these tissues lie in a *matrix* of non-living material which they have secreted. Unlike epithelia, connective tissues have a rich *blood supply* and the cells are not closely packed. *Fibres* are always present in the matrix. The nature of the matrix largely determines the properties of the various types of connective tissue which are *binding* or *supporting* in function.

- **Areolar** connective tissue is smooth and moist with a semi-fluid matrix containing *hyaluronic acid* which has moisturising properties. Running through the matrix are bundles of white fibres composed of *collagen* protein which strengthen the tissue, and a network of yellow fibres composed of *elastin* protein to give elasticity. The living cells of the tissue are of three types. Large flat *fibroblasts* secrete the matrix and fibres. *Mast* cells secrete *histamine,* a substance which enlarges small blood vessels, and *heparin,* an anti-coagulant. *Macrophages* destroy bacteria and tissue debris. This *loose* connective tissue binds together the various tissues and organs eg it attaches the skin to the underlying muscle;

Figure 2.7
Areolar tissue

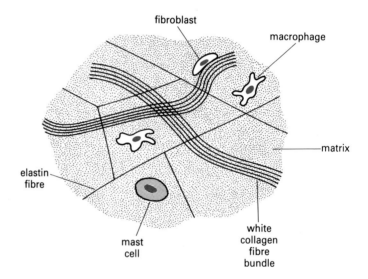

fibroblast

macrophage

matrix

elastin fibre

mast cell

white collagen fibre bundle

- **Adipose** tissue is a form of *loose* connective tissue in which the fibroblasts are modified for storing *fat*. The nucleus of each adipose cell is flattened against the plasma membrane by the large fat droplet, giving the cells a 'signet-ring' appearance. Adipose tissue forms the subcutaneous layer below the skin, and occurs around the heart and kidneys. It acts as an *insulating* layer, reducing heat loss from the body. It also acts as a major *food reserve;*
- **White fibrous** tissue is a *dense* connective tissue where many bundles of firm *collagen* fibres run through the matrix, pushing the fibroblasts into rows between the bundles. The tissue appears silvery-white and is very tough. It occurs in the cord-like *tendons* and broad *aponeuroses* which connect muscles to bones;
- **Yellow elastic** tissue has a branching network of *elastin* fibres in the matrix which gives the tissue its yellowish

Figure 2.8
Adipose tissue

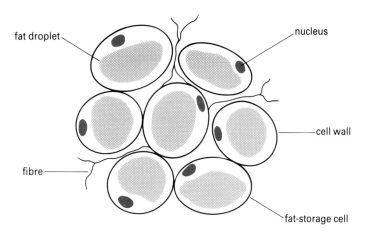

fat droplet

nucleus

cell wall

fibre

fat-storage cell

colour. The fibroblasts occur in the gaps between the fibres. This elastic connective tissue occurs in the walls of arteries and lungs;

- **Lymphoid tissue** (see Chapter 12), **blood** (see Chapter 10), **cartilage** and **bone** (see Chapter 4) are connective tissues also.

Muscular tissue

This tissue brings about *movement* by its ability to contract and relax (see Chapter 5).

Nervous tissue

This tissue transmits *messages* (see Chapter 6).

Membranes

The combination of an epithelial layer with an underlying connective tissue layer is known as a membrane. *Mucous* and *serous* membranes are of this type:

- **Mucous membranes** line the body cavities that open to the outside, such as the food canal and air passages. *Mucus* is a thin slimy fluid which lubricates surfaces and prevents them from drying out. It is secreted by *goblet* cells in the epithelial layer;
- **Serous membranes** line body cavities that do not open to the outside. They also cover the organs lying in those body cavities, allowing them to slide smoothly over one another. They consist of a thin layer of areolar connective tissue covered by an epithelial layer of flattened cells through which a watery fluid oozes. The pleural membranes lining the chest cavity and outer surfaces of the lungs are serous membranes;

● **Synovial membranes** line joint cavities and secrete a thick fluid to lubricate the movement of bones. They are composed of connective tissue with elastic fibres, but do not contain epithelium.

Table 2.2
Summary of types of tissues

Main type	Subclasses		Occurrence
EPITHELIAL covers surfaces basement membrane present	Simple single layer of cells	Squamous Cubical Columnar Ciliated Glandular	Wall of blood capillary Thyroid gland Wall of stomach and intestine Lining windpipe Mucous membrane of nose
	Compound several layers of cells	Transitional Stratified squamous Stratified cubical	Wall of bladder Skin epidermis Ducts of sweat glands
CONNECTIVE binding or supporting non-living matrix fibres present highly vascular	Areolar – matrix semi-fluid Adipose – cells store fat White fibrous – dense collagen fibres Yellow elastic – elastin fibre network Lymphoid – fluid matrix. Fibres on clotting Blood – fluid matrix. Fibres on clotting Cartilage – matrix gel-like Bone – matrix hardened with calcium salts		Dermis of skin Subcutaneous layer Tendons and aponeuroses Lungs and artery walls Lymph in lymphatic vessels In blood vessels Ends of bones Bones and teeth
MUSCULAR bring about movement	Cardiac Skeletal Smooth (visceral)		In heart Muscles of arms and legs In walls of food canal
NERVOUS conduct impulses	Neurons and neuroglia		In brain, spinal cord, and nerves

Organs and body systems

In the body different kinds of tissues combine together to form **organs** which have one, or a related group of functions. The heart, for example, is an organ with the function of pumping blood round the body. It contains muscular and nervous tissues and the connective tissue, blood.

Body systems consist of a group of organs which are concerned with one of the body's living processes. These living processes involve the use and supply of chemicals and energy, and the removal of waste. They are collectively known as *metabolism,* and include the activities of *nutrition, respiration, excretion, movement, growth, repair,* and *reproduction.* These activities must continue in spite of changes inside and outside the body, or death eventually occurs. The body must therefore be *sensitive* to these internal and external changes, and able to respond to them.

Table 2.3
Body systems

System	Main organs/tissues	Functions in the body
Integumentary	Skin; hair; nails	Protection; temperature regulation; sensitivity to external changes
Skeletal	Cartilages; bones; joints	Supports, protects, and gives shape to the body; forms blood cells, and stores minerals
Muscular	Skeletal muscles; tendons	Causes movement, maintains posture; produces heat
	Visceral and cardiac muscles	See below
Nervous	Brain; spinal cord; nerves; sense organs	Co-ordinates the body's activities; perceives stimuli
Digestive	Alimentary canal; liver; pancreas; gall bladder	Physical and chemical breakdown of food; removal of solid waste
Respiratory	Lungs; respiratory ducts	Supplies oxygen and removes carbon dioxide
Urinary	Kidneys; urinary ducts; bladder	Regulates composition of the blood; maintains the salt/water (osmotic) balance
Vascular	Heart and cardiac muscles; blood vessels; blood	Transports materials round the body to the living cells; collects up waste products
Lymphatic	Lymphatics; lymph nodes; lymph; spleen; thymus; tonsils	Removes materials from the tissues and returns them to the blood, eg protein and water; protects against disease
Endocrine	Glands producing hormones	Regulates growth and development and other body processes
Reproductive	Ovaries, testes and their ducts	Produces new generations of human beings

Body cavities

The spaces within the body that contain internal organs are called **body cavities**. Inside these cavities the organs are protected. Close to the back, or posterior surface of the body, are the *cranial* cavity in the skull containing the brain, and the *spinal canal* formed by the vertebrae containing the spinal cord. These two cavities together form the **dorsal body cavity**.

Figure 2.9
Body cavities (side view)

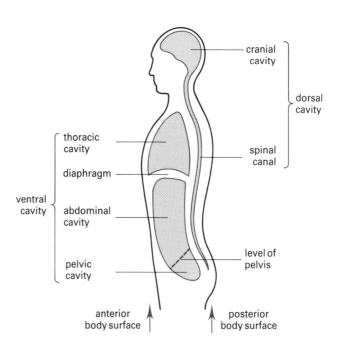

The **ventral body cavity** occurs nearer the front, or anterior surface of the body. It consists of the *thoracic* cavity in the chest, and the *abdominal* cavity below the diaphragm. The lower part of the abdominal cavity is known as the *pelvic* cavity. The thoracic cavity is subdivided into two *pleural* cavities, one round each lung, and a *pericardial* cavity round the heart. The cavities are lined by serous membranes known as the *pleurae* and *pericardium* respectively. The abdominal cavity contains most of the alimentary canal below the oesophagus (gullet), and the two kidneys with their ducts. The pelvic cavity contains the bladder, the lower colon and rectum of the alimentary canal, and the reproductive organs. The serous membrane lining the cavity and binding the organs to each other, is the *peritoneum*. The organs inside the ventral body cavities are collectively called the *viscera*.

Anatomy and physiology

The *anatomy* of the body refers to its *structure*, and the arrangement of the organs of the body systems. Definitions of *anatomical terms* will be found in *Appendix I. Physiology* is the study of the way the organs *function* in the body.

Self-assessment questions

I Where in the body do the following structures occur:

(a) organelles; (b) goblet cells?

2 Give **one** important structual difference between exocrine and endocrine glands.

3 List **three** characteristics of connective tissue.

4 Explain the difference between 'semi-permeable' and 'selectively permeable' when applied to membranes.

5 Give the scientific name for the cellular structures known as:

(a) suicide bags;
(b) sperm tails.

6 Name the process by which white blood cells engulf harmful bacteria.

7 Where in the body would you find the following:

(a) stratified squamous epithelium;
(b) compound tubular acinar glands?

8 Name the type of secretion release method found in:

(a) sebaceous gland cells;
(b) salivary gland cells.

9 In which tissues do the following materials occur:

(a) elastin; (b) fat droplets;
(c) hyaluronic acid?

10 Give **two** functions of the adipose tissue in the subcutaneous layer.

CHAPTER 3

The Skin

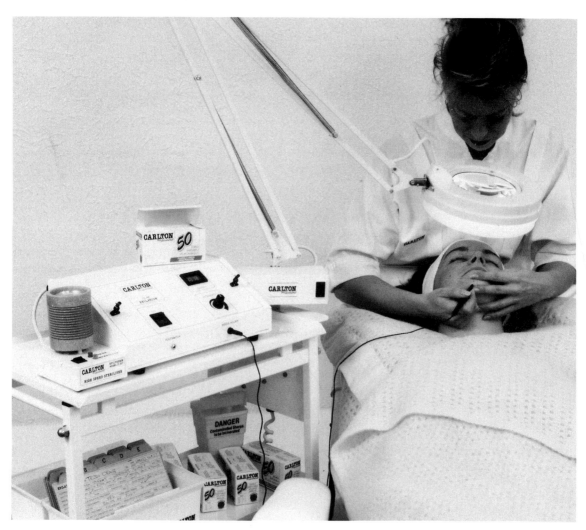

Epilation by diathermy

Structure of the skin

The skin is a large *organ* covering the outside of the body. Its *thickness* varies between 0.05 and 3 mm, dorsal surfaces having thicker skin than ventral surfaces, except where ventral surfaces are subjected to considerable wear, as on the palms of the hands. A vertical section through the skin shows two distinct layers, an outer **epidermis** and an inner thicker **dermis**.

Epidermis

The tissue forming the epidermis is *stratified squamous epithelium* in which five distinct layers can be recognized. The two inner layers are composed of *living* cells, and together form the *stratum germinativum*. In the three outer layers the cells are *dying* or *dead* as a result of *keratinization*. During this process the cells become filled with a horny waterproof protein called *keratin*.

The innermost layer or **stratum basale** consists of a single row of columnar cells resting on a basement membrane which separates the epidermis from the dermis. The cells are capable of *dividing* continuously to produce new cells, and are stimulated into rapid division by friction on the skin surface. At intervals between the columnar dividing cells are large star-shaped *melanocytes* which form the skin pigment *melanin*.

Above the stratum basale is a layer composed of eight to ten rows of rounded cells fitting closely together. Short projections emerge from these cells (prickle cells) to make contact with neighbouring cells, and so the layer is called the **stratum spinosum**. The living cells of this layer remain capable of dividing.

The next layer, or **stratum granulosum,** consists of two or three rows of rather flattened cells that contain granules of *keratohyalin* produced as the first stage of keratinization in these dying cells.

A fourth layer, the **stratum lucidum,** is pronounced in the thick hairless skin on the palms of the hands and soles of the feet, but is not present in hairy skin. It consists of three or four rows of flat dead cells which look translucent as they contain *eleidin* droplets, produced as a further stage in keratinization.

The **stratum corneum** is the outer 25 to 30 rows of dead scaly cells which contain *keratin* granules.

The skin *melanocytes* produce two types of pigment, *eumelanin* which is black or brown, and *phaeomelanin* which is yellowish-brown or red. The amount and distribution of these melanin pigments is responsible for the variation in skin colour. In the *Caucasian* (white) races, eumelanin is present in relatively small amounts in the basale, spinosum, and granulosum strata. In the *Negroid* (black) races much more eumelanin is present, and it occurs in all the epidermal layers.

Dermis

The dermis is composed of *connective tissue* containing cells, and both *collagen* and *elastin* fibres in the matrix. The outer region of the dermis is called the **papillary layer** and its outer ridged surface pushes up into the epidermis as the *dermal papillae*. The papillary layer is continued round the hair follicles as a *connective tissue sheath*.

The inner region of the dermis is the **reticular layer**. It contains more *collagen* fibres, making the tissue both strong and flexible. *Hyaluronic acid* in the matrix of the dermis has excellent moisturizing properties.

Figure 3.1
Vertical section through the skin

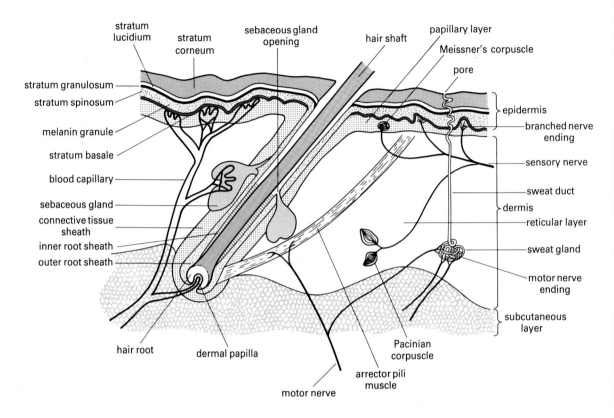

The dermis contains a number of structures which have grown down into it from the epidermis. These are the *pilosebaceous units* consisting of a hair follicle and its associated sebaceous glands, and the *sweat glands*. Blood vessels, nerves, and muscles are all dermal structures:

- **Blood vessels:** Unlike the epidermis, the dermis is highly *vascular*. Arterioles (small arteries) enter the dermis from below and branch into networks of blood capillaries round active or growing structures. Such networks occur in the *dermal papillae* to provide the stratum basale of the epidermis with food and oxygen. A network forms the *dermal hair papilla* at the growing root of each hair. Similar networks surround the sweat glands, and the arrector pili muscles which pull the hairs upright. The capillary networks drain into venules (small veins) which carry the blood away from the skin;
- **Nerves** run through the dermis, terminating in nerve endings of various types. *Branched* nerve endings which are *sensory* occur in the papillary layer and hair root, and

respond to touch and temperature changes. More complex nerve endings also occur such as *Meissner's corpuscles* in the dermal papillae, sensitive to gentle pressure, and Pacinian corpuscles in the reticular layer, responsive to deep pressure. The nerve endings in the sweat glands and arrector pili muscles are *motor*, affecting the rate of secretion and state of contraction respectively. Motor nerve endings in the walls of the dermal blood vessels cause them to contract or dilate;

- The **arrector pili muscles** are attached to hair follicle walls at one end, and to the papillary layer just below the epidermis at the other end. When these muscles contract they pull the hair follicles vertical and pinch up the surrounding skin to produce 'gooseflesh';
- **Sweat glands** (eccrine or sudoriferous glands) are *simple coiled exocrine* glands. The glandular region is deeply embedded in the reticular layer and the long duct passes to the skin surface, opening at a *pore*. In the dermis the duct is straight, but becomes coiled where it passes through the epidermis, as an adaptation to skin stretching. The pores occur on the top of the epidermal ridges to aid the evaporation of sweat. Very large numbers of pores occur on the palms of the hands, soles of the feet, armpits, and forehead.

Figure 3.2
Pores in skin indicated by sweat droplets

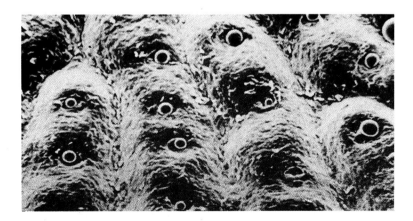

The blood capillaries supply the water and solutes which are secreted as sweat. *Sweat* contains *water* and *sodium chloride* as its main components together with small amounts of *urea, uric acid, ammonia,* and *lactic acid,* which are waste products. There are also traces of *amino-acids, sugar,* and *ascorbic acid* (Vitamin C) in sweat, which provide materials for bacterial growth on the skin surface. The activity of sweat secretion is under *nervous* control.

Apocrine sweat glands (odoriferous glands) are slightly larger than eccrine sweat glands, and produce a milky fluid containing small amounts of organic substances ie fats, sugars, proteins, and *pheromones* (sexual attractants). They occur in the *axillae* (armpits) and *pubic* region associated with hair follicles into which they usually open. Bacterial breakdown of apocrine sweat produces an unpleasant smell. The activity of these glands begins at *puberty*, and is under both *nervous* and *hormonal* control;

- **Sebaceous glands** are *simple branched acinar exocrine glands* which lie on the outside of the hair follicles and open into them. The sebaceous glands are particularly large in the skin of the face, neck, breasts, and upper part of the back. The fatty *sebum* secreted by these glands contains fats, cholesterol, proteins, and some salts, providing material for bacterial and fungal growth on the skin and hair. The activity of the sebaceous glands is controlled by *hormones* brought by the blood. Secretion of sebum is increased at *puberty* by male sex hormones, and reduced during *pregnancy* by the higher level of female sex hormones;

Figure 3.3
Pilosebaceous unit

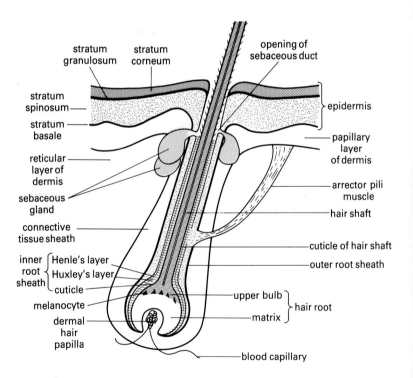

- **Hair follicles** have a two-layered *wall* formed by the outer and inner root sheaths. The *outer root sheath* is formed from, and continuous with, the epidermis, and narrows down to the single stratum basale layer at the hair root. The *inner root sheath* is three-layered and extends only two-thirds of the way up the follicle, being absent above the sebaceous gland opening. On its outer edge, where it is in contact with the outer root sheath, is *Henle's layer*, a single row of cuboid cells with flattened nuclei. In the middle is *Huxley's layer*, consisting of one or two rows of flattened cells. On the inside, and pressed against the hair, is the *cuticle*, a single layer of flattened cells. The inner root sheath is formed from the matrix of the hair root.

At its base the follicle is enlarged to form the *bulb* or *hair root*. The bulb is pushed in from below, the space formed being occupied by the capillary network of the *dermal hair papilla*. The hair root consists of two regions, the *matrix* and the *upper bulb*. The matrix is the lower region where the unpigmented cells are all alike and *dividing* rapidly. The matrix lies over the dermal hair papilla, whose blood capillaries supply the food and oxygen needed for hair growth. Above the matrix is the upper bulb where the cells formed by the matrix are *differentiating* into cells of the inner root sheath, and cuticle, cortex, and medulla of the hair shaft. The inner root sheath interlocks with the cuticle of the hair shaft, so that hair and sheath grow up together. Between the matrix and the upper bulb is a layer of *melanocytes* which secrete the hair pigment granules, and pass them into the developing cortex cells of the hair shaft.

Hair

Two types of hair occur on the body. Short fair **vellus hair** covers most of the body except the palms of the hands, soles of the feet, lips, nipples, terminal joints of the fingers, and regions occupied by the second type or terminal hair. **Terminal hair** occurs on the scalp, face (eyebrows, eyelashes, moustache and beard), axillae, pubic region, chest (in men), and round the nipples (in women).

The *hair shaft* is a dead structure composed of keratin. The first centimetre of the hair emerging from the scalp is not fully keratinized and hardened. The *diameter* of the hair shaft in terminal hairs varies with the individual, and there are racial differences also. Coarse terminal hairs may have a diameter eight times that of the finest hairs. The *Caucasoid* races have hair which is oval in cross-section, while that of *Negroid* races is much more flattened. The yellow skinned *Mongoloid* races have hair which is round in cross-section.

The cells making up the hair shaft are arranged in three layers in coarse terminal hair, but fine terminal and vellus hair have only two layers, the central medulla being absent. The outer protective *cuticle* consists of seven to ten layers of irregular scaly bands composed of colourless transparent keratin. These bands are short and overlapping, and each one extends sideways approximately one-third of the distance round the hair shaft. The cuticle bands have their free edge towards the tip of the hair.

Figure 3.4
Hair showing cuticle bands

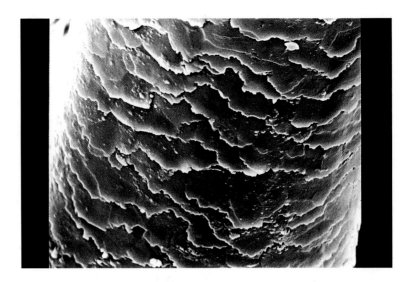

The *cortex* is originally composed of long interlacing spindle-shaped cells full of keratin. The walls of the cells soon break down leaving the long parallel keratin fibres which give the cortex its strength. Between the fibres are pigment granules of eumelanin and phaeomelanin which give the hair its natural colour.

The *medulla,* when present, contains large air spaces and loosely packed cells containing eleidin granules. It forms a soft spongy tissue in the centre of the hair shaft.

Subcutaneous layer

Beneath the dermis is a layer of *areolar* and fat-storing *adipose* tissues called the *superficial fascia.* The boundary between the dermis and superficial fascia is irregular in outline, the two layers being held together by *collagen* fibres. Small blood vessels and lymphatic vessels occur in the subcutaneous tissue and hair follicles project down into it from the dermis.

The superficial fascia is attached to underlying muscle or bone by its areolar connective tissue. The adipose tissue reduces heat loss through the skin. Below the waist in the region of the hips and buttocks, the subcutaneous layer may contain regions of lumpy dimpled fat called *cellulite.* The presence of cellulite indicates lack of exercise and a poor diet.

Growth of skin and hair

Skin growth

Skin growth is due to *mitosis* in the cells of the stratum basale of the epidermis. New cells are produced towards the outside and are continuously pushed upwards by subsequent cell divisions in the stratum basale. It takes between 40 and 56 days for a new cell to complete its *migration* to the skin surface, where it forms part of a skin scale, and is finally removed by friction. Blood capillary networks in the dermal papillae provide the food and oxygen for skin growth. Ultra-violet radiation *increases* the *rate* of skin growth and thickens the stratum corneum.

Hair growth

Growth at the hair root is initiated by *mitosis* in the cells of the *matrix*. As the cells are pushed outwards by further divisions, *differentiation* occurs. The cells in the upper bulb therefore become altered structurally according to the region of the hair or inner root sheath in which they will ultimately occur. Apart from changes in shape, the differentiating cells undergo *keratinization* and die. On the scalp the average *rate* of hair growth is 0.35 mm per day.

A *hair growth cycle* occurs in each hair follicle. A period of hair growth is followed by a resting period after which the hair is shed as a new hair develops in the follicle. The *life span* of a scalp hair is between one and a quarter and seven years, with three years being an average growing period. Eyelashes and eyebrows are replaced every four to five months, while vellus hairs have a life span of around six months. A *hair loss* of between 50 and 100 hairs daily is normal for the scalp. Pregnancy reduces hair loss temporarily, but after the birth the drop in sex hormone level causes many more hairs to fall out at once.

The growing phase of a hair is known as **anagen**. During this phase the cells of the hair matrix are dividing rapidly. Anagen is followed by a short transition period lasting two weeks called **catagen**. During catagen the bulb and lower part of the hair follicle break down, except for a column of epithelial cells which remain in contact with the dermal papilla. The hair has now become a *club hair* in the shortened follicle, and remains in this condition throughout the resting phase or **telogen**. Telogen lasts for three to four months in terminal hairs, and two and a half months in vellus hairs. At the end of telogen the epithelial column becomes active, forming a new hair root at its lower end and lengthening the follicle at its upper end. The club hair is shed as a new hair develops below it, and a new anagen phase begins. *Plucking* a hair out of the follicle starts the growth of a new hair from a resting follicle. It takes 61 days for a plucked eyebrow hair to be replaced.

The *rate* of hair growth is *slowed* down by illness and malnutrition, and by pregnancy and using the oral contraceptive pill.

Functions of the skin

Protection

The skin protects the body against *mechanical damage* due to friction, as cells lost from the stratum corneum are replaced by the stratum basale. As the stratum corneum is waterproof and the dermis contains natural moisturizing factors such as hyaluronic acid which binds water, the skin protects the body against *water loss*. The slightly acid and salty film known as the 'acid mantle' which coats the skin surface has a pH of between 5.6 and 5.8 and prevents *micro-organisms* from multiplying rapidly on the skin surface. The horny stratum corneum prevents micro-organisms becoming established on, or penetrating, the skin to cause disease. Macrophages in the dermis connective tissue will also destroy micro-organisms by phagocytosis.

The *melanin* in the epidermis protects underlying tissues from *radiation damage* by the *ultra-violet* (UV) rays, and from burning by the *infra-red* rays in sunlight. *UVA* (wavelength 320–400 nm) and *UVB* (wavelength 290–320 nm) rays reach the skin. *UVC* (wavelength shorter than 290 nm) rays, however, are unable to penetrate the earth's atmosphere to reach the skin. Both UVA and UVB stimulate the formation of more melanin, with UVA exposure darkening melanin.

UVB is the cause of most radiation damage as it penetrates to the DNA and proteins in the underlying tissues of the skin which absorb the rays. Furthermore UVB causes increased growth of the cells of the stratum basale which thickens the skin, thereby reducing the amounts of UVA and UVB which penetrate to the deeper layers. UVB exposure, if sufficiently frequent and prolonged, can cause *skin cancer* particularly in white-skinned people.

Figure 3.5
Part of the electromagnetic spectrum affecting the skin

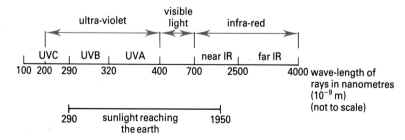

Regulating body temperature

The skin has a major role in regulating the body temperature so that it is maintained around 37 °C. The *adipose* tissue in the dermis and subcutaneous layer *insulates* the body against heat loss. The *evaporation* of *sweat* from the skin surface lowers the skin temperature by removing the *latent heat* required for evaporation, and so cools the body. The removal of latent heat is also the cause of the cold sensation when perfume or toilet water on the skin evaporate rapidly.

Variations in blood flow due to changes in diameter of the skin *blood vessels* regulate the heat lost by *radiation* from the skin surface.

Sensitivity

The skin is sensitive to changes in the body's external environment. Nerve endings detect temperature changes, and indicate the nature of objects in contact with the skin (see Chapter 6).

Nutrient supply

Vitamin D is formed in the skin by the action of UVB rays on a substance derived from cholesterol present in the adipose layer. The *stored fat* in the dermis and subcutaneous layer acts as an energy source. It is continually released from storage and transported by the blood to be used in cell metabolism.

Excretion

The skin also functions as a minor excretory organ. *Sweat* contains small amounts of waste products (urea, uric acid, ammonia and lactic acid) which are therefore removed from the body.

Special features of black skin

The *stratum corneum* of the *epidermis* is much thicker in black skins, and the surface tends to *desquamate*, giving a greyish scaly appearance. The scales contain melanin granules, as melanin is present in all five epidermal layers. The number of *melanocytes* in black skin is approximately the same as in white skin, but the *melanin granules* secreted are four times larger.

Figure 3.6
Epidermis in black and white skins
(a) Black skin
(b) White skin

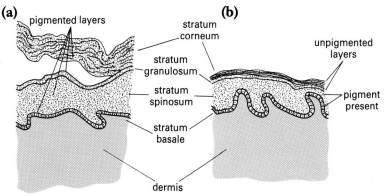

There are more *collagen* fibres in the dermis of black skin making it very tough. Degeneration of collagen due to ageing is much slower in black skins which retain their elasticity for a longer time.

Black skin contains many more apocrine and eccrine *sweat glands*, and they are larger than those of white skin. The glands and ducts of eccrine sweat glands are pigmented and have large *pores. Sebaceous glands* are also more numerous, and a greater proportion open directly onto the skin surface instead of into a hair follicle. Although the *sebum* secreted is richer in fats, black skins are not greasy even though the surface is shiny. *Woolly hair* is flattened in cross-section, and a medulla is absent.

The epidermis of black skin absorbs 70% of the *ultra-violet* radiation reaching it, while white skin absorbs only 25%. However the heavy pigmentation allows only 5% to pass through it to reach the dermis. In white skins 15% reaches the dermis. The damaging effect of ultra-violet radiation on the deeper tissues is thus much less in black skins, and skin *cancers* occur less frequently. The melanic pigment increases the absorption of near *infra-red* heating rays from sunlight (wavelength 700–2500 nm), but the greater sweat secretion of black skin reduces the heating effect. The reduced ultra-violet penetration in a less sunny climate causes lower *Vitamin D* production, and this can cause a dietary problem in immigrants with black skins.

Diseases and disorders of the skin

A damaged area of skin is known as a **lesion,** and is a symptom of a disease or disorder. Diseases of the skin arise because there is both a *causal agent* known as a *pathogen,* and a *predisposition* in the person to succumb to the disease due to lowered skin resistance. The diseases caused by pathogenic living organisms can be passed from one person to another, and are said to be **infectious**. Where a disease is passed on by contact with the lesion, or with infected material, it is said to be **contagious.** Where the causal agent is a small *animal parasite,* the disease is known as an **infestation**. Infectious diseases are often *acute,* having a rapid onset but lasting for a short time only. When an infectious skin disease is present beauty therapy treatments are *contra-indicated,* ie not advisable.

Non-infectious diseases are not caused by pathogens and cannot be transmitted to other people. They are often *chronic* (long term) disorders, which are difficult to treat effectively.

Table 3.1
Infectious skin diseases and
infestations

Name	Pathogen	Effects on the skin
Carbuncle	*Staphylococcus aureus* (bacterium)	Forms large red painful lumps involving a group of hair follicles and discharges pus
Conjunctivitis	*Staphylococcus* (bacterium)	Inflammation of the mucous membrane covering the eye and lining the eyelids
Face mites	*Demodex folliculorum* (animal parasite)	Infestation of hair follicles of eyelashes, nose, and chin; usually harmless; may cause irritation
Favus (honeycomb ringworm)	*Trichophyton* (fungus)	Forms saucer-shaped yellow crusts 1 cm in diameter; causes hairs to break off
Fleas	*Pulex irritans* (insect parasite)	Sucks blood; bites appear as groups of small red spots which itch intensely
Folliculitis	*Staphylococcus aureus* (bacterium)	Pustules develop at the opening of the hair follicles; whole scalp may be affected
Furuncle (boil)	*Staphylococcus aureus* (bacterium)	Forms an inflamed lump round a hair follicle and discharges pus
Herpes simplex (cold sore)	A virus living in the skin of the lips	Red itchy spots form round the mouth which blister, ooze, and then form crusts
Herpes zoster (shingles)	Modified chickenpox virus	Vesicles develop along the pathway of a nerve, often on face, neck, or waist; pain persists after lesions heal
Impetigo contagiosa	*Streptococcus pyogenes* *Staphylococcus aureus* (bacteria)	Blisters develop where skin is damaged, then dry to form yellow crusts; often occurs round the mouth and ears
Pediculosis capitis (head lice)	*Pediculus capitis* (insect parasite)	Infestation of the scalp starts behind the ears; blood sucking causes irritation leading to scratching and secondary infections, eg impetigo
Pediculosis corporis (body lice)	*Pediculus humanus* (insect parasite)	Lives in the underclothing and sucks blood; bites are small red spots with dried blood in the centre
Pediculosis pubis (crab lice)	*Phthirus pubis* (insect parasite)	Infests the pubic area sucking blood; it clings to the pubic hair
Scabies (itch mites)	*Sarcoptes scabiei* (animal parasite)	An infestation where the mite burrows into loose skin at joints, eg wrist; a very irritant disease

Name	Pathogen	Effects on the skin
Stye	*Staphylococcus* (bacterium)	Infection of the sebaceous gland of an eyelash follicle, which discharges pus
Sycosis barbae (barbers itch)	*Staphylococcus aureus* (bacterium)	Infection of the hair follicles of the beard, forming pustules; a form of folliculitis
Tinea capitis (scalp ringworm)	*Microsporum* (fungus)	Infects the epidermis and hair shafts of the scalp forming grey scaly areas with short broken hairs
Tinea corporis (body ringworm)	*Microsporum* or *Trichophyton* fungi	Infects the epidermis forming red scaly patches which heal at the centre and spread outwards
Tinea pedis (Athletes foot)	*Epidermophyton* (fungus)	Infects the skin between the toes forming red patches which blister and scale; itchy or sore
Verrucae (warts)	Papova virus	Infects the skin causing rapid cell division in the epidermis forming a small raised papilloma; plantar warts on the feet grow inwards and are painful

Among their *causes* are physiological and growth disorders, external skin irritation by chemicals and climatic conditions, and abnormalities of pigmentation. Only some of these conditions *contra-indicate* beauty therapy treatments.

Table 3.2
Non-infectious skin disorders

Name	Cause	Effects on the skin
Achrochordon (skin tag)	Localized hypertrophy (excessive growth)	Small, greyish, projecting fibrous growth usually on the neck or eyelids
Acne vulgaris	Overactivity of the sebaceous glands	Inflammation of the sebaceous glands due to blocking of hair follicles by sebum; infected sebum plugs form pustules (spots)
Bromidrosis (body odour)	Overactive sweat glands	Very unpleasant smell particularly from the feet, due to bacterial breakdown of copious sweat
Callosity (callus)	Hypertrophied area of skin	Thickened and hardened skin on hands, feet, knees, and elbows due to external pressure
* Cancer of skin (tumour)	Excessive exposure to strong sunlight – UVB is the most damaging	It may begin as a small pearly lump, or an ulcer that does not heal; melanoma is a cancer due to the growth of a dark mole

Name	Cause	Effects on the skin
Chilblains (Erythema pernio)	Abnormal vascular response to cold	Reddish-blue swellings on exposed skin which itch intensely
Comedo (blackhead)	Blocked hair follicle	A plug of sebum oxidizes at the skin surface forming a small black spot
Corn	Localized hypertrophy of skin of the foot	A cone of hard skin pointing inwards on the foot which is painful under pressure
*Dermatitis (contact dermatitis)	External skin irritant	Reddening, blistering, oozing or swelling of the skin soon after contact with the irritant
*Eczema	Allergy with a genetic cause	Red patches which itch, blister, ooze and form crusts, or become scaly; no form of water therapy (Sauna, Jacuzzi) should be undertaken
Erythema	Vascular disorder usually due to UV or infra-red rays	Blood capillaries dilate making the skin red; it occurs with any skin injury or inflammation
Freckles	Hyperactive scattered melanocytes in the skin	Small darker-coloured areas of the skin, level with its surface (macules)
Hyperidrosis	Overactive sweat glands	Localized excessive sweating of hands, feet and axillae
Keratosis	Skin hypertrophy, one cause being excessive exposure to sunlight	Thick stratum corneum forms firm dry adherent scales; surrounding skin is red, and pigmentation is patchy
Milia (whiteheads)	Blocked hair follicle	A plug of sebum is covered by stratum corneum so no oxidation occurs; small spots are pearly-white
Naevus (birthmark)	Abnormal skin pigmentation often present at birth	Flat or raised areas of skin varying in colour; red (strawberry mark), purple (portwine stain), or brown (mole)
*Psoriasis	General skin hypertrophy; may be inherited	Reddish slightly raised patches, on any part of the body, which are covered with silvery scales
*Sunburn	Prolonged exposure to sunlight or UV lamps	Painful erythema with blistering; rapid growth of stratum corneum, followed by desquamation (peeling)
Vitiligo	Groups of melanocytes in skin stop functioning	Absence of any pigment in small defined skin areas

Those contra-indicating beauty therapy treatments are marked *

Table 3.3
Hair and scalp disorders

Name	Cause	Effect on the hair and scalp
Alopecia areata (patchy hair loss)	Nervous disorder	Round bald patches on the scalp with smooth glossy skin and no broken hairs
Alopecia totalis	Nervous disorder	Total baldness of the scalp
Fragilitas crinium (split ends)	Mechanical or chemical damage to hair shaft	Loss of cuticle on ends of hairs allows splitting of the cortex layer
Hypertrichosis or Hirsuties (superfluous hair)	Terminal hair grows in follicles normally producing vellus hair	Facial hair in women in beard and moustache regions; it is often related to hormone imbalance
Male patterned baldness	Male sex hormones and increasing age in men; an inherited condition	Baldness starting at the temples and crown on the scalp
Monilethrix (beaded hair)	Uneven rate of hair growth in a follicle	Hair shafts are constricted at intervals along their length and break easily
Pityriasis simplex (dry dandruff or scurf)	Normal skin growth of scalp, where scales are small and dry	Itchy scalp, with the accumulation of dry powdery scales which are trapped by the hairs
Pityriasis steatoides or *Seborrhoeic dermatitis*	Overactive sebaceous glands on the scalp	Scalp scales have a greasy covering of sebum and stick together; the underlying skin is erythematous
Seborrhoea	Overactive sebaceous glands	Very greasy hair and scalp
Sebaceous cyst (wen)	Blocked sebaceous gland	Sebum is held in a sac under the skin, and may become a large projection devoid of hair on the scalp
Trichonodosis (knotted hair)	Hair follicle damage often after unskilled electrolysis treatment	Hairs become looped or knotted just above the skin
Trichorrhexis nodosa	Chemical or mechanical damage to the hair shaft	Rough swellings on the hair shaft where cuticle damage leaves the cortex exposed
Trichotillomania	Nervous disorder	Tugging at the hair causes irregular bald patches with a few short hairs

Allergies

An *allergy* is a condition of sensitivity to a substance, the *allergen*, to which most other people do not react. Allergens are usually *proteins*, and when taken internally, or touching the skin, cause tissue damage in *hypersensitive* people. A hypersensitive skin prone to allergic reaction *contra-indicates* facial massage.

External *allergens* (primary irritants) cause *contact dermatitis* or *eczema* in the skin. Allergens in certain *foods* such as shellfish, strawberries, eggs, and cheese, cause *rashes*. Certain *drugs*, particularly penicillin and aspirin, may cause the allergic reaction called *urticaria* (nettlerash).

The response of dermal mast cells to the allergen is to release *histamine*. This causes tissue inflammation with heat and reddening due to dilation of blood capillaries, and increases the permeability of the blood vessel walls, so that more fluid enters the tissue causing *oedema* (swelling).

The first contact with an allergen may leave the body cells *sensitized*, although it may not cause tissue damage. Later contact with the allergen then results in tissue damage not confined to the area of contact. *Cross-sensitization* may occur where the person has previously been in contact with another, different drug or chemical (eg a food azo dye or saccharine) and then has a first contact with the allergen (eg a para-dye used to tint the hair) which causes tissue damage (eg dermatitis).

Certain chemicals become activated in the body by *sunlight*, and become allergens. Typically, a rash appears on skin areas exposed to the sun, and the condition is called *photosensitization*. Some drugs (eg tetracycline), food constituents (eg Vitamin B2), and perfume oils (eg oil of bergamot) are photosensitizers. Foods which can cause photosensitivity if eaten in large amounts are lemons, figs, fennel, parsley, celery, and carrots.

Effects of ageing on the skin

Wrinkling

Wrinkling of the skin is due to loss of elasticity, so that stretched skin does not immediately return to its original area when stretching stops. This effect is due to changes in the *collagen* and *elastin* fibres of the dermal connective tissue, and to progressive *dehydration* of the skin, as water is required to keep the collagen pliable.

Collagen *synthesis* starts in the dermal *fibroblast* cells with the formation of procollagen molecules. These consist of three chains of amino-acids (polypeptide chains) coiled round each other, and known as a *triple helix*. The amino-acids in these chains are mainly *glycine, proline,* and *hydroxyproline*. The three polypeptide chains are held together by *hydrogen bonds*, giving considerable tensile strength to the procollagen.

The procollagen molecules pass out of the fibroblast cells into the *matrix* of the dermal connective tissue. Groups of five procollagen molecules become arranged lengthways to form *microfibrils* in which the procollagen molecules are staggered, but held together by firm cross-links. There are gaps between adjacent ends of the procollagen molecules, which give a banded appearance when collagen is seen under an electron microscope. Microfibrils are themselves coiled, and combined into larger fibrils.

Figure 3.7
Structure of collagen
(a) Procollagen molecule
(b) Collagen microfibril
(c) Collagen fibril

(a)

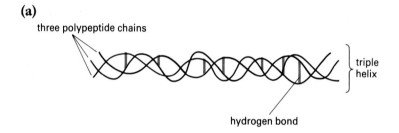

three polypeptide chains

triple helix

hydrogen bond

(b)

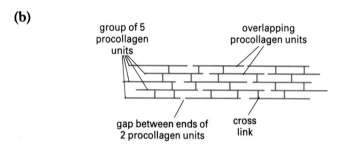

group of 5 procollagen units

overlapping procollagen units

gap between ends of 2 procollagen units

cross link

(c)

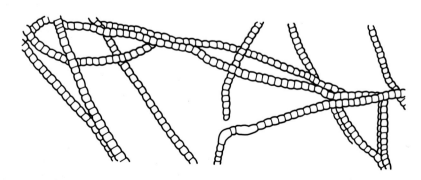

An increase in the number of *cross-links* in collagen with increasing age is thought to be the cause of its reduced solubility, increased hardness and loss of flexibility which reduces skin *elasticity*. Degeneration of collagen is considerably slower in *black* skin.

The amount of *hyaluronic acid* in the dermis declines with increasing age, so the skin is less able to bind water and prevent its loss to the atmosphere.

The number of functioning *melanocytes* decreases in skin and hair, so the skin colour becomes lighter and white terminal hairs develop. The mixture of white and coloured hairs on the scalp is called *canities*. Localized groups of melanocytes in the skin may become more active causing pigmented areas known as *'liver spots'*, which occur commonly on the back of the hand.

With ageing, the blood flow to the skin is reduced, and the rate of *mitosis* in the stratum basale slows down. The stratum corneum is therefore *thinner*, making the skin more fragile. The skin looks thinner, especially on the backs of the hands. The *basement membrane* below the stratum basale becomes flattened and broken. *Sebaceous* and *sweat* glands are less active, and loss of subcutaneous *fat* often occurs.

Nails

Nails are *protective* structures on the end joints of fingers and toes which have developed from the skin *epidermis*.

Nail structure

Each nail is a curved sheet of the protein *keratin* called the **nail plate**. This has a **root** which is buried in the epidermis, and a *body* with a distal free edge, forming the visible part of the nail. The horizontal insertion of the nail root splits the *epidermis*, so part is above the nail plate and part is below it. The *upper* part representing the stratum corneum forms the **cuticle** and **nail fold** around the base and sides of the nail. The furrow between the nail body and the nail fold is the **nail groove**. The *lower* part, representing the strata basale and spinosum, forms the **matrix** which extends below the **lunula** (half-moon). The nail plate is a thickening of the *stratum lucidum*. Below the body of the nail the epidermis is called the **nail bed**. The dermis below the nail is very strongly *ridged*, which holds the nail plate firmly to the nail bed.

The *matrix* is the region from which the nail grows. The lateral walls of the nail fold and the nail bed also contribute to the growth of the nail. The *cuticle* prevents infection of the nail matrix by closing the space between the nail plate and the roof of the nail fold.

The *colour* of the blood in the dermal capillaries below the nail bed shows through the nail plate producing its pink colour.

Figure 3.8
Nail structure
(a) Cross section of finger nail
(b) Longitudinal section of finger nail

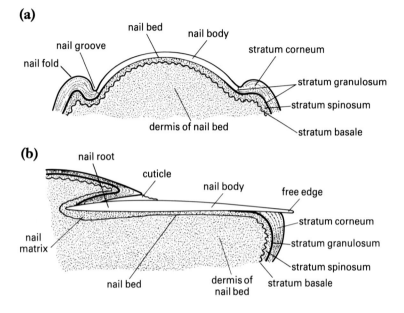

The average weekly *growth* in length of finger nails is 1 mm, while that of toe nails is only 0.5 mm. The dermis below the nail bed and matrix contains the blood capillaries supplying the *food* and *oxygen* needed for nail growth.

Diseases and disorders of the nails

The three main *causes* of nail defects are mechanical damage, physiological disorders, and infections. During manicure, hygienic working practices and the use of sterilized implements are important in preventing nail diseases and disorders. Where manicure is contra-indicated, the following diseases and disorders are marked with a *.

- *Agnail* (hang nails) occur when narrow strips of horny epidermis split away from the lateral nail fold. They should be cut away with sharp scissors. They may be the result of damage during a manicure and are common in nail-biters;

- *Atrophy* may occur in nails which were normal at birth, but become progressively ridged and deformed, and the whole nail plate decreases in size. Ultimate loss of the nail, with scarring, often occurs;

- *Beau's lines* are single transverse furrows running across the nail plates of all the fingers. They are a growth disorder due to a damaged matrix, possibly resulting from an illness such as measles, or from trapping the fingers in a door;

- *Blueish colouration* of the nail plate is due to circulatory defects where the blood contains insufficient oxygen (cyanosis). It can also be due to a bruise below the nail;

- *Clubbing* where the nails are strongly curved downwards over the top of the fingers, is an indication of chronic chest disorders;

- **Eczema* of the nails is shown by irregular ridges and coarse pitting, and part of the nail may be shed;

- *Fragilitas unguium* (brittle nails) is the effect of dehydration of the nail plate causing the free edge to break or split. Frequent use of detergents and non-oily nail varnish remover are common causes of this disorder. It does not respond to dietary supplements;

- *Hypertrophy* is the thickening and lengthening of the nail plate, usually as a result of physical damage (trauma);

- **Ingrowing nails* occur only on the toes, and are the effect of pressure by badly fitting shoes, or by cutting away the corners of the toe nails. The skin below the free edge of the nail becomes inflamed and painful, requiring medical attention. Toe nails should be cut straight across to prevent this disorder;

- *Koilonychia* is a condition where the nails are concave (spoon-shaped) due to abnormal growth of the nail matrix. It may be a symptom of anaemia;

- *Leuconychia* is the presence of white spots on the nail plate. These are the result of injury to the nail matrix separating small areas of the nail plate from the nail bed. Refraction of light from abnormal keratin in these areas may cause the white colour;

- **Onycholysis* is the gradual separation of the nail plate from the nail bed beginning from the free edge. It can be caused by accidental tearing, or by using sharp metal implements for cleaning below the nail. Psoriasis or ringworm infections may also cause this disorder;

- **Onychomycosis* (nail ringworm) is due to the Trichophyton fungus infecting the nail plate. White patches may form, and the free edge of the nail crumbles as it becomes brittle. Yellow streaks develop in the nail plate, and Onycholysis may occur. Medical treatment for several months is required;

- **Paronychia* is an acute infection round the sides and base of the nail plate. Pain, redness and swelling occur with pus oozing below the cuticle, and the condition requires medical treatment. It can be due to nail biting injury;

- *Psoriasis* of the nails may result in the nail plate becoming pitted, resembling the surface of a thimble. Alternatively the nail may become roughened and the free edge begin to crumble. Onycholysis often occurs, with a yellow margin between the pink nail and the white separated region;

- *Pterygium unguis* results when the cuticle grows forward over the nail plate splitting it into two side pieces, and continuing to grow until the nail is eventually lost. The epidermis of the nail fold fuses to the matrix and nail bed. It may result from poor circulation in the hands;

- *Traumatic nail dystrophy* is seen as a depression about 2 mm wide down the centre of the thumb nail bearing a series of parallel cross ridges. It may occur on one or both of the thumb nails. It is due to overactive pushing back of the cuticle during manicuring, or repeated pressure on the nail plate by rubbing with another finger;

- **Whitlow* is an abscess which develops following infection of the nail fold, and causes the terminal joint of the finger to be hot, swollen and inflamed. This condition is very painful and requires medical treatment.

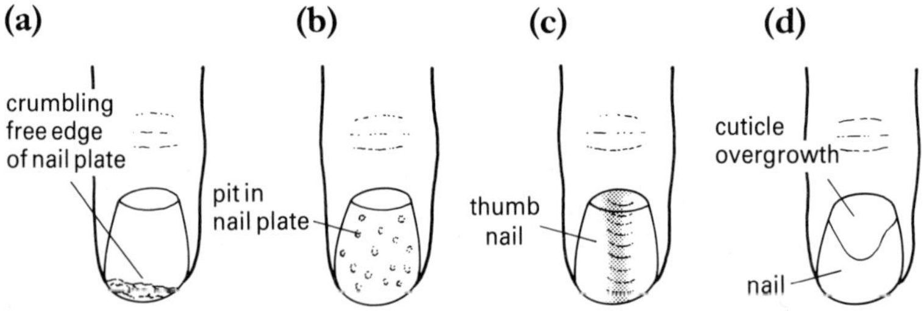

Figure 3.9
Examples of diseases and disorders of the nail
(a) Nail showing Onychomycosis
(b) Nail showing Psoriasis
(c) Traumatic nail dystrophy
(d) Nail showing Pterygium

(a) crumbling free edge of nail plate
(b) pit in nail plate
(c) thumb nail
(d) cuticle overgrowth — nail

Self-assessment questions

1 List the structures which together form a pilosebaceous unit.

2 In which layers of the skin epidermis do the following processes occur:

(a) keratinization;   (b) mitosis;
(c) desquamation?

3 What is the function of Meissners and Pacinian corpuscles?

4 What controls the rate of secretion in:

(a) eccrine sweat glands;
(b) sebceous glands?

5 Explain the difference in origin of the inner and outer root sheaths of the hair follicle.

6 Distinguish between the terms 'anagen' and 'alopecia'.

7 State the wavelength limits of the following types of radiation:

(a) UVB;   (b) near IR;
(c) visible light.

8 State **three** ways in which the epidermis of black and white skins differ.

9 Describe how body tissues respond to the presence of an allergen.

10 Which layers of the skin epidermis form the following nail structures:

(a) cuticle;   (b) nail plate;
(c) nail matrix?

CHAPTER 4

The Skeletal System

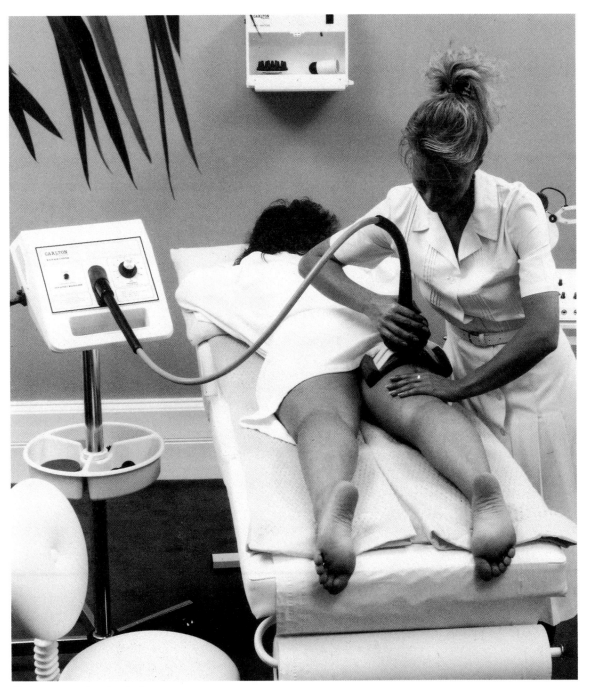

Body massage (mechanical)

The body has an *endoskeleton*, which is under the skin, covered and moved by the muscles. The skeleton is made of the connective tissues bone and cartilage and consists of a large number of separate structures (the bones) which *articulate* (meet at a joint) with one another.

The *functions* of the skeletal system include **support, protection,** and **movement.** The skeleton raises the body from the ground, maintains body shape, and suspends some of the internal organs, in its *supportive* role. It *protects* delicate organs by surrounding them with a hard covering. Bones act as levers, and when muscles pull on bones, parts of the body undergo *movement.* Locomotion, or movement from place to place, is the result of the co-ordinated action of muscles on the bones. Movements of the skeleton require a system of *joints* and *muscle attachments.* Muscles are usually attached to bones by *tendons* composed of tough fibrous non-elastic connective tissue.

Bone tissue

Bone is a porous connective tissue containing living cells, nerves, and blood vessels, and has a matrix hardened by the minerals *calcium phosphate* and *calcium carbonate*. *Collagen* fibres in the matrix form a scaffolding on which the minerals are deposited. The collagen makes bone tissue less brittle.

In **compact bone** the *osteocytes* (bone cells) are arranged in concentric rings called *Haversian* systems, round a branching system of Haversian canals which contain the nerves and blood vessels. The osteocytes secrete the hard matrix, which fills the

Figure 4.1
Compact bone tissue

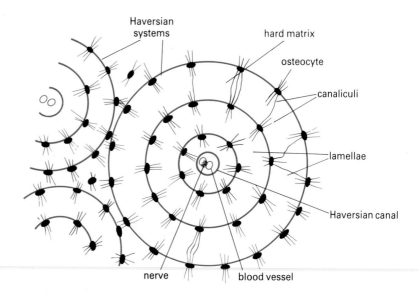

spaces between the rings of bone cells. Narrow canals called *canaliculi* pass through the layers of matrix allowing tissue fluid to pass between the rings of bone cells. The layers of hard matrix between the rings of osteocytes are called *lamellae*. A small space or *lacuna* surrounds each osteocyte.

Cancellate (spongy) **bone** tissue does not have the concentric ring structure of compact bone. It consists of a meshwork of thin plates of bone called *trabeculae* containing the osteocytes. The large spaces between the trabeculae are filled with *bone marrow*. *Red* bone marrow consists of cells which make new red blood cells. *Yellow* bone marrow contains fat cells, and makes certain types of white blood cells.

Cartilage tissue

Cartilage is a more flexible connective tissue than bone. Single cells, or groups of two or four cells, are embedded in a tough matrix containing a dense network of collagen and elastic fibres. The cells are surrounded by a small space or lacuna. There are three types of cartilage, hyaline, fibro, and elastic, which have different properties.

- **Hyaline cartilage** (gristle) is a blueish glossy tissue which covers the ends of bones. Separate cartilages of this tissue occur in the nose, and trachea (windpipe), and join the ribs to the sternum (breastbone);
- **Fibrocartilage** contains many bundles of collagen fibres, making it strong and rigid. It occurs in the discs between the vertebrae, and in the knee (menisci);
- **Elastic cartilage** contains more elastic fibres, making it more flexible. It occurs in the larynx (voice box), and the external part of the ear. It also forms the epiglottis which closes the trachea when swallowing.

Figure 4.2
Hyaline cartilage

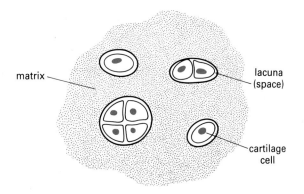

matrix

lacuna (space)

cartilage cell

Classification of bones

Bones are divided into four types according to their shape:

- **Long bones** have a long shaft or *diaphysis*, and two wider ends or *epiphyses*. The shaft is slightly curved, and they have more compact than cancellate bone, which makes them stronger. Red bone marrow occurs in their ends, and yellow bone marrow in their hollow shafts. The thigh and upper arm bones are long bones;
- **Short bones** are roughly cube-shaped, and are mainly composed of cancellate bone, with only a thin surface layer of compact bone. The bones of the wrist and ankle are short bones;
- **Flat bones** consist of two thin surface layers of compact bone surrounding a central layer of cancellate bone, in which red bone marrow occurs. Most of the skull bones, and the scapulae (shoulder blades) are flat bones;
- **Irregular bones** have a more complicated shape, and do not fit into any of the other three groups. The vertebrae and the zygomatic (cheek bone) are irregular bones.

Sesamoid bones are a special type which develop in tendons. The patella (knee cap) is of this type.

Growth and development of a long bone

In a developing baby each long bone is represented by a rod of cartilage which is replaced by bone tissue during the process of *ossification*. The cartilage rod is surrounded by a vascular membrane called the *perichondrium*. A *primary ossification centre* develops in the cartilage rod at the centre of the diaphysis (shaft). Later, *secondary ossification centres* develop in the two epiphyses (ends). The cartilage that remains between the epiphysis and the ossifying diaphysis is called the *epiphysial plate*. This allows the bone to grow, as its cartilage cells divide to thicken the epiphysial plate and lengthen the diaphysis.

There are three stages in the ossification process:

- In the *first stage*, starting in the middle region of the diaphysis, the cells of the inner layer of the perichondrium membrane develop into *osteoblasts*, which form a region or *collar* of compact bone. Where this occurs the perichondrium becomes the *periosteum*, and the bone collar lies just within it. At the same time changes occur in the primary ossification centre. Cartilage cells arranged in columns enlarge, and calcium salts are deposited in the matrix to form *calcified cartilage*. The cartilage cells then die;

- In the *second stage*, cartilage-destroying cells called *osteoclasts* penetrate inwards from the periosteum and resorb the calcified cartilage in the centre of the diaphysis. This process forms spaces which later become part of the *marrow cavity*;
- In the *third stage*, osteoblasts and blood capillaries invade the spaces in the diaphysis centre and bone tissue is formed. Bone tissue continues to form towards the epiphyses, eventually reaching the epiphyseal plates. A layer of osteoclast cells breaks down the bone matrix in the centre of the diaphysis to maintain the marrow cavity, into which the blood vessel ramifies.

Later, blood vessels enter each epiphysis, and secondary ossifications occur there, forming cancellate bone in place of cartilage. A thin layer of articular cartilage remains unossified over the ends of the bones, where they form joints. The epiphysial plate between the primary and secondary ossifications does not ossify at this time. Its cartilage cells continue to divide, allowing the bone to continue growing in length.

Finally, the epihysial plate begins to ossify due to the influence of the *sex hormones*. The cartilage of the epiphyseal plate is completely replaced by bone at around 18 years in women, and 20 years in men, when growth of the bone stops.

Figure 4.3
Development of a long bone
(a) Embryonic cartilage rod
(b) Ossification

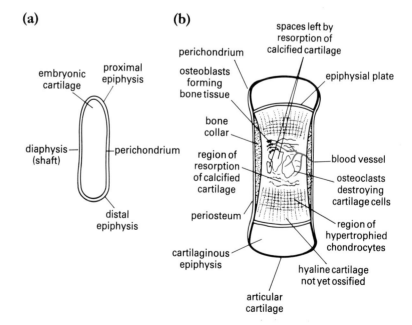

Bones of the skeleton

The adult human skeleton usually consists of 206 bones arranged in two groups known as the **axial** and **appendicular skeletons**. The axial skeleton of 80 bones comprises the skull, hyoid, vertebral column, sternum, ribs, and the auditory ossicles in the ears. The appendicular skeleton of 126 bones comprises the shoulder and hip girdles, and the limb bones. For the terms used in *describing bones*, see *Appendix II*.

The axial skeleton

The skull

The skull encloses and protects the brain and sense organs. It consists of two regions, the cranium and the face.

Figure 4.4
Skull (side view)

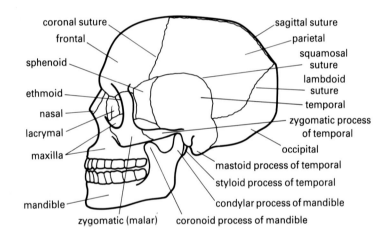

coronal suture
frontal
sphenoid
ethmoid
nasal
lacrymal
maxilla
mandible
zygomatic (malar)

sagittal suture
parietal
squamosal suture
lambdoid suture
temporal
zygomatic process of temporal
occipital
mastoid process of temporal
styloid process of temporal
condylar process of mandible
coronoid process of mandible

- **Cranium**

There are eight flat bones forming the cranium, which articulate at interlocking joints called *sutures,* and surround the brain:

- The **frontal** bone forms the forehead and upper wall of the orbits (eye-sockets). It contains two *frontal sinuses* above the nose, which are air chambers giving resonance to the voice;
- The two **parietal** bones form the sides and roof of the cranium;
- Two **temporal** bones form the lower part of the sides of the cranium. Each temporal bone has a projection behind the ear called the *mastoid process*, and an anterior *zygomatic process* which forms part of the *zygomatic arch* (cheek bone);
- The **occipital** bone forms the back and base of the cranium. It contains a large hole, the *foramen magnum*, through which the spinal cord, blood vessels, and nerves pass. On each side of the foramen are the *occipital condyles* which articulate with the first vertebra (Atlas);

- The single **sphenoid** bone forms the anterior part of the base of the cranium. It binds the cranial bones together, articulating with the frontal, temporal, occipital, and ethmoid bones. It is bat-shaped, with a central *body*, greater and lesser *wings*, and two *pterygoid processes*. It forms part of the floor and sides of the orbits. The *optic foramen* for the optic nerve from the eye occurs between the body and lesser wing of the sphenoid bone;
- The single **ethmoid** bone is anterior to the sphenoid, forming part of the cranial floor, and the medial wall of the orbits. It roofs the nasal cavities and forms part of the nasal septum. The region of the ethmoid bone between the nasal cavity and the orbits contains several air spaces known as the *ethmoidal sinuses*. On either side of the nasal septum, the ethmoid bone has two thin scroll-like *conchae* which project into the nasal cavity.

The four main *sutures* of the cranium are the **coronal** (frontal/parietal), the **sagittal** (parietal/parietal), the **lambdoidal** (parietal/occipital), and the **squamosal** (parietal/temporal).

Figure 4.5
Skull from below (mandible removed)

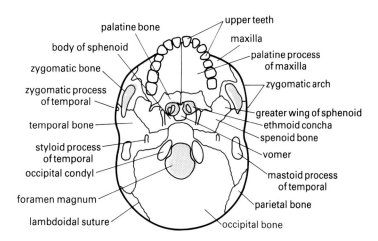

- Face

The face consists of 14 bones, most of which are *irregular* in type:

- The paired **nasal** bones are small and oblong, and form the upper part of the bridge of the nose. The lower portion of the nose is supported by more flexible cartilage. The nasal bones articulate with the frontal bone, and the maxillae;
- The two **maxillae** unite to form the upper jaw and carry the upper teeth. They articulate with all the other bones of the face except the mandible. They also form part of the floor of

the orbits and nasal cavities, and a horizontal projection, the *palatine process*, forms part of the roof of the mouth (hard palate);

- Two irregular **zygomatic** or *malar* bones occur on the outside of the orbits forming their outer rim and walls, and part of their floor. Each zygomatic bone has a *temporal process* which articulates with the zygomatic process of the temporal bone to form the zygomatic arch of the cheek;
- The single **mandible** is the only movable facial bone, and forms the lower jaw and chin. Its *condylar process* articulates with the temporal bone, forming a condyloid joint below the ear. Its *coronoid process* provides the attachment for the temporalis muscle which moves the lower jaw. The mandible carries the lower teeth. The *movements* of the mandible include raising and lowering, protrusion and retraction (forwards and backwards), and slight side-to-side movements;
- The paired **lacrymal** bones which are only the size of a finger nail, form the inner walls of the orbits. They each have a vertical groove for the *tear duct*.
- Two **palatine** bones, which are L-shaped, form the back part of the hard palate, and walls of the nasal cavities;
- Two **turbinate** bones occur in the lateral wall of the nasal cavities below the ethmoid conchi. They are scroll-like bones and, like the conchi, are covered with mucous membrane, to filter and warm the air before it passes into the lungs.
- The single triangular **vomer** forms part of the nasal septum, articulating with the ethmoid bone and cartilage which form the rest of the nasal septum.

The hyoid bone

This single U-shaped bone is unique as it does not articulate with any other bone. It is suspended from the styloid process of the temporal bone of the skull by ligaments. It occurs in the neck between the mandible and the larynx, and supports the tongue.

The vertebral column

A series of 26 bones in the posterior wall of the trunk forms a strong flexible vertebral column. Its *functions* are to *protect* the spinal cord while allowing nerves to pass out between the vertebrae, to *support* the head, and to provide *attachment* for the ribs and muscles of the back. Between successive vertebrae are *intervertebral discs* of fibrocartilage which have a cushioning effect. If one of these discs is *ruptured*, the condition known as 'slipped disc' occurs.

The vertebral column has five distinct regions in which the vertebrae show small structural differences. There are:

- seven **cervical** vertebrae in the neck;

- twelve **thoracic** vertebrae articulating with the ribs in the thorax;
- five strong **lumbar** vertebrae in the lower back;
- five **sacral** vertebrae fused into one *sacrum* in the pelvic region;
- four bones fused into one **coccyx** at the base of the vertebral column.

Viewed laterally, the vertebral column has four *curves* which are alternately *concave* and *convex* in the posterior view. The upper concave *cervical* curve develops as a baby learns to hold its head up. The concave *lumbar* curve develops as a baby learns to walk. The *thoracic* and *sacral* curves retain the foetal convexity. These curves increase the strength of the vertebral column, help to maintain balance in the upright position, and absorb mechanical shocks when walking or running.

• Structure of a typical vertebra

All vertebrae have a basically similar structure. They are irregular bones consisting of a *body* (centrum), a posterior *vertebral (neural) arch* with a *spinous process* and two *transverse processes,* and four *articulating* processes that form joints with the two adjacent vertebrae. A *vertebral foramen* for the spinal cord occurs between the centrum and the vertebral (neural) arch.

Figure 4.6
Typical vertebra (from above)

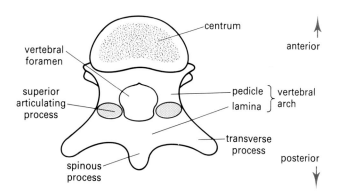

In the different regions of the vertebral column the vertebrae have special features. **Cervical** vertebrae have a small centrum and a large arch with a forked spinous process. Each transverse process has a foramen for the vertebral blood vessels. The first cervical vertebra or *atlas* is ring-shaped, being without a centrum or spinous process. Its superior surface has two concave articular surfaces to receive the occipital condyles of the skull, which allows the nodding movement of the head. The second cervical vertebra or *axis* has a centrum from which an *odontoid process* projects up through the ring-shaped atlas to allow the small rotary head movements.

Figure 4.7
Thoracic vertebra (side view)

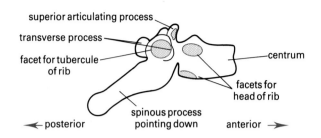

Thoracic vertebrae have long spinous processes directed downwards, and their transverse processes have facets for articulating with the tubercles of the ribs. Facets on the centrum articulate with the heads of the ribs. **Lumbar** vertebrae are large and strong with short thick processes for the attachment of the large back muscles. A considerable amount of bending (flexion) occurs in the lumbar region of the vertebral column, but almost no rotation.

The **sacrum** is triangular, articulating on both sides with the pelvic girdle which it supports. The anterior surface has four pairs of *pelvic foramina*, and the posterior surface has four pairs of *dorsal foramina*. Nerves and blood vessels pass through the foramina. The **coccyx** is a very small triangular bone at the apex of the sacrum, which represents the vestige of a tail. It is easily displaced by falling heavily onto the buttocks.

The thoracic cage

The skeleton supporting the thorax is cone-shaped, narrowing towards the neck. It comprises the centra of the thoracic vertebrae, the ribs and costal cartilages, and the sternum (breast bone). Its *functions* are to protect the heart and lungs, and to support the pectoral (shoulder) girdle. It is essential for breathing, and provides attachment for many of the muscles moving the arm.

There are 12 pairs of *ribs*, each pair articulating with a thoracic vertebra by synovial gliding joints at the *head* and *tubercle*. The first seven pairs of ribs are connected to the sternum by *costal cartilages* and are called *true ribs*. The remaining five pairs are *false ribs*. In the eighth to tenth pairs of ribs, the costal cartilages connect with those of the seventh pair. The short eleventh and twelfth pairs are called *floating ribs* as they have no attachment to the sternum.

Figure 4.8
Typical rib

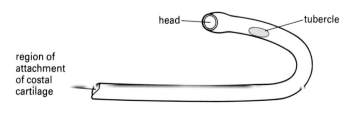

Figure 4.9
Sternum (anterior view)

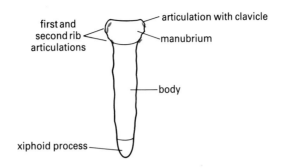

first and
second rib
articulations
articulation with clavicle
manubrium
body
xiphoid process

The *sternum* is a flat bone lying medially in the anterior wall of the thorax. It consists of three parts; an upper wider *manubrium* articulates with the first two pairs of ribs, a *body* articulates with the second to tenth pairs of ribs, and it terminates in a *xiphoid process*. The manubrium also articulates superiorly with the two clavicles (collar bones) of the pectoral girdle.

The appendicular skeleton

The pectoral (shoulder) girdle

The pectoral girdle connects the arm bones to the axial skeleton, and is formed by two *clavicles* and two *scapulae* (shoulder blades). It is incomplete posteriorly as the scapulae do not articulate with the vertebral column. Anteriorly the clavicles articulate with the sternum.

The **clavicles** are long bones with a slight S-shaped curvature, and are placed horizontally at the top of the anterior thoracic wall. Their medial end is rounded where it articulates with the manubrium. Their lateral end is flattened and articulates with the acromion process of the scapula. Both lateral and medial articulations are gliding joints. The *coracoid tuberosity* on the inferior surface of the clavicle is for attachment of ligaments from the coracoid process of the scapula. The clavicles provide the only attachment of the pectoral girdle to the axial skeleton, and are the most frequently fractured bones in the body.

The **scapulae** are two large triangular, flat bones in the upper part of the posterior thoracic wall between the second and seventh ribs. A ridge, the *scapular spine*, runs diagonally across

Figure 4.10
Clavicle (anterior view)

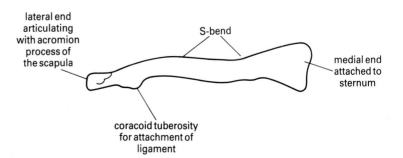

lateral end
articulating
with acromion
process of
the scapula
S-bend
medial end
attached to
sternum
coracoid tuberosity
for attachment of
ligament

Figure 4.11
Scapula (posterior view)

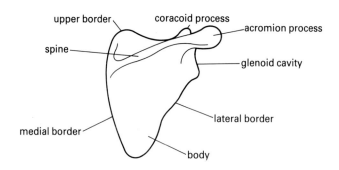

the posterior face of the bone. The end of the spine projects as the *acromion process* at the shoulder, and the scapula has a *coracoid process* just anterior to it. Just below these two processes the scapula has a depression, the *glenoid cavity*, which articulates with the humerus of the upper arm. The acromion process articulates with the clavicle.

The pelvic (hip) girdle or pelvis

The pelvis is basin-shaped and consists of two **coxal** bones joined anteriorly at the *symphysis pubis*. Posteriorly, the coxae articulate with the sacrum at a gliding joint where movement only occurs during childbirth. The *functions* of the pelvis are to provide a strong support for the legs which carry the weight of the body, to protect the organs in the pelvic cavity, and to provide a surface for attachment of the muscles of locomotion.

Each *coxal bone* has three regions, a superior *ilium*, an inferior posterior *ischium*, and an inferior anterior *pubis*. The three regions meet at the *acetabulum*, where the femur (thigh bone) articulates with the pelvis at a hip joint. The ischium has a posterior *ischial tuberosity* for muscle attachment. The ischium and pubis surround the *obturator foramen*, a large gap in the coxal bone occupied by a fibrous membrane. Nerves and blood vessels supplying the legs pierce this fibrous membrane.

Figure 4.12
Pelvis (anterior view)

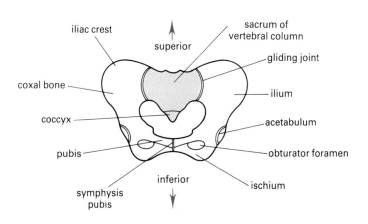

The fore limb or arm

The arm contains 30 bones arranged on a *pentadactyl* (five-fingered) plan. Most are long bones. (For the nature of the joints, see later section.)

The **humerus** is the bone of the upper arm between the shoulder and the elbow. At the proximal end is the *head*, a lateral *greater tubercle*, and an anterior *lesser tubercle*. Between the tubercles is a *sulcus*, the *bicipital groove*. The distal end of the humerus at the elbow has a *capitulum* articulating with the radius of the forearm, and a *trochlea* articulating with the ulna of the forearm. The medial and lateral *epicondyles* are rough projections on either side of the distal end of the humerus.

Figure 4.13
Right humerus (anterior view)

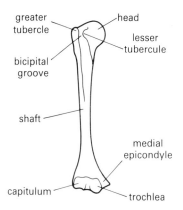

greater tubercle — head — lesser tubercule — bicipital groove — shaft — medial epicondyle — capitulum — trochlea

The **ulna** is the medial bone of the forearm, on the little finger side. Its proximal end has a projecting *olecranon process* forming the elbow;

The **radius** is the lateral bone of the forearm, on the thumb side. Its distal end has a lateral *styloid process*, and articulates with the proximal carpals. Its proximal end articulates with the humerus and the ulna.

Figure 4.14
Right radius and ulna (anterior view)

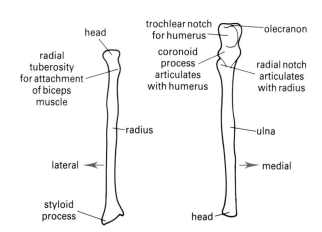

head — radial tuberosity for attachment of biceps muscle — radius — lateral — styloid process — trochlear notch for humerus — coronoid process articulates with humerus — olecranon — radial notch articulates with radius — ulna — medial — head

The wrist is composed of eight small **carpal** bones arranged in two rows of four. The carpals are of the short bone type. The *proximal* row of carpals comprise the *scaphoid* (on the thumb side), *lunate, triquetral* and *pisiform*. The *distal* carpals comprise the *trapezium* (on the thumb side), *trapezoid, capitate,* and *hamate*. The bones are joined together by ligaments.

The hand has five **metacarpal** bones in the palm, and 14 *phalanges* in the digits. The *pollex* (thumb) has two phalanges, while each finger has a proximal, middle, and distal phalanx.

Figure 4.15
Bones of right wrist and hand
(palmar surface)

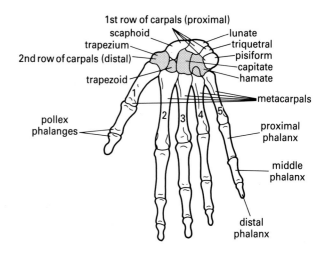

The hind limb or leg

The leg is built on the same plan as the arm, and it also contains 30 bones. (For the nature of the joints, see later section.)

- The **femur** (thigh bone) is the largest and strongest of the long bones of the limb. Its shaft *inclines* medially towards the knee, particularly in women, who have wider hips than men. This line brings the knee joint closer to the mid-line. Although it gives a narrower base to support the body's weight, making the body less stable, it allows easier body movements. The proximal *head* of the femur articulates with the acetabulum of the coxal bone at the hip joint. Proximally, there is a lateral *greater trochanter* and a medial *lesser trochanter* for attachment of buttock and thigh muscles. There is a narrow *neck* between the head and the trochanters, which may fracture in elderly people. The distal end of the femur has medial and lateral *condyles* which articulate with the tibia (shin bone) and patella (knee cap). The *patellar surface* is a triangular area between the condyles.
- The **patella** is a *sesamoid* bone which develops in the *tendon* of the quadriceps femoris muscle, and lies anterior to the knee joint.

Figure 4.16
Right femur (anterior view)

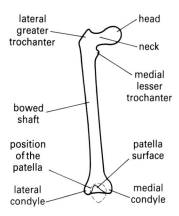

Figure 4.16
Right femur (anterior view)

- The **tibia** (shin bone) is the larger medial bone of the lower leg, and bears the body weight. Its proximal end has lateral and medial *condyles* articulating with the femur. The *tibial tuberosity* on its anterior surface is where the *patellar ligament* is attached. The distal end of the tibia has a *medial malleolus* forming the projection on the inner side of the ankle. A *fibular notch* articulates with the end of the fibula.
- The **fibula** bone lies parallel to the tibia in the lower leg. It is lateral to the tibia, and does not articulate with the femur. At its proximal end, the *head* of the fibula articulates with the lateral condyle of the tibia. Its distal end has a *lateral malleolus* forming the projection on the outside of the ankle.

Figure 4.17
Right tibia and fibula (anterior view)

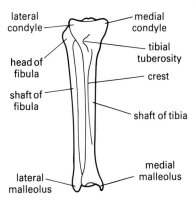

- The *ankle* consists of seven **tarsal** bones. The *talus* and *calcaneum* are posterior, the *cuboid, navicular*, and three *cuneiform* tarsals are anterior. The talus is the only tarsal that articulates with the tibia and fibula, and thus bears the weight of the leg. The calcaneum forms the *heel*.
- The *foot* has five **metatarsal** bones, which, with the tarsals,

support the *arches* of the foot. The metatarsals articulate proximally with the three cuneiform tarsals and the cuboid, and distally with the phalanges. There are 14 *phalanges* in the toes, two in the *hallux* (big toe), and three in each of the other toes.

Figure 4.18
Bones of right ankle and foot (side view)

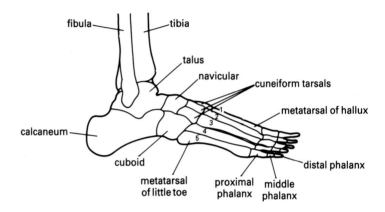

● **The arches of the foot**

The bones of the foot form arches to support the body weight and provide leverage when walking. They yield slightly when weight is applied, and spring back when the weight is lifted. Two of the arches run *longitudinally* along the foot, while the other two are *transverse:*

● The *medial longitudinal* arch on the big toe side is the highest of the arches, and is formed by the calcaneum, navicular, three cuneiform, and first three metatarsal bones. Only the calcaneum and metatarsal bones should make contact with the ground;

● The *lateral longitudinal* arch is formed by the calcaneum, cuboid, and last two metatarsal bones. The cuboid is the 'keystone' of the arch;

● The *posterior transverse* arch is formed by the calcaneum, navicular, and cuboid tarsals;

● The *anterior transverse* arch is formed by the posterior parts of the five metatarsals.

Movements of bones

All movements that change the position of the bones occur at joints. Several different kinds of movement may occur.

● *Flexion* is a movement which bends a limb, eg at the elbow when the forearm and hand moves towards the face, or when bending the head forward onto the chest;

- *Extension* is a movement which straightens a limb, or the spine, and is the reverse of flexion;

- *Hyperextension* involves bending further back than the vertical position, eg bending the head backwards to look up at the ceiling;

- *Abduction* is a movement away from the mid-line of the body, eg when the arms are raised horizontally sideways;

- *Adduction* is a movement towards the mid-line of the body, eg lowering the arms to the sides;

- *Circumduction* is a circular movement in which the moving bone describes a cone in the air, eg circling the extended arm at the shoulder;

- *Dorsiflexion* is the upward movement of the top of the foot towards the tibia at the ankle joint;

- *Plantar flexion* is the movement of the sole of the foot downwards, extending the foot at the ankle joint, eg when standing on tip-toe;

- *Eversion* is turning the sole of the foot outwards at the ankle, so that the body weight is on the inner edge of the foot;

- *Inversion* is turning the sole of the foot inwards at the ankle, so that the body weight is on the outer edge of the foot;

- *Pronation* is a movement of the flexed forearm, turning the palm to face downwards by rotating the radius on the ulna;

- *Supination* is a movement of the flexed forearm, turning the palm of the hand upwards;

- *Rotation* is the movement of a bone turning about its long axis, either towards or away from the mid-line of the body eg the atlas is rotated on the odontoid process of the axis when shaking the head, producing rotation on a horizontal plane.

Joints

Joints occur where bones *articulate*, and are *classified* according to the amount and type of movement between them.

- **Fibrous** joints are immovable, as the bones are held together by fibrous connective tissue, and there is no joint cavity. The sutures between the bones of the skull, and the joints between the teeth and jawbones are examples of fibrous joints;

- **Cartilaginous** joints are only slightly movable, the articulating bones being held together by a pad of cartilage, and there is no joint cavity. The joints between the centra of successive vertebrae are cartilaginous. A symphysis, such as the joint between the two pubic bones of the pelvis, has a broad flat disc of fibrocartilage between the bones.

- **Synovial** joints are freely movable, and a joint cavity is present, as there is a space between the articulating bones. The articulating surfaces at the ends of the bones are covered with a thin layer of smooth hyaline cartilage to reduce friction. In the space between the bones is the lubricating *synovial fluid* secreted by a *synovial membrane* lining the joint cavity. Outside the synovial membrane is a *fibrous capsule* continuous with the periosteum of each bone. The synovial membrane and fibrous capsule together make up the *articular capsule,* which is strong and flexible and retains the synovial fluid. The bones are held in position at the joint by additional accessory elastic *ligaments*, which prevent dislocation during normal movement.

Synovial joints are divided into several types according to the kind of movement which occurs:

(a) **Ball-and-socket** joints allow rotation and movement in all three planes (one *horizontal,* and two *vertical* at right angles). The rounded head of one bone fits into a cup-shaped socket in another bone. The head of the humerus fits into the glenoid socket in the scapula at the shoulder, and the head of the femur fits into the acetabulum of the pelvis at the hip. Thus there is great freedom of movement at the shoulder and hip joints;

(b) **Hinge** joints allow flexion and extension, which are movements in one plane only. The cylindrical end of one bone fits into a notch in another bone. The elbow is a hinge joint, where the lower end of the humerus fits into the trochlear notch in the ulna. Hinge joints also occur at the knee, and between the phalanges of the fingers and toes;

(c) **Gliding** (sliding) joints only allow side-to-side and back-and-forth movements in two planes. The articulating surfaces of the bones are flat. The joints between the carpals in the wrist, and between the tarsals in the ankle are gliding joints;

(d) **Condyloid** joints occur where an oval condyle projecting from one bone fits into an oval cavity on another bone, allowing side-to-side and back-and-forth movements. The occipital condyles of the skull fit into concavities on the atlas vertebra. Condyloid joints occur between the meta-carpals and proximal phalanges in the hands, and at the wrist between the ulna and radius and the proximal row of carpals. A condyloid joint occurs between the skull and the lower jaw;

(e) **Saddle** joints allow movements which are slightly freer than those of condyloid joints. The articular surfaces of the bones are saddle-shaped, concave on one side, and convex on the other. The convexity on one bone fits the concavity in the other. In the thumb joint the trapezium articulates with the first metacarpal by a saddle joint;

(f) **Pivot** joints allow rotation only. The radius and ulna rotate round one another at the elbow, and the odontoid peg of the axis vertebra rotates in a ring-shaped socket in the atlas vertebra;

Inside some synovial joints, discs of fibrocartilage (*menisci*) lie between the articular surfaces of the bones. They help to stabilize the joint, and are found in the knee joint. A 'torn cartilage' in the knee is due to damage to the menisci;

- **Ligaments** are fibrous or fibroelastic bands of dense connective tissue which are silvery in appearance. The majority of ligaments are found at joints, where they hold the bones in position.

Table 4.1
Major joints of the body

Name	Type	Structure	Movements
Shoulder	Synovial Ball-and-socket	Head of the humerus fits into the glenoid cavity of the scapula. The acromion process of the scapular spine articulates with the clavicle. The tendon of the biceps runs through the articular capsule; ligaments and deep shoulder muscles strengthen the joint	Flexion/extension; abduction and adduction; rotation outwards; rotation inwards; circum-duction
Elbow	Synovial Hinge	The capitulum of the humerus articulates with the head of the radius. The trochlea of the humerus fits into the trochlear notch of the ulna, behind which is the olecranon forming the elbow (funny bone)	Flexion/extension
	Pivot	The radius articulates with the radial notch of the ulna	Pronation and supination
Wrist	Synovial Condyloid	The radius articulates with the scaphoid lunate and triquetral carpals. It is strengthened by ligaments and surrounded by a capsule	Flexion/extension; abduction and adduction; circumduction

Table 4.1 (cont)

Name	Type	Structure	Movements
Wrist	Gliding	Joints between the carpals	Flexion/extension; abduction and adduction
Hip (bears 66% of body weight)	Synovial Ball-and-socket	The head of the femur articulates with the acetabulum of the coxal bone of the pelvis. The articular capsule is very strong and there are ligaments and muscles which strengthen the joint	Flexion/extension; abduction and adduction; rotation outwards; rotation inwards; circumduction
Knee (bears 88% of the body weight)	Synovial Hinge	Between the femur and tibia. Cruciate ligaments hold the bones together. Menisci occur between tibial and femoral condyles	Flexion/extension; some rotation
	Gliding	Between femur and patella. The patella is supported by the patellar ligament and the tendon of the quadriceps femoris. There is no complete articular capsule but a large number of ligaments strengthen the joint	Abduction and adduction
Ankle (bears whole weight of the body)	Synovial Hinge	The talus articulates with the malleoli of the tibia and fibula. A very strong deltoid ligament passes from the tibial malleolus to the talus, navicular and calcaneum binding the leg to the foot. Several smaller ligaments also occur	Dorsiflexion; plantar flexion
Intervertebral	Cartilaginous Symphysis	A broad flat intervertebral disc of fibrocartilage occurs between the centra of adjacent vertebrae. All movements are very small, but are additive	Flexion/extension; lateral flexion; rotation; circumduction

Figure 4.19
Synovial joint (vertical section)

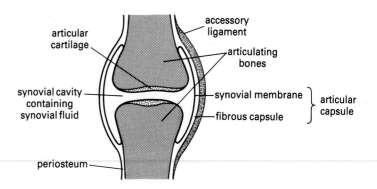

Figure 4.20
Shoulder joint

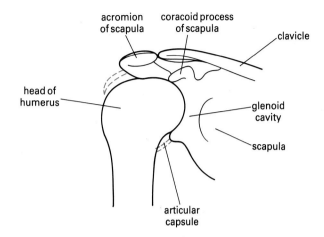

Figure 4.21
Elbow joint

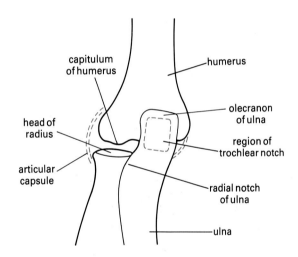

Figure 4.22
Hip joint (vertical section)

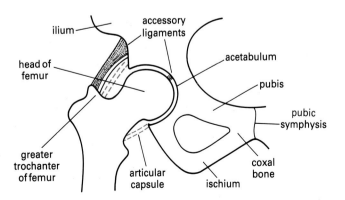

Figure 4.23
Knee joint (vertical section)

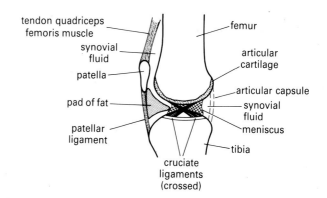

Figure 4.24
Intervertebral joint (side view)

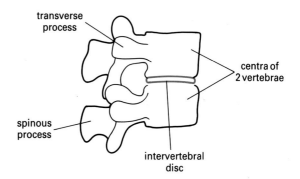

Effects of ageing on the skeletal system

With increasing age, especially menopausally, *osteoporosis,* a decrease in bone mass, occurs and there is a shortening of the legs due to compression of the softened bone. An average height loss of 1.5 cm occurs between the ages of 30 and 60 years in women.

Arthritis is a degenerative inflammatory condition of the joints. There are several types of arthritis, *osteoarthrosis* and *rheumatoid arthritis* commonly affecting women. In *osteoarthrosis* the ends of the bones slowly degenerate, starting with the crumbling of the articular cartilage. It commonly affects hip, knee, shoulder, and terminal finger joints, and is found in many women over 60 years of age. *Rheumatoid arthritis* is an *autoimmune* disease (where the defence mechanism attacks the body's own normal tissues) which usually starts between the ages of 35 and 40 years. There is a thickening of the synovial membrane of the joint, crumbling of the articular cartilage, and over-production of connective tissue. The joint eventually becomes fixed.

Self-assessment questions

1 State the functions of the vertebral column.

2 Where in the body would you find the following structures:

(a) Haversian systems;
(b) zygomatic arches;
(c) costal cartilages?

3 What is the function of:

(a) synovial fluid;
(b) red bone marrow;
(c) the hyoid bone?

4 Distinguish between plantar flexion and dorsiflexion.

5 List the functions of the pelvis.

6 In each case, name the bone on which the particular feature occurs:

(a) bicipital groove;
(b) greater trochanter;
(c) medial malleolus;
(d) olecranon process.

7 State the functions of:

(a) tendons;   (b) foramina;
(c) ligaments.

8 Name the bones forming:

(a) the median longitudinal arch of the foot;
(b) the cranium.

9 List the parts of a typical vertebra.

10 Give **four** functions of the human skeletal system.

CHAPTER 5

The Muscular System

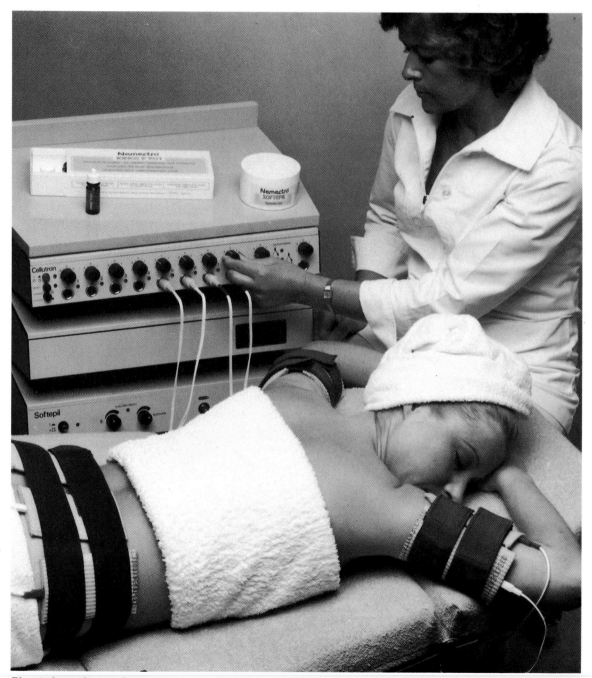

Electrical muscle stimulation

The muscular system consists of the **skeletal muscle tissue** and **connective tissue** that make up the individual muscles which are attached to the bones of the skeleton. These muscles form the *flesh*, covering the bones on the outside, and helping to give the body its shape.

The muscular system has three main *functions*, those of causing *movement* (see below), maintaining *posture* (see p 104) and producing *heat* (see p 103). It brings about movement by exerting a pull on *tendons* which move bones at joints. The pulling force is due to the *contraction* or shortening, of the muscle. Parts of the body, such as the limbs, are moved in this way. When the entire body moves from one place to another, *locomotion* is said to occur.

Usually muscles are attached by their tendons to two articulating bones on either side of the joint. When a joint is moved, one of the two articulating bones remains *stationary* while the other one *moves*. The attachment of the muscle to the stationary bone is the muscle *origin*, ie the anchorage end of the muscle. The attachment to the bone that moves is the *insertion*, ie the pulling end of the muscle. In the limb muscles the origin is usually proximal, while the insertion is distal.

During movement bones act as **levers**, hinged at the joint which acts as the *fulcrum* (F). The muscle provides the *effort* (E), while the weight of the part being moved is the *load* (L). The positions of the fulcrum, effort, and load determine the type of lever action:

- In a **first class** lever, the fulcrum is placed between the effort and the load. The movement of the head on the vertebral column is an example of first class lever action. When the head is lifted, the muscles at the back of the neck provide the effort, while the weight of the facial region of the skull is the load. The joint between the skull and atlas vertebra is the fulcrum;
- In a **third class** lever, the fulcrum is at one end, the load is at the other end of the lever, and the effort is between them. Flexing the arm at the elbow is an example of third class lever action. The elbow joint is the fulcrum, the biceps muscle provides the effort, and the weight of the forearm and hand is the load. The body movements usually involve lever action of these two types;
- In a **second class** lever, the fulcrum is at one end and the effort at the other, with the load in between. An example of this type of lever action is raising the body onto the toes. The weight of the body is the load, the ball of the foot is the fulcrum, and the contraction of the calf muscles provides the effort which lifts the heel off the ground.

The *mechanical advantage* which lever action provides is

greatest when a large weight (load) can be moved by a small muscular effort. This occurs in the second class lever action where the body is raised onto the toes. In the third class lever action at the elbow joint great muscular power develops in the biceps muscle to move the small weight of the hand, so the mechanical advantage is small.

Figure 5.1
Lever action in body movements
(a) First class lever
(b) Second class lever
(c) Third class lever

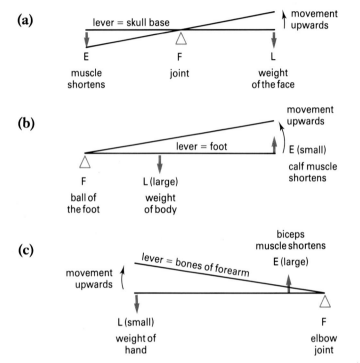

In most cases movements are brought about by several muscles acting in groups. Many muscles work in *antagonistic pairs*, where one contracts to move the bone one way, and the other contracts to move the bone back. The calf and shin muscles form an antagonistic pair which lower and raise the foot. *Isotonic* contractions develop *tension*, and the muscle *shortens* (eg the raising of the arm at the elbow by the biceps muscle, which bulges outwards as it shortens). *Isometric* contractions develop *tension*, but the muscle does not shorten (eg carrying a weight on the hand with the arm extended, when the biceps muscle does not bulge).

Muscle tissue

Muscle tissue has four main *characteristics*:

● It has the ability to shorten or *contract;*
● It can be stretched when it is relaxed, so it is *extensible;*

- After contraction or extension it can return to its original shape, so it has *elasticity*;
- Muscle tissue *responds to stimuli* provided by nerve impulses.

By contracting, muscle tissue performs the *functions* of causing *movements*, maintaining *posture*, and producing *heat* which helps to maintain normal body temperature. Muscular movements aid the flow of blood and lymph through the veins and lymphatics respectively.

There are three types of muscle tissue, skeletal, cardiac and smooth:

- **Skeletal** muscle is attached to the bones of the skeleton and is under *voluntary conscious* control by the brain and nerves. Viewed under a microscope, transverse stripes are visible, so the muscle is said to be *striated*. It is red in colour due to the presence of an oxygen-storing pigment called *myoglobin*. Skeletal muscle tissue consists of bundles of parallel muscle *fibres*. Each fibre has an outer membrane enclosing cytoplasm containing contractile protein fibrils and many nuclei. Skeletal muscle can do a great deal of work, but will tire easily. Postural muscles contain more slow-acting fibres (red), while primary movers contain more fast-acting fibres (pale);

Figure 5.2
Muscle tissue
(a) Sketetal muscle
(b) Cardiac muscle
(c) Smooth muscle

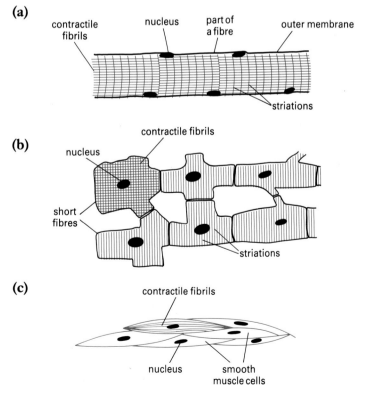

- **Cardiac** muscle is found only in the wall of the heart. The muscle fibres are *striated*, but short, and have a single nucleus. Cardiac muscle contracts *automatically* and *rhythmically* without any nervous stimulation, but its rate of contraction can be regulated by the autonomic nervous system and the hormone adrenalin. It does not tire readily, but works continuously throughout life;

- **Smooth** muscle is found in the walls of the food canal, blood vessels, and urinary system. It consists of spindle-shaped cells which interlock. Each cell has one nucleus, contains contractile fibres, but is unstriated. Smooth muscle is regulated by the autonomic nervous system and adrenalin but exhibits rhythmic contraction in the absence of nervous stimulation. Smooth muscle is capable of slow but sustained contraction, and does not tire readily.

All muscle tissue must be well supplied with *nerves* and *blood vessels*. In *skeletal* muscle, nerves bring the impulses which stimulate the muscle tissue to contract according to the *all-or-none* principle, where the muscle fibre either contracts fully or not at all. Blood vessels bring glucose and oxygen to supply energy, and the calcium ions necessary for normal contraction. They also remove waste-products such as carbon dioxide and lactic acid (see Chapter 8). Blood also brings adrenalin, which causes some muscle tissue to contract. Muscle tissue contains molecules of ATP which store energy produced from food, and release it to the tissue as it contracts.

Muscle tone

If all the skeletal muscles relaxed at once, the body would crumple. All the muscles must be slightly contracted for the body to remain upright. At any one time some of the muscle fibres in skeletal muscle tissue are contracted, while the rest are relaxed. This small amount of contraction will *tense* a muscle without causing movement. Different groups of fibres contract at different times to spread the work load. This continuous slight tension of the muscle tissue is involuntary, and is known as muscle tone. It is essential for maintaining *posture*.

Effect of temperature

When muscle tissue is *warmer*, the process of contraction occurs faster due to the speeding up of the chemical reactions involved. However, muscle tone is reduced as the body temperature rises, so more of the skeletal muscle fibres are relaxed. *Massage* is more easily carried out when the muscle tissue is warm and relaxed. *Heat cramps* will occur in muscles which are active at high temperature. Increased sweating causes loss of salt, resulting in a lower concentration of sodium ions in the blood supplying the muscle. *Cramp* is a sudden involuntary contraction of the muscle which is painful.

As muscle tissue is *cooled* the chemical reactions slow, so the contraction takes longer to occur. There is an involuntary increase in muscle tone, eventually resulting in *shivering*. *Hypothermia* finally occurs, when the muscles become rigid, and shivering stops as the reflex actions slow down. Once this stage is reached, the person is unable to move, and survival is unlikely without external warming.

Muscle fatigue

When skeletal muscle is continuously stimulated, its contraction becomes progressively weaker, and eventually ceases. This condition is *muscle fatigue*, and is due both to the accumulation of the *toxic waste* products lactic acid and carbon dioxide, and the shortage of ATP (adenosine triphosphate, an energy-rich compound), glucose, and oxygen, which provide the *energy* for contraction. When all the skeletal muscles are fatigued, the muscles exert very little balancing effect, so the ligaments and tendons must support the body and may become *strained*.

Mechanism of muscle contraction

The longitudinal *fibrils* in skeletal muscle consist of two kinds of protein filaments one type being thicker than the other. The thinner filaments are composed of *actin*, and the thicker ones of *myosin*, and the two types of filaments are arranged in alternating bands, which gives the fibre its *striated* appearance. As contraction of the muscle fibre proceeds, the thinner actin filaments *slide* further and further in-between the myosin filaments. The *energy* for this sliding movement comes from ATP in the muscle fibre.

Figure 5.3
Relaxed and contracted muscle fibres

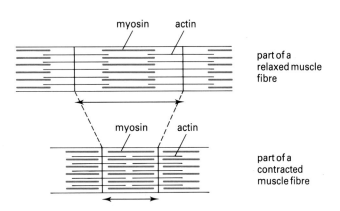

A skeletal muscle fibre will only contract if a *stimulus* is applied to it by a *motor nerve cell* or neuron. A long fibre of the neuron called the *axon* carries the stimulus to the muscle fibre, and transmits it at a *neuro-muscular junction*. Here the axon ends in fine knobbed branches resting on the muscle fibre membrane, which are known as *motor end plates*. A single motor neuron may transmit stimuli to one or two muscle fibres, or to as many as 150. The point at which a motor nerve enters a muscle is called the *motor point*.

Muscles

Within a muscle, the skeletal muscle fibres are arranged in bundles called *fasiculi*. Each bundle of fibres is surrounded by a sheath of connective tissue (*perimysium*). The entire muscle is surrounded by a layer of fibrous connective tissue (*epimysium*) which is an extension of the deep fascia. The *deep fascia* is a layer of dense inelastic connective tissue lining the body wall and limbs, which holds the muscles together, and divides them into functioning groups. It contains no fat (unlike the superficial fascia) but carries nerves and blood vessels. The *fascia lata* is the deep fascia of the thigh thickened laterally as the *iliotibial tract*. The epimysium and perimysium continue into the *tendons* which attach the muscle to bones. Skeletal muscles are well-supplied with nerves and blood vessels, and blood capillaries occur between the muscle fibres in each fasiculus.

Some of the muscles are *superficial,* lying just below the skin and superficial fascia. Others lie beneath the superficial muscles, and are said to be *deep* muscles.

Table 5.1
Muscles of mastication

Name	Position	Origin	Insertion	Action
Masseter	Lateral region of cheek between the cheekbone and angle of the jaw	Zygomatic arch	Mandible	Raises the lower jaw and clenches the teeth
Temporalis	On the side of the head above and in front of the ear, to the lower jaw	Temporal bone	Mandible	Raises the lower jaw and retracts it if it is protruding
Lateral and medial ptergyoids	On the lateral region of the cheek beneath the masseter muscle	Sphenoid and maxilla	Mandible	Open the mouth and protrude the lower jaw. Move the jaw from side to side

All these muscles of mastication are supplied by the mandibular branch of the fifth (trigeminal) cranial nerve

Muscles of the head

The muscles of the head fall into two groups. One group comprises the muscles of **mastication,** used in chewing. The muscles of the other group are responsible for **facial expression,** and may be attached to *skin* instead of bone. The wrinkling of the skin which occurs when they contract results in the various facial expressions.

Table 5.2
Muscles of facial expressions

Name	Position	Origin	Insertion	Nerve supply	Action
Occipitalis	Back of skull	Occipital	Epicranial aponeurosis	Auricular VII	Moves scalp back-wards
Frontalis	Forehead	Epicranial aponeurosis	Skin above orbits	Temporal VII	Moves scalp forwards, raises eyebrows and wrinkles forehead; expresses fright
Corrugator	Below eyebrow	Orbit and inner edge of eyebrow ridge	Skin of eyebrow	Temporal VII	Forms vertical wrinkles between the eyebrows when frowning
Orbicularis oculi	Surrounding the eye	Rim of the orbit	Skin of the eyelid	Temporal and zygomatic VII	Closes the eyelids. Used in blinking and winking. Forms 'crows feet' folds from outer angle of the eyes
Nasalis	At the side of the nose	Maxilla	Nasal bone	Buccal VII	Compresses and dilates the nostril. Expresses anger
Procerus	At the top of the nose between the eyes	Nasal bone	Skin between the eyebrows	Buccal VII	Forms transverse wrinkles over the bridge of the nose. Also expresses distaste
Quadratus (Levator) labii	Radiates from the upper lip	Lower rim of orbit	Skin of upper lip and nose	Buccal VII	Raises the lip and flares the nostril; forms the nasolabial furrow giving a sad expression
Orbicularis oris	Surrounding the mouth	Skin, and other muscles round the mouth	Skin at the corners of the mouth	Buccal VII	Closes and puckers the lips; shapes the lips during speech

Table 5.2 (cont)

Name	Position	Origin	Insertion	Nerve supply	Action
Buccinator	At the side of the face	Maxilla and mandible	Skin at the angle of the mouth, and orbicularis oris	Buccal VII	Compresses the cheek; keeps food between the teeth when chewing; used in sucking and blowing
Zygomaticus, major and minor	Radiates from the upper lip	Zygomatic arch	Skin at the angle of the mouth, and orbicularis oris	Buccal VII	Draws the angle of the mouth upwards when smiling and laughing
Risorius	Radiates laterally from the corner of the mouth	In fascia over the masseter muscle	Skin at the angle of the mouth	Buccal VII	Draws the mouth sideways and outwards in the 'grin of death'
Triangularis (depressor anguli oris)	Radiates from the lower lip over the chin	Lower margin of the mandible	Skin at the angle of the mouth	Mandibular VII	Draws the angle of the mouth down giving a sad expression
Depressor labii inferioris	Radiates from the lower lip over the chin	Base of mandible	Skin of the lower lip	Mandibular VII	Pulls down the lower lip giving a sulky expression
Mentalis	Radiates from lower lip over centre of the chin	Mandible	Skin of chin and lower lip	Mandibular VII	Lifts and protrudes the lower lip, and wrinkles the chin when expressing doubt
Platysma	Side of the neck and chin	Skin and fascia of pectoral and deltoid muscles	Skin of the lower face	Cervical VII	Depresses the mandible and draws the lip up when annoyed; loss of muscle tone causes crepey neck

Muscles of the neck

The muscles of the neck are responsible for moving the head. The **platysma** muscle of facial expression rises obliquely from the side of the neck to below the centre of the chin, and up onto the lower jaw. It is superficial to the muscles moving the head.

Figure 5.4
Muscles of mastication (side view)

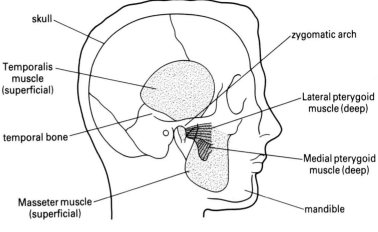

Figure 5.5
Muscles of facial expression (side view)

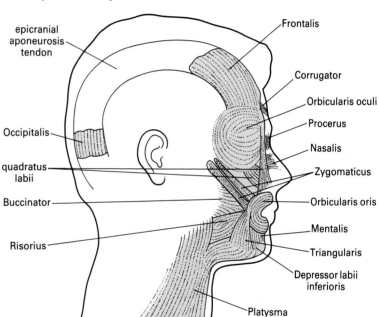

Figure 5.6
Muscles of the neck (side view)

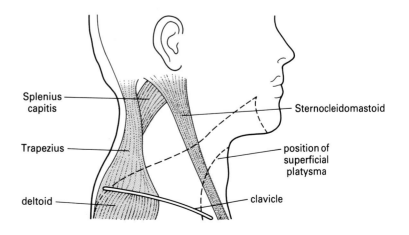

Table 5.3
Muscles of the neck

Name	Position	Origin	Insertion	Nerve supply	Action
Sternocleido-mastoid	Obliquely down the side of the neck from below the ear to the breastbone	Sternum and clavicle	Mastoid region of the temporal bone	XI cranial	When both contract together, the chin is pulled down onto the chest; when only one contracts, the head turns to the opposite side
Trapezius	Down the back of the neck onto the shoulders	Occipital and seventh cervical, and all the thoracic vertebrae	Clavicle and scapula	XI cranial	Lifts the clavicle and rotates the scapula upwards; it extends the head (hyperextension)
Splenius capitis	Up the back of the neck beneath the trapezius to just behind the ear	Spines of seventh cervical and first four thoracic vertebrae	Occipital, and mastoid process of the temporal	Cervical spinal	When both contract together the neck is lengthened to hold the head upright; contraction of one muscle rotates the head to the same side

Muscles of the shoulder moving the shoulder joint

Key: ☐ Origin
      ☐ Insertion

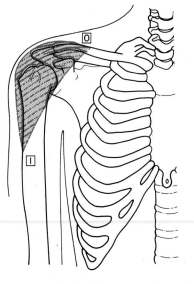

Deltoid

position:
caps top of shoulder and upper arm
origin:
clavicle, scapula spine, and acromion process
insertion:
shaft of humerus on lateral side, below its head
nerve supply:
axillary nerves of brachial plexus
action:
abducts arm, and draws it backwards and forwards

Latissimus dorsi

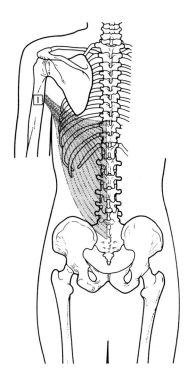

Pectoralis major

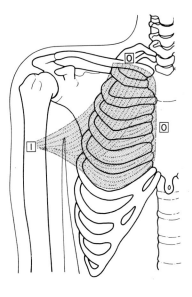

nerve supply:
pectoral nerves of brachial
plexus
action:
draws shoulder down and
forwards

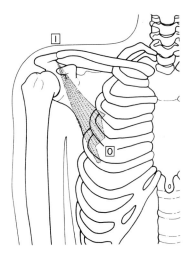

Levator scapulae

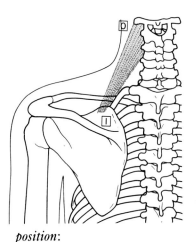

position:
a large sheet of muscle down
back of lower thorax and
lumbar region
origin:
lower thoracic vertebrae,
lumbar vertebrae, sacrum and
rim of pelvis
insertion:
shaft of humerus below its
head
nerve supply:
from brachial plexus
(thoracodorsal branch)
action:
draws shoulder downwards
and backwards; adducts and
rotates arm; with both arms
fixed when climbing, helps
pull body upwards

position:
across front of upper part of
thorax, beneath breasts
origin:
clavicle, sternum, and rib
cartilages
insertion:
shaft of humerus below its
head (greater tubercle)
nerve supply:
pectoral nerves of brachial
plexus
action:
adducts arm, and rotates it
inwards (throwing action)

Pectoralis minor

position:
across front of upper part of
thorax beneath pectoralis
major
origin:
third to fifth ribs
insertion:
coracoid process of scapula

position:
at back and sides of neck,
onto shoulder
origin:
upper four cervical vertebrae
insertion:
upper edge of scapula
nerve supply:
cervical spinal nerves
action:
lifts scapula and shoulder

Other muscles of the shoulder and chest

Serratus anterior

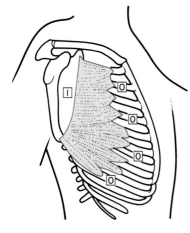

position:
sides of ribcage below armpits
origin:
upper ribs
insertion:
medial edge of scapula
nerve supply:
cervical spinal nerves
action:
draws scapula forwards and
rotates it upwards; used in
pushing movements

Rhomboids

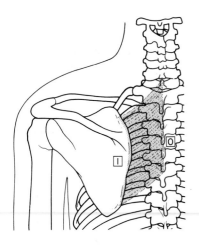

position:
on back of thorax between
shoulders
origin:
thoracic vertebrae
insertion:
medial edge of scapula
nerve supply:
cervical spinal nerves
action:
braces shoulder, and rotates
scapula

Teres major

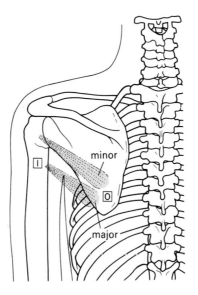

position:
across back of shoulders; a
deep muscle
origin:
lateral edge of the scapula
insertion:
shaft of humerus just below
lesser tubercle
nerve supply:
lower subscapular nerves of
brachial plexus
action:
rotates humerus inwards
(medially) in its socket, and
assists in drawing arm
downwards

Teres minor

position:
across back of shoulders; a
deep muscle
origin:
lateral edge of scapula
insertion:
greater tubercle of humerus
nerve supply:
axillary nerve of brachial
plexus
action:
rotates humerus outwards
(laterally) in its socket

Supraspinatus

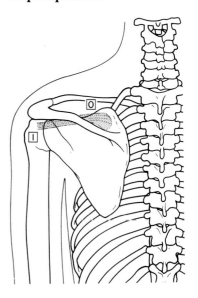

position:
across back of shoulders; a
deep muscle
origin:
upper edge of the spine of
scapula
insertion:
greater tubercle of humerus
nerve supply:
suprascapular nerve of
brachial plexus
action:
abducts humerus, assisting
deltoid muscle

Infraspinatus

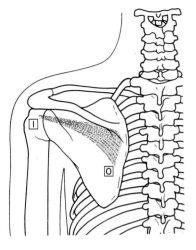

position:
across back of shoulders; a
deep muscle
origin:
lower edge of spine of scapula
insertion:
greater tubercle of humerus
nerve supply:
suprascapular nerve of
brachial plexus
action:
rotates humerus outwards
(laterally)

Coracobrachialis

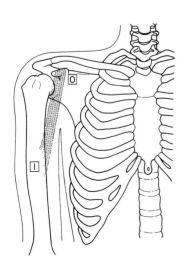

position:
at the upper medial part of
arm, beneath deltoid
origin:
coracoid process of scapula
insertion:
middle of shaft of humerus on
medial side
nerve supply:
from brachial plexus
(musculocutaneous branch)
action:
flexes arm and adducts it,
drawing it forward and
towards mid-line of body

Muscles of respiration of the thorax

Diaphragm

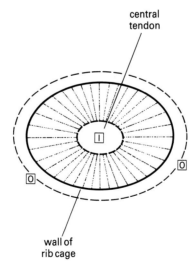

central
tendon

wall of
rib cage

position:
separating thoracic and
abdominal cavities
origin:
xiphoid, cartilages of last six
ribs, and lumbar vertebrae

insertion:
central tendon forming
membranous part of
diaphragm
nerve supply:
phrenic nerves of cervical
plexus
action:
flattens diaphragm to increase
thoracic cavity for inspiration

External intercostals

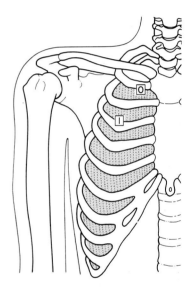

position:
between ribs, running
obliquely downwards
origin:
lower edge of rib above
insertion:
upper edge of rib immediately
below
nerve supply:
intercostal nerves
action:
raise ribs to increase thoracic
cavity for normal inspiration

Internal intercostals

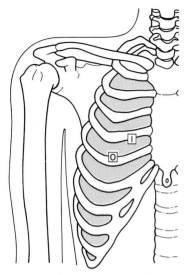

position:
between ribs, beneath external intercostals
origin:
upper edge of rib below
insertion:
lower edge of rib immediately above
nerve supply:
intercostal nerves
action:
pull ribs down during forced expiration

Muscles of the abdominal wall

Anterior muscles

Rectus abdominis

position:
extends whole length of front of abdomen, and is divided into four sections by three fibrous bands
origin:
pubic bone of pelvis

insertion:
cartilages of fifth to seventh ribs, and xiphoid
nerve supply:
intercostal nerves (seventh to twelfth)
action:
both acting together bend trunk forwards, flexing spine; alone, compresses abdomen, pushing internal organs towards spine to keep centre of gravity over arches of feet; is therefore an important muscle in maintaining posture; draws front of pelvis upwards

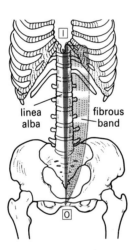

linea alba   fibrous band

External oblique

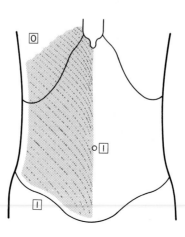

position:
extends laterally down the front of the abdomen
origin:
lower eight ribs
insertion:
linea alba (tendon from xiphoid process to pubic symphysis) and iliac crest of pelvis
nerve supply:
intercostal nerves (eight to twelfth), and upper nerves of lumbar plexus
action:
both acting together compress abdomen; one acting alone twists trunk, turning front of abdomen towards opposite side

Internal oblique

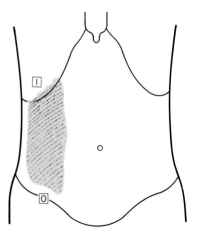

position:
laterally on front of abdomen, deep to external oblique muscle, running diagonally in the opposite direction to it
origin:
iliac crest of the pelvis
insertion:
cartilages of the last four ribs

nerve supply:
intercostal nerves (eighth to
twelfth) and upper nerves of
the lumbar plexus
action:
both acting together compress
abdomen; one acting alone
twists trunk turning front of
abdomen towards same side;
works with external oblique
muscle of opposite side

Transversus abdominis

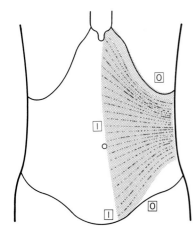

position:
laterally on front of abdomen,
deep to internal oblique
muscle
origin:
ilium of pelvis, lumbar fascia,
and last six ribs
insertion:
xiphoid, linea alba, and pubis
of the pelvis
nerve supply:
intercostal nerves (seventh to
twelfth) and upper nerves of
lumbar plexus
action:
compresses abdomen

Posterior muscles

Quadratus lumborum

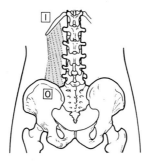

position:
medially, on the lower part of
back
origin:
iliac crest of pelvis
insertion:
twelfth rib and upper four
lumbar vertebrae
nerve supply:
last thoracic and first lumbar
nerves
action:
flexes spine laterally

Erector spinae (three groups of muscles)

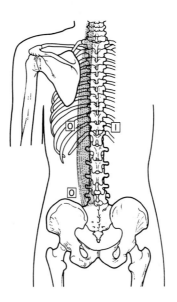

position:
medially on posterior surface
of neck, thorax, and abdomen
origin:
iliac crest, lumbar vertebrae,
ribs and thoracic vertebrae
insertion:
ribs, cervical and lumbar
vertebrae
nerve supply:
cervical, thoracic, and lumbar
nerves
action:
extends spine; the main
postural muscle holding the
body upright

Psoas (part of iliopsoas)

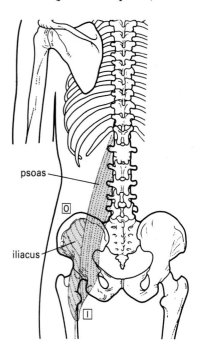

position:
in lumbar region from spine
to rim of pelvis, and across
hip joint
origin:
transverse processes of
lumbar vertebrae
insertion:
lesser trochanter of femur

nerve supply:
second and third lumbar
nerves
action:
flexes and rotates thigh
laterally, and flexes spine
when rising from a lying to a
sitting position

Iliacus (part of iliopsoas)

position:
laterally, inside the pelvis, and
across the hip joint
origin:
iliac bone of pelvis
insertion:
lesser trochanter of femur,
with tendon of the psoas
nerve supply:
femoral nerve of lumbar
plexus
action:
flexes and rotates thigh
laterally; acts as a postural
muscle helping to keep body
erect at hip joint

Muscles of the buttocks

Gluteus maximus

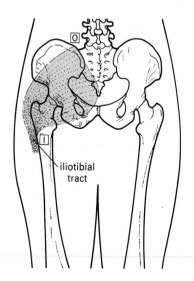

iliotibial
tract

position:
lower part of back forming
buttocks
origin:
ilium of pelvis, sacrum, and
coccyx
insertion:
posterior surface of shaft of
femur iliotibial tract
nerve supply:
gluteal nerve of sacral plexus
action:
extends and rotates thigh
laterally; used in running and
jumping, and raises body after
stooping; through the
iliotibial tract it steadies the
femur on the tibia during
standing

Gluteus medius

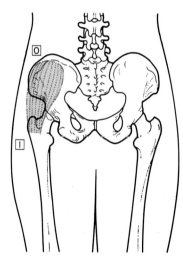

position:
lateral area of the buttocks, its
posterior part covered by
gluteus maximus
origin:
ilium of pelvis
insertion:
greater trochanter of femur
nerve supply:
gluteal nerve of sacral plexus

action:
abducts and rotates thigh
medially; used in walking and
running; it maintains the
balance when standing on one
leg

Gluteus minimus

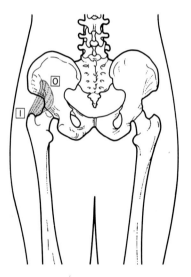

position:
immediately deep to gluteus
medius, on lateral area of the
buttocks
origin:
ilium of pelvis
insertion:
greater trochanter of femur
nerve supply:
gluteal nerve of sacral plexus
action:
abducts and rotates thigh
laterally; used in walking and
running; it maintains the
balance when standing on one
leg

Muscles of the pelvic floor

The muscles of the pelvic floor, together with their fasciae, are known as the *pelvic diaphragm.* They support the organs in the pelvic cavity, including the bladder. Damage to these muscles during childbirth can result in prolapse of the uterus or stress incontinence. The muscles can also be damaged by inappropriate exercise.

Levator ani

position:
forms funnel-shaped floor of pelvic cavity; contains openings through which the anal canal, urethra and vagina pass
origin:
pubis and ischium of the pelvis
insertion:
coccyx, urethra and anal canal
nerve supply:
from the fourth sacral nerve and the sacral plexus (pudendal branch)
action:
supports and slightly raises the floor of the pelvis, resisting any downward pressure in the abdomen; constricts lower end of vagina and rectum

Coccygeus

position:
behind Levator ani muscle
origin:
ischium of pelvis
insertion:
coccyx and lower part of sacrum

nerve supply:
fourth and fifth sacral nerves
action:
supports and slightly raises floor of pelvis, resisting any downward pressure in abdomen; pulls coccyx forward after it has been pushed back during defaecation or childbirth

Muscles that move the forearm at the elbow joint

Biceps brachii

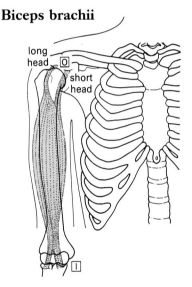

position:
down anterior surface of the humerus) has two heads
origin:
long head – above glenoid cavity; short head – on coracoid process of scapula
insertion:
on radius, just below elbow
nerve supply:
from brachial plexus (musculocutaneous nerve)
action:
flexes and supinates (turns palm upwards) forearm

Brachialis

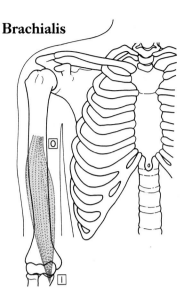

position:
anterior surface of lower part of humerus, deep to biceps, and across elbow joint
origin:
halfway down shaft on the anterior surface of humerus
insertion:
coronoid process of ulna
nerve supply:
From brachial plexus (musculocutaneous and radial nerves)
action:
flexes the forearm

Triceps brachii

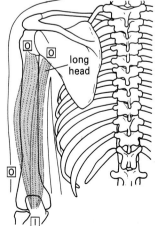

position:
posterior surface of humerus; has three heads
origin:
long head on scapula; other two heads on humerus
insertion:
olecranon process of the ulna
nerve supply:
from brachial plexus (radial nerve)
action:
extends the forearm

Brachioradialis

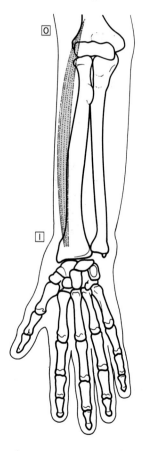

position:
on radial (thumb) side of forearm
origin:
shaft of humerus above lateral condyle

insertion:
distal end of radius above styloid process
nerve supply:
from brachial plexus (radial nerve)
action:
flexes forearm

Pronator teres

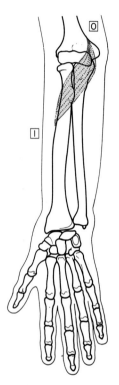

position:
on anterior side of forearm across elbow joint
origin:
distal end of humerus, and coronoid process of ulna
insertion:
lateral surface of radius
nerve supply:
from brachial plexus (median nerve)
action:
pronates (turns palm downwards) forearm, and flexes it at the elbow

Supinator

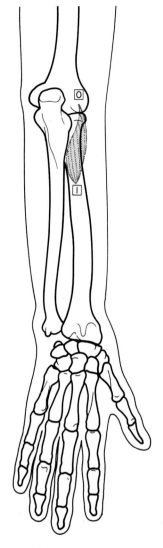

position:
surrounds upper part of radius
origin:
lateral epicondyle of humerus, and ridge on ulna
insertion:
lateral surface of radius
nerve supply:
from brachial plexus (radial nerve)
action:
supinates the forearm

Muscles of the arm that move the wrist and fingers

Anterior muscles

Pronator quadratus

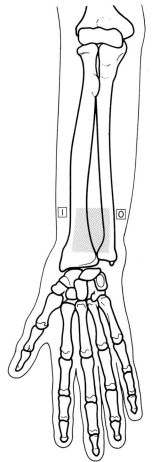

position:
crosses lower part of front of forearm
origin:
lower part of ulna just above wrist
insertion:
lower part of radius just above wrist
nerve supply:
from brachial plexus (median nerve)

action:
pronates forearm, and prevents separation of lower ends of radius and ulna when falling on wrist

Palmaris longus

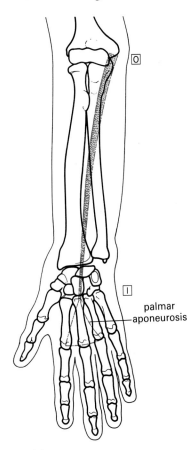

palmar aponeurosis

position:
down anterior medial side of forearm
origin:
medial epicondyle of humerus
insertion:
palmar aponeurosis in palm of hand
nerve supply:
from brachial plexus (median nerve)
action:
flexes wrist

Flexor carpi radialis

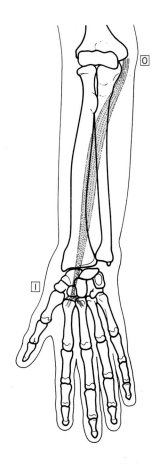

position:
down anterior side of forearm from inside elbow joint towards thumb
origin:
medial epicondyle of humerus
insertion:
second and third metacarpals
nerve supply:
from brachial plexus (median nerve)
action:
flexes and abducts wrist (moving hand away from the body)

Flexor carpi ulnaris

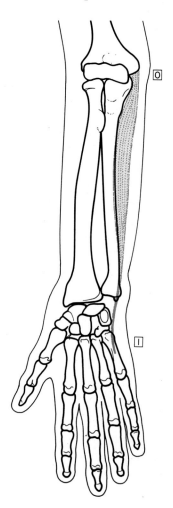

Flexor digitorum sublimis (superficialis)

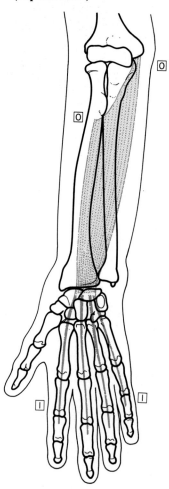

Flexor digitorum profundus

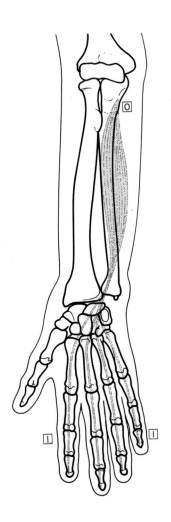

position:
along ulnar (little finger) side of forearm
origin:
medial epicondyle of humerus
insertion:
fifth metacarpal, and pisiform and hamate carpals
nerve supply:
from brachial plexus (ulnar nerve)
action:
flexes and adducts wrist (moving the hand in towards body)

position:
down medial side of forearm, deep to palmaris longus
origin:
medial epicondyle of the humerus, coronoid process of ulna, and shaft of the radius
insertion:
the middle phalanx of each finger
nerve supply:
from brachial plexus (median nerve)
action:
flexes middle phalanx of each finger

position:
along ulnar side of forearm; a deep muscle
origin:
upper part of ulna
insertion:
bases of distal phalanges
nerve supply:
from brachial plexus (median and ulnar nerves)
action:
flexes distal phalanx of each finger

Posterior muscles

Extensor carpi radialis longus

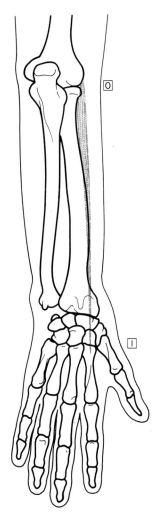

Extensor carpi radialis brevis

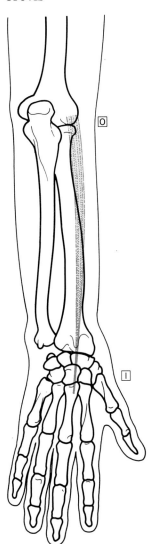

Extensor carpi ulnaris

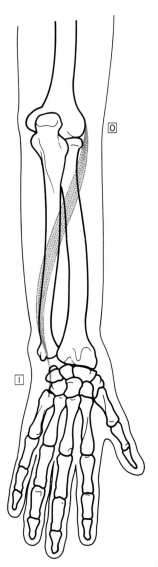

position:
along radial (thumb) side of forearm
origin:
lateral epicondyle of humerus
insertion:
second metacarpal
nerve supply:
from brachial plexus (radial nerve)
action:
extends and abducts wrist

position:
along radial side of forearm; a deep muscle
origin:
lateral epicondyle of humerus
insertion:
base of third metacarpal
nerve supply:
from brachial plexus (radial nerve)
action:
extends and abducts wrist

position:
along back of forearm on ulnar side
origin:
lateral epicondyle of humerus
insertion:
fifth metacarpal
nerve supply:
from brachial plexus (radial nerve)
action:
extends and adducts wrist

Extensor digitorum

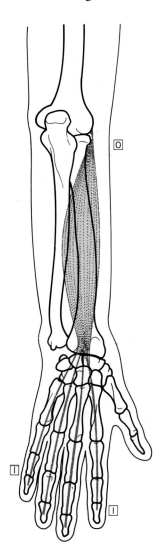

Muscles of the thigh

Acting at the hip joint

Adductors brevis, longus, and magnus

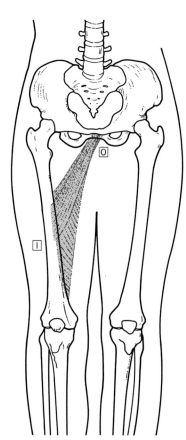

Pectineus

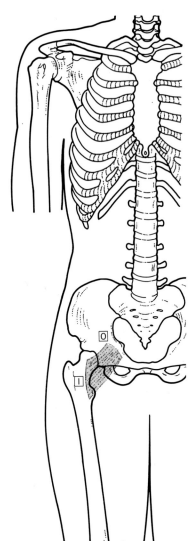

position:
along back of forearm on radial side
origin:
lateral epicondyle of humerus
insertion:
middle and distal phalanges of each finger
nerve supply:
from brachial plexus (radial nerve)
action:
extends fingers

position:
on medial side of thigh; longus is the most superficial
origin:
pubis of pelvis
insertion:
shaft of femur
nerve supply:
from lumbar plexus (obturator nerve)
action:
adduct, rotate, and flex thigh at hip

position:
crosses front of thigh at top, from the medial to lateral side
origin:
front of pubis
insertion:
lesser trochanter of femur
nerve of supply:
femoral nerve of lumbar plexus
action:
flexes, adducts, and rotates thigh laterally

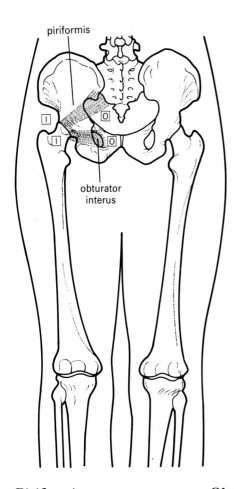

Tensor fasciae latae

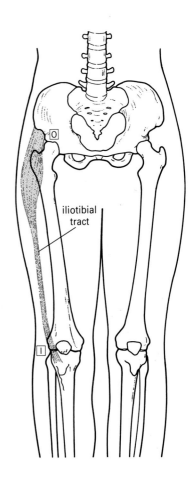

Piriformis

position:
crossing top of thigh below
buttocks; a deep muscle
origin:
sacrum
insertion:
greater trochanter of the
femur
nerve supply:
from the sacral plexus (1 and
2 sacral nerves).
action:
rotates the thigh laterally, and
abducts it. It is a postural
muscle controlling the
position of the neck of the
femur

Obturator internus

position:
crosses top of thigh below
buttocks; occurs partly within
pelvis and partly at back of hip
joint
origin:
margin of obturator foramen
of pelvis
insertion:
greater trochanter of femur
nerve supply:
from sacral plexus (obturator
nerve)
action:
rotates thigh laterally, and
abducts it; is a postural
muscle assisting piriformis
and other lateral rotators

position:
along lateral side of thigh
origin:
iliac crest of pelvis
insertion:
tibia, by iliotibial tract
nerve supply:
from sacral plexus (gluteal
nerve)
action:
flexes and abducts thigh

Acting at both the hip joint and the knee (two-joint muscles)

Rectus femoris (*part of the Quadriceps femoris*)

Biceps femoris (one of the hamstrings)

Semitendinosus and Semimembranosus (hamstrings)

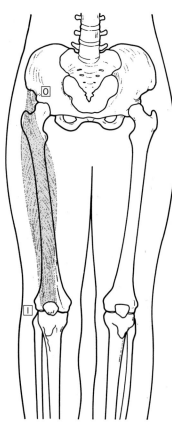

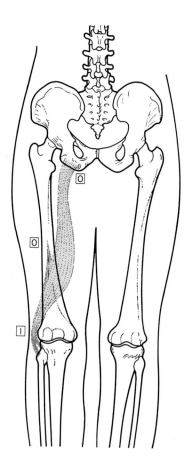

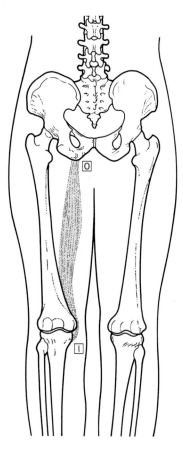

position:
down front of thigh
origin:
ilium of pelvis
insertion:
upper border of patella, and head of tibia via patellar ligament
nerve supply:
femoral nerve of lumbar plexus
action:
flexes thigh, and extends leg at knee

position:
down back of thigh
origin:
femur and ischium of pelvis
insertion:
head of fibula and lateral condyle of tibia
nerve supply:
sciatic nerve of sacral plexus
action:
extend thigh, and flex leg at knee

position:
down posterior medial side of thigh
origin:
ischium of pelvis
insertion:
tibia
nerve supply:
sciatic nerve of sacral plexus
action:
extend thigh, and flex leg at knee

Sartorius

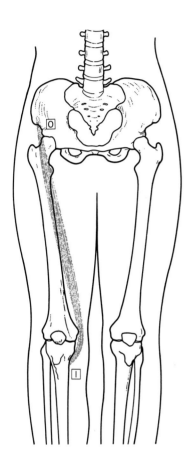

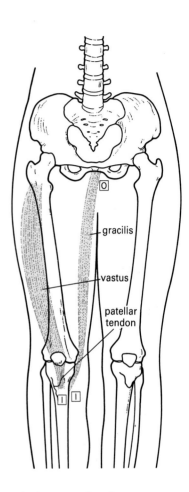

gracilis

vastus

patellar
tendon

Acting at the knee

position:
crosses front of thigh from
lateral to medial side
origin:
ilium of pelvis
insertion:
medial side of tibia
nerve supply:
femoral nerve of lumbar
plexus
action:
flexes hip and knee as when
sitting cross-legged

Gracilis

position:
down medial side of thigh
origin:
pubis of pelvis
insertion:
medial side of tibia
nerve supply:
from lumbar plexus
(obturator nerve)
action:
adducts thigh, and flexes leg
at knee

Quadriceps femoris (Vastus
lateralis, medialis, and
intermedius parts)

position:
down front of thigh
origin:
femur
insertion:
patella, and tibia via patellar
tendon
nerve supply:
femoral nerve of lumbar
plexus
action:
extend leg at knee

Muscles of the leg that move the foot and toes

Anterior muscles

Tibialis anterior

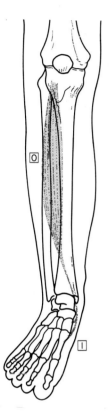

Peroneus tertius

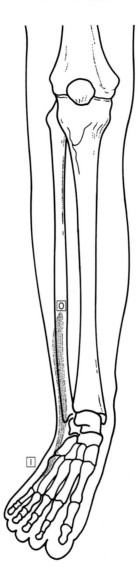

Extensor digitorum longus

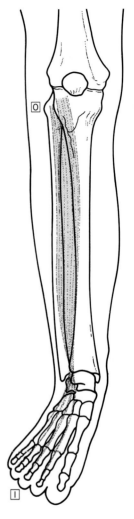

position:
down shin, on lateral side of tibia
origin:
lateral condyle and upper half of shaft of tibia
insertion:
first cuneiform tarsal and first metatarsal
nerve sypply:
from sciatic nerve (deep peroneal branch)
action:
dorsiflexes (bends ankle to pull foot up) and inverts (soles facing one another) foot

position:
lower lateral part of shin
origin:
lower part of shaft of fibula
insertion:
fifth metatarsal
nerve supply:
from sciatic nerve (deep peroneal branch)
action:
dorsiflexes and everts (soles facing outwards) foot

position:
lateral part of shin
origin:
lateral condyle of tibia, and shaft of fibula
insertion:
middle and distal phalanges of four outer toes
nerve supply:
from sciatic nerve (deep peroneal branch)
action:
dorsiflexes and everts foot, and extends toes

Extensor hallucis longus

Posterior muscles

Gastrocnemius

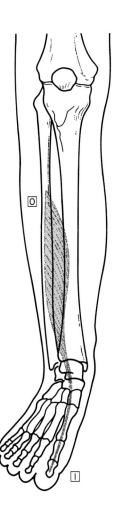

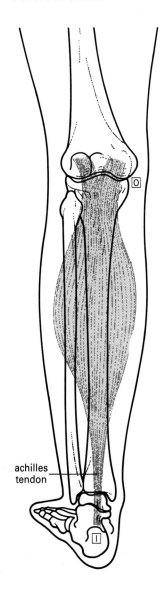

achilles tendon

position:
down shin, partly beneath
Tibialis muscle
origin:
middle region of shaft of
fibula
insertion:
base of distal phalanx of big
toe
nerve supply:
from sciatic nerve (deep
peroneal branch)
action:
extends big toe

position:
at back of lower leg, forming
calf
origin:
lateral and medial condyles of
femur
insertion:
calcaneum, via Achilles
tendon

nerve supply:
from sciatic nerve (tibial
branch)
action:
plantar flexes foot (pointing
the toes), and propels the
body in walking and running

Soleus

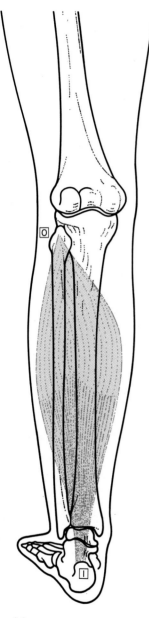

Plantaris

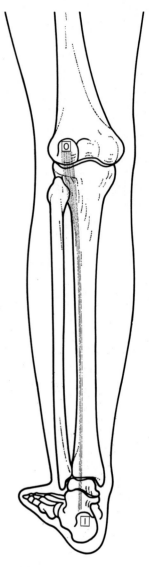

position:
at back of lower leg, deep to gastrocnemius
origin:
head of fibula, and upper part of tibia shaft
insertion:
calcaneum, via Achilles tendon

nerve supply:
from sciatic nerve (tibial branch)
action:
plantar flexes foot; has postural function steadying leg

position:
down back of lower leg, beneath gastrocnemius
origin:
above lateral condyle of femur
insertion:
calcaneum
nerve supply:
from sciatic nerve (tibial branch)
action:
plantar flexes foot

Tibialis posterior

Peroneus longus

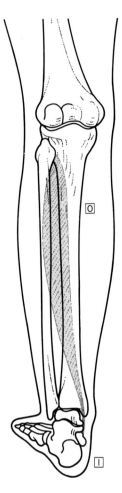

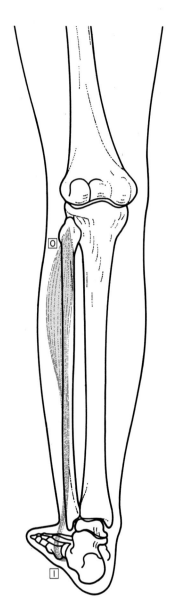

position:
deepest muscle on back of lower leg
origin:
shafts of tibia and fibula
insertion:
second, third and fourth metatarsals, navicular, third cuneiform, and cuboid tarsals
nerve supply:
from sciatic nerve (tibial branch)
action:
plantar flexes and inverts foot; supports inner medial longitudinal arch of foot

position:
down outside of upper part of back of lower leg
origin:
head and upper shaft of fibula
insertion:
first metatarsal and first cuneiform tarsal on sole of foot

nerve supply:
from sciatic nerve (superficial peroneal branch)
action:
plantar flexes and everts foot; supports transverse and outer longitudinal arches of foot

Peroneus brevis

Flexor digitorum longus

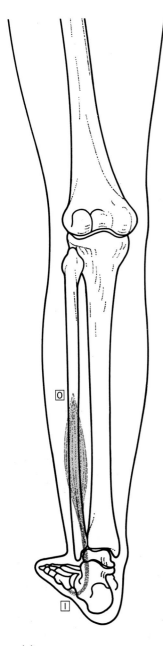

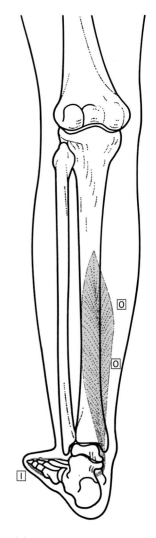

position:
on inside of back of lower leg
origin:
shaft of tibia
insertion:
distal phalanges of four outer
toes
nerve supply:
from sciatic nerve (tibial
branch)
action:
plantar flexes and inverts foot;
flexes the toes; supports inner
longitudinal arch of foot

position:
down outside of lower part of
back of lower leg
origin:
lower part of shaft of fibula
insertion:
fifth metatarsal

nerve supply:
from sciatic nerve (superficial
peroneal branch)
action:
plantar flexes and everts foot;
supports longitudinal arches
of the foot

Flexor hallucis longus

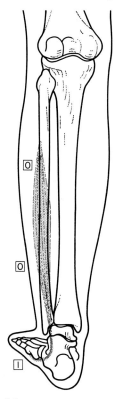

position:
on outer side of back of lower leg
origin:
shaft of lower part of fibula
insertion:
on underside of distal phalanx of big toe

nerve supply:
from sciatic nerve (tibial branch)
action:
plantar flexes and inverts foot; flexes the big toe; supports inner longitudinal arch of foot

Muscles and tendons of the hand

The flexor and extensor muscles which bend and straighten the fingers occur in the forearm and not in the hand. The long tendons from these muscles pass to the ends of the fingers. The tendons are surrounded by protective *synovial sheaths,* and held in place by fibrous bands or fasciae, called the *transverse* and *dorsal carpal ligaments.* The **palmar aponeurosis** is a flat wide tendon into which the tendon of the Palmaris longus muscle is inserted. The palmar aponeurosis is traiangular in shape and occupies the middle of the palm.

The hand contains only very small muscles. The flexor of the thumb, and the adductor and abductor muscles moving the thumb and fingers occur in the hand. The **thenar eminence** consists of the muscles moving the thumb while the hypothenar eminence on the medial side consists of the muscles moving the little finger. The *adductor* muscles of the eminences enable the hand to *grip* objects. Although these muscles are small they have a very rich nerve supply allowing very fine control. This allows the variety of grips needed to handle both small and large objects. They are supplied by the median nerve.

Figure 5.7
Front of hand (palmar surface)

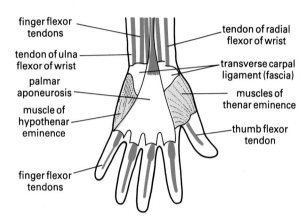

finger flexor tendons

tendon of radial flexor of wrist

tendon of ulna flexor of wrist

transverse carpal ligament (fascia)

palmar aponeurosis

muscles of thenar eminence

muscle of hypothenar eminence

thumb flexor tendon

finger flexor tendons

Figure 5.8
Back of hand

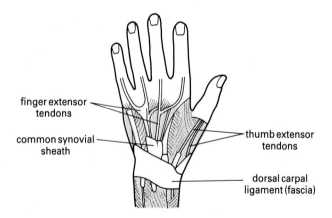

finger extensor tendons

thumb extensor tendons

common synovial sheath

dorsal carpal ligament (fascia)

Muscles and tendons of the foot

As the tendons from the flexor and extensor muscles in the leg cross the ankle into the foot, they are held in place by fasciae known as the *transverse crural* and *cruciate crural ligaments*. Each toe has an extensor tendon on its upper (dorsal) surface. There is also an extensor muscle to the four larger toes on the upper surface, or *dorsum*, of the foot. This extensor muscle has its origin on the upper surface of the calcaneum. Each toe has a flexor tendon on the sole, or *plantar surface*, of the foot.

The *spring ligament* connects the calcaneum to the navicular tarsal. It resists the flattening of the inner longitudinal arch of the foot. The long *plantar ligament* attaches the calcaneum to the metatarsals, and resists the flattening of the outer longitudinal arch. These ligaments take the strain when walking, and are aided by the short plantar muscles. The **plantar** muscles make up the fleshy part of the sole of the foot, and are the flexors, adductors, and abductors of the toes. *Clawed toe* results from loss of control of the flexors and extensors of the foot. Deep peroneal and plantar nerves supply the foot muscles.

Figure 5.9
Foot (dorsum)

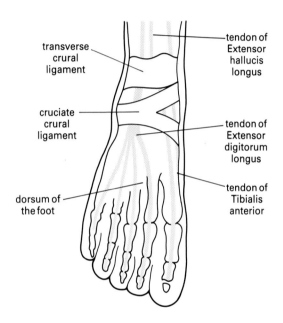

Figure 5.10
Foot (plantar surface)

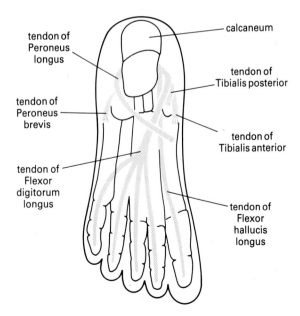

Effects of exercise on muscles

Exercising muscles stimulates blood and lymph flow, as it generates *heat* which dilates blood capillaries and causes *movements* which push the fluid along veins and lymph vessels. This improved circulation removes *toxic waste* products and supplies nutrients more rapidly, allowing the muscle to function more effectively.

Exercising a muscle increases the number of *mitochondria* in the muscle fibres. Mitochondria are the cell organelles which produce ATP, the immediate source of energy for contracting muscle fibres.

Muscle which is not regularly exercised will *atrophy* (waste away). Exercise increases the strength of muscles and the flexibility of joints. It improves posture, and can help to prevent low back pain. Excessive or unsuitable exercising causes muscle fatigue and minor injury to muscles, tendons and ligaments.

Effects of massage on muscles

Massage produces *frictional heat* which warms the skin and dilates the blood capillaries. This speeds up the circulation of blood and supplies nutrients to the muscle more rapidly. During massage the stroking movements towards the heart assist the return of venous blood and lymph to the heart. Toxic waste products in the muscle tissue are therefore removed more rapidly, so massage reduces muscle fatigue. Massage will increase muscle *relaxation*, releasing muscular tension which may be straining ligaments or tendons. Because massage does not cause muscular contractions it does not strengthen muscle.

Contra-indications to massage

The presence of inflammation in a muscle or in the skin covering it, highly vascular skin conditions, or a hypersensitive skin prone to allergic reactions all contra-indicate massage treatment. Painful joints where there could be structural damage to a tendon or ligament, should not be massaged.

Self-assessment questions

1 Which muscle is used in:

(a) sucking;   (b) smiling;
(c) frowning;   (d) blinking?

2 Define, in relation to muscular movement, the terms:

(a) insertion;
(b) tendon;
(c) origin;
(d) antagonistic pair.

3 Give **two** similarities and **two** differences between skeletal and smooth muscle.

4 List the muscles involved in breathing. What actions do they have when they contract?

5 Explain the meaning of:

(a) adduction;   (b) abduction;
(c) pronation;   (d) dorsiflexion.

Give the name of one muscle in each case which causes this type of movement.

6 List the muscles of the anterior abdominal wall and describe their positions in relation to one another.

7 Give the origin, insertion, and action of the following muscles:

(a) Brachialis;
(b) Extensor digitorum longus;
(c) Gastrocnemius;
(d) Trapezius.

8 List the muscles which cause movement at both the hip and knee joints. For each muscle, name the type of movement they perform at each joint.

9 Which muscles move the mandible? Give the origin of each muscle and the name of the nerve which supplies them all.

10 Which are the principal muscles used to:

(a) raise the shoulders;
(b) sit cross-leged;
(c) bend the big toe;
(d) propel the body when running;
(e) push objects?

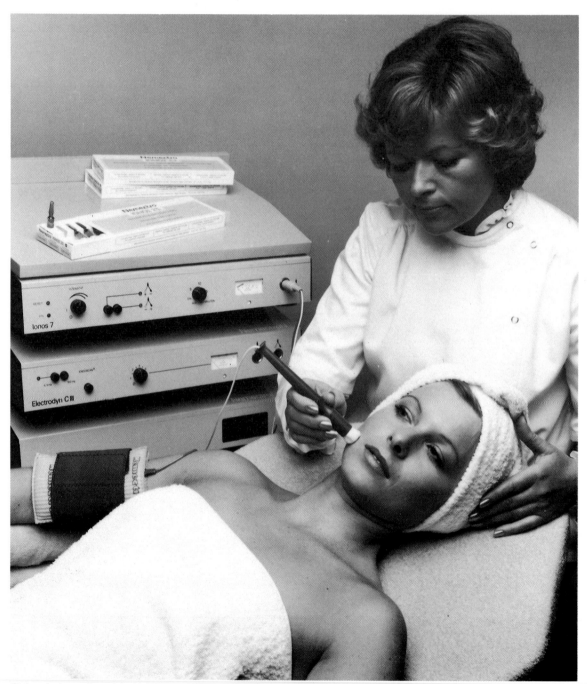

Galvanic iontophoresis

The nervous system provides the most rapid means of *communication* between the various parts of the body. It stimulates muscular movements, and co-ordinates all the body's activities. *Co-ordination* requires feedback, so that the level of response is related to the strength and direction of the stimulus. The nervous system combines with the endocrine system to maintain *homeostasis*, ie keeping the body in a steady state. It *senses* changes outside and inside the body by means of its sense organs, *interprets* the changes in the central nervous system, then *initiates* actions to maintain homeostasis.

Nervous tissue

Nervous tissue is composed of two types of cells, **neurons** and **neuroglia.** The neurons are the structural and functional units, while the neuroglia has a supporting and protective function.

The *neurons* conduct nerve impulses. Each neuron consists of a *cell body* from which impulse-conducting processes extend. The cell body has a central nucleus, and granular cytoplasm containing mitochondria and a Golgi body. The rough endoplasmic reticulum and ribosomes form characteristic *Nissl granules* in neurons. The cytoplasm also contains thin fibres called *neurofibrils.*

The slender processes extending from the neuron cell body are of two types, *dendrons,* and *axons.* **Dendrons** have short branches called *dendrites,* and conduct impulses inwards towards the cell body. One or many dendrons may be present in a single neuron. An **axon** is a longer process branching at the end, which conducts impulses outwards away from the cell body. Each neuron has a single axon composed of *axoplasm,* which may be surrounded by a fatty non-conducting sheath of *myelin* secreted by *Schwann cells* of the neuroglia. Such axons are said to be *myelinated.* The myelin sheath insulates the axon to prevent loss of the electrical impulse, and increases the speed at which the impulse is conducted. At intervals there are gaps in the myelin sheath called *nodes of Ranvier.* On the outside of the myelin sheath is a membrane called the *neurilemma.* An axon and its sheaths is known as a *nerve fibre.*

The axons from a large number of neurons are arranged in bundles and covered with connective tissue sheaths, forming *nerves.* Neurons are unable to undergo cell division and reproduce themselves. When destroyed they cannot be replaced, although some damaged neurons can be repaired. There are three types of neurons, *sensory, motor,* and *interneurons.*

- **Sensory neurons** carry impulses from sensory receptors to the brain and spinal cord. They usually have one process from the cell body which divides into an axon and a dendron, and are said to be *unipolar*.

- **Motor neurons** carry impulses from the brain and spinal cord to effectors (muscles and glands). They have several branched dendrons and a single axon, and are said to be *multipolar*.

- **Interneurons** (association or connector neurons) carry impulses from sensory neurons to motor neurons, and occur only in the brain and spinal cord. They are multipolar, often with a short axon (stellate).

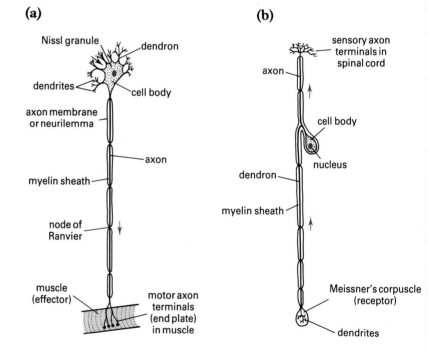

Figure 6.1
Types of neurons
(a) Motor neuron (multipolar)
(b) Sensory neuron (unipolar)
(c) Interneuron (stellate)

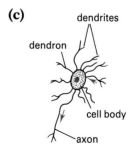

The nerve impulse

A nerve impulse is electrical in nature, and is produced when a neuron is stimulated. When a neuron is not conducting an impulse, the inside of the cell membrane is negatively charged, while the outside of the cell membrane is positively charged. Thus there is a *potential difference* between the two sides of the cell membrane, which is said to be *polarized.*

The electrical charges are due to the proportions of negatively and positively charged *ions* inside and outside the neuron. The ions are derived from two salts, *sodium chloride* and *potassium chloride*, which split up, or ionize, in solution to form positive sodium (Na^+) and potassium (K^+) ions, and negative chloride (Cl^-) ions. There are also many negatively charged protein ions inside the neuron. The potassium ions are mostly inside the neuron, while the sodium ions are mostly outside. The non-conducting condition of a neuron is known as *resting potential.*

Figure 6.2
Resting potential in an axon

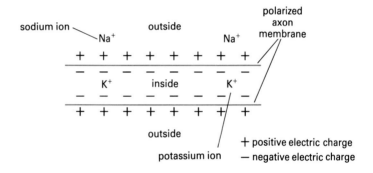

If a stimulus of sufficient strength is applied to a neuron, an impulse passes through it along the axon. As the impulse passes, the charges on the membrane at that point are momentarily reversed, so the membrane *depolarizes*. The outside of the cell membrane becomes negatively charged, and the inside becomes positively charged. This reversal is due to the movements of sodium and potassium ions through the cell membrane. The

Figure 6.3
Action potential in an axon

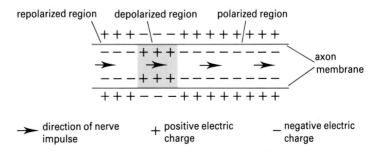

conducting condition of the neuron is known as *action potential*.

After the impulse has passed, the membrane becomes polarized again. The time taken for the membrane to repolarize is the *refractory period* of the neuron and is about 3 millisecs. Until the end of the refractory period the neuron is unable to transmit another impulse.

Properties of nerve impulses

The speed of transmission of a nerve impulse is greater in axons with a larger diameter, and where they are myelinated. The response of a neuron to a stimulus follows the *all-or-none law*. Below a particular strength of stimulus or threshold, no action potential is generated. Above the threshold there is a full-sized action potential. If a series of below-threshold stimuli are applied to a neuron in quick succession, an impulse may be generated by their cumulative effect. This property is known as *summation*.

Conduction across synapses

The junction between two neurons is called a *synapse*. It occurs where the end of the axon of one neuron lies close to a dendrite of the other neuron, leaving a narrow gap, the *synaptic cleft*, between the two. This gap has to be crossed for the impulse to pass from one neuron to the other. Electrical impulses are unable to cross the gap, and must be converted into *chemical transmitters*. The end of the axon bears a *synaptic knob* containing mitochondria to provide energy, and many vesicles containing the chemical transmitter substance, usually *acetylcholine*. The synaptic knob ends in a *presynaptic* membrane bounding the synaptic cleft. On the opposite side of the cleft is the *postsynaptic* membrane of the dendrite of the next neuron.

Figure 6.4
Conduction of nerve impulse across synapse

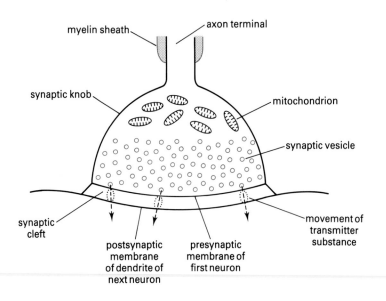

The arrival of an electrical impulse at the synaptic knob causes the release of *transmitter substance* from vesicles which become attached to the presynaptic membrane. The transmitter substance crosses the synaptic cleft and becomes attached to *receptor sites* on the postsynaptic membrane and *depolarizes* it. Thus an action potential is generated, and an electrical impulse passes through the neuron to the next synapse. Synapses cause nerve impulses to pass in one direction only through the neuron. A special kind of synapse occurs at a nerve-muscle junction known as a *motor end plate.*

The reflex arc

The simplest type of nervous activity is a *reflex action.* This is an automatic rapid response to a particular stimulus, with no conscious involvement of the brain. *Examples* of reflex actions are the knee jerk when the patellar ligament is tapped, and the contraction of the pupil in response to a bright light shining on the eye. Coughing, sneezing, and the secretion of saliva are also reflex actions.

The conduction pathway of the impulse causing a reflex action is called a *reflex arc,* and one simple type involves just three neurons. A sensory *receptor* picks up a stimulus and triggers an impulse in a *sensory neuron.* The impulse crosses the synapse to an *interneuron* in the spinal cord. A second synapse passes the impulse to a *motor neuron* whose motor end plate synapse passes on the impulse which makes the *muscle* contract. There are thus five parts to a simple reflex arc: a receptor, three conducting neurons, and an effector (the muscle).

Figure 6.5
Patellar reflex (knee jerk)

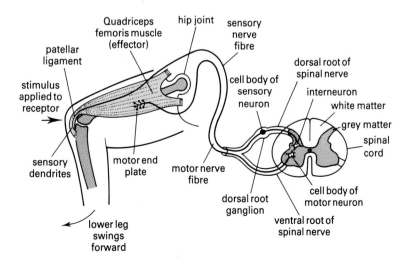

Where the interneuron is in the spinal cord, a *spinal reflex* occurs, eg the patellar reflex. Reflexes are the body's main method of maintaining homeostasis, as they give a rapid countering response to changes in the internal and external environment.

Voluntary actions are more complicated than reflex actions, as the control centres of the brain modify the response. From the spinal cord the sensory impulse passes up to the brain, which may inhibit the immediate reflex response in the light of stored memory and intelligence. A motor response then passes down the spinal cord, and appropriate muscles are stimulated to produce a conscious reasoned reaction to the original stimulus.

The sensory system

The ability to sense stimuli is vital for an individual's survival. **Sensation** is a state of awareness of the external and internal environment of an individual. **Perception** is the conscious knowledge of a sensory stimulus.

Stimuli are picked up by receptors and converted into nerve impulses. Stimuli may be light rays, sound waves, temperature changes, touch, pressure or chemical substances. All sense receptors contain the dendrites of sensory neurons, and respond to a stimulus of relatively low intensity. Receptors may be single cells as in the skin, or may be part of a complex sense organ like the eye.

Many sensory nerve impulses pass to the brain to produce a conscious sensation. Some sensory impulses that end in the spinal cord can initiate muscle contractions, but do not produce conscious sensations. Conscious sensations undergo *projection*; although they are perceived by the brain, they appear to come from the point of stimulation. Thus, one appears to feel heat on the area of skin warmed by an infra-red lamp, but the feeling of warmth is actually in the brain.

The perception of a sensation may disappear if the stimulus is prolonged. On entering a bath of hot water the skin feels to be burning, but this sensation quickly decreases. This is known as *adaptation*, and is due to synapse fatigue. The sensation of wearing clothes and jewellery is also quickly lost as a result of adaptation.

Receptors may be classified according to their position in the body:

● *Exteroceptors* occur near the body surface and detect changes in the external environment;

- *Visceroceptors* occur in blood vessels, the food canal, and other internal organs (viscera). Sensations from these receptors are felt as pain, pressure, hunger, thirst and nausea;
- *Proprioceptors* occur in muscles, joints, tendons, ligaments, and the internal ear (organ of balance). They give information about the state of muscular contraction, the position of bones, and tension of the joints, so defining body position and movements. This is known as the *kinesthetic* sense.

General senses

General senses involve a simple receptor and occur throughout the body. **Cutaneous** (skin) **sensations** and the **kinesthetic sense** are general senses. *Cutaneous* sensations include light touch, deep pressure, cold, heat, and pain (see Chapter 3). Some parts of the skin contain many more receptors than others. The most sensitive areas with the greatest density of receptors are the eyelids, finger tips, lips, and nipples. Cutaneous receptors are simple consisting of the dendrites of sensory neurons that may or may not be enclosed in a *capsule*. In the hair root the dendrites form a network but are not enclosed in a capsule. Meissners and Pacinian corpuscles have connective tissue capsules enclosing the dendrites.

Pain receptors are the dendrites of certain sensory neurons which respond to excessive stimuli of any type as a sensation of pain. They do not undergo adaptation, unlike the receptors for touch and temperature sensations, as pain sensations must not be ignored in order to identify danger. The sensory impulses for pain all pass to the brain.

Anaesthesia is the loss of feeling. It may occur over a limited area of skin due to nervous disease, 'freezing' by solid carbon dioxide, or by local anaesthetics. When only loss of the sense of pain is meant, the correct term is *analgesia,* and pain-killing drugs are *analgesics*. The brain can produce natural analgesics known as *endorphins* which inhibit pain impulses.

Hyperaesthesia is over-sensitiveness to touch and contra-indicates beauty therapy treatments. It is a symptom of certain nervous diseases such as *neuralgia*. The pain occurs in the skin above a sensory nerve, eg in the skin above the trigeminal cranial nerve of the face following an attack of shingles.

Special senses

Special senses involve complex receptors called **sense organs** which are localized in the head. The *eye* supplies information about the shape, size, and colour of objects, and their movements. It also informs the brain about the direction and intensity of the light reaching the eye. The chemical senses of smell and taste are perceived by the *nose* and *taste buds* of the tongue respectively. The *ears* contain sound receptors for hearing, as well as the receptors concerned with balance.

The central nervous system

The central nervous system comprises the *spinal cord* and *brain*, the *meninges* (membranes surrounding the brain and spinal cord), and the *cerebro-spinal fluid*.

The spinal cord

The spinal cord has several *functions*. It allows spinal reflex actions, forming part of the conducting pathway or reflex arc. It also conveys sensory impulses from one region of the spinal cord to another, and from the skin and muscles of the trunk and limbs to the brain.

The spinal cord is a long cylindrical organ with a tapering end. It runs from the brain to the second lumbar vertebra. It passes through the *vertebral foramina* of the vertebrae, which give protection to the delicate nervous tissue. The cord is divided into right and left halves by two grooves: the *anterior median fissure* is a deep wide groove, while the *posterior median sulcus* is shallower and narrow. The cord has a central cavity, the *spinal canal*, continuous with the cavities of the brain, and containing *cerebro-spinal fluid*.

Round the spinal canal is an area largely composed of the cell bodies of neurons which is H-shaped in cross-section. This is the *grey matter*, and at intervals it connects with spinal nerves. Pairs of *spinal nerves* emerge from the spinal cord between adjacent vertebrae, each nerve being formed by the fusion of a *dorsal* and a *ventral root*. Surrounding the grey matter is the *white matter* composed of the myelinated axons of both motor and sensory neurons. These axons form sensory ascending and motor descending *tracts* to and from the brain. Other shorter tracts convey impulses from one level in the spinal cord to another level.

Figure 6.6
Spinal cord (cross-section)

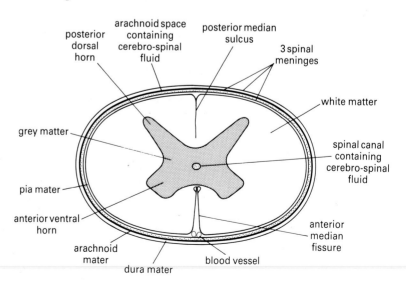

The meninges

The meninges are three membranes covering the outside of the spinal cord and brain. The spinal meninges consist of an outer thick fibrous *dura mater,* a middle thinner *arachnoid mater* of more delicate connective tissue, and an inner thin *pia mater* which is a transparent fibrous membrane containing the blood vessels which nourish the nervous tissue.

Between the dura mater and the bony wall of the vertebral canal is the *epidural space.* It contains adipose tissue to pad the cord, and blood vessels. Local anaesthetics can be injected into this space during childbirth to relieve severe labour pains. Between the arachnoid and the pia mater is the *subarachnoid space* where the cerebro-spinal fluid circulates.

The *functions* of the spinal meninges are to form a protective covering round the spinal cord, and to retain the cerebro-spinal fluid.

Cerebro-spinal fluid

This fluid circulates through the ventricles (cavities) of the brain, the spinal canal, and the arachnoid space between the arachnoid and pia mater of the cranial and spinal meninges. It is a clear colourless watery fluid containing white blood cells, and dissolved glucose, salts, proteins, and urea. It diffuses out of the blood contained in networks of capillaries called choroid plexuses present in the ventricles of the brain.

The *functions* of the cerebro-spinal fluid are to supply nutrients from the blood to the brain cells, to act as a shock absorber for the brain and spinal cord, and to keep the cranial volume constant.

The brain

The brain is the enlarged front end of the spinal cord developing in three regions as fore, mid, and hindbrain. It is protected by the cranial bones of the skull, and covered by the cranial meninges which are continuous with the spinal ones and have the same names. The subarachnoid space contains cerebro-spinal fluid.

The *functions* of the brain are those of a nervous *control centre.* It receives impulses from all the sense receptors and interprets them in its sensory association centres. It also sends motor impulses to the effector organs (muscles and glands). Its association and motor centres co-ordinate the body's movements, allowing it to function efficiently as a whole, and develop skills. The brain controls feeding, sleeping, temperature regulation, drinking, and the salt/water balance of the body. It stores information in the memory, so that behaviour can be modified by past experience. It also has association centres concerned with emotional and intellectual processes.

Figure 6.7
Brain (vertical section)

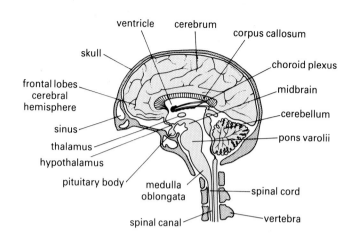

Structure of the brain

The brain is divided into four main parts, the *brain stem*, the *cerebellum*, the *diencephalon*, and the *cerebrum*. The brain contains a number of cavities called *ventricles* that communicate with one another, with the subarachnoid space, and with the spinal canal. The cerebro-spinal fluid circulates through all these cavities. A superficial layer of nerve cells known as a *cortex* occurs in the cerebrum and cerebellum. The brain is well supplied with *blood vessels* in the pia mater, as it needs a continuous supply of oxygen and glucose to maintain consciousness and life.

- The **brain stem** consists of the *medulla oblongata*, the *pons varolii*, and the *midbrain*. The medulla and pons are part of the hindbrain.
  (a) The *medulla* is a continuation of the spinal cord above the foramen magnum of the skull, and is about 2.5 cm long. It contains all the ascending and descending tracts from the spinal cord in its white matter. It contains three vital reflex centres in its grey matter, the *cardiac, respiratory*, and *vasomotor* centres, which regulate the heart, breathing, and diameter of the blood vessels respectively. The medulla also controls coughing, sneezing, swallowing, vomiting, and hiccuping, all of which are involuntary reflex actions;
  (b) The *pons varolii* lies immediately above the medulla. It forms a bridge 2.5 cm long carrying the longitudinal tracts from the spinal cord and medulla to upper regions of the brain. It also contains transverse nerve fibres which connect the two halves of the cerebellum;
  (c) The *midbrain* extends anteriorly from the pons, and is also 2.5 cm long. It contains two *cerebral peduncles* (fibre bundles) carrying the longitudinal tracts from the pons to upper regions of the brain. It also contains the *corpora quadrigemina*, which are a group of four rounded bodies.

The upper two bodies control the movements of the eyeballs and head related to sight, while the lower two bodies control reflex movements of the head and trunk related to hearing;

- The **cerebellum** is the largest part of the hindbrain, and occurs posteriorly at the level of the pons and medulla. It is separated from the cerebrum by a *transverse fissure*. The cerebellum has a narrow central *vermis*, and two lateral *wings*. Its superficial *cortex* is composed of grey matter arranged in parallel ridges. Below the grey matter, white matter tracts occurs in a tree-like pattern. The cerebellum is connected with the brain stem by three paired bundles of nerve fibres called the *cerebellar peduncles*.

  The cerebellum is the motor co-ordinating centre of the brain. It maintains posture, and allows the co-ordinated movements required in muscular skills. It receives motor impulses from the cerebrum, and sensory impulses from the proprioceptors in the muscles and joints. Information about the position of the head in relation to the rest of the body reaches the cerebellum from the inner ear receptors. The cerebellum is then able to generate the muscle contractions needed to maintain balance;

- The **diencephalon**, consisting of the thalamus and hypothalamus, is part of the forebrain.
  (a) The *thalamus* is an oval structure 3 cm long which lies above the midbrain. It consists of two masses of grey matter covered by a thin layer of white matter. It functions as the relay station for all sensory impulses reaching the brain, except those of smell. These sensory impulses are relayed to the appropriate region of the cerebrum;
  (b) The *hypothalamus* lies between the thalamus and the pituitary gland, and controls many of the body's homeostatic mechanisms. It controls the autonomic nervous system which regulates the heart rate, the emptying of the bladder, and the movement of food through the food canal. It links the functioning of the nervous and endocrine systems via the pituitary gland. The hypothalamus controls normal body temperature, acting as a thermostat, and has centres controlling the body's water content (osmoregulation centre), thirst, and appetite. It also maintains the pattern of wakefulness and sleep;

- The **cerebrum** forms the major part of the forebrain, and is the largest of the brain regions. Its surface is composed of a layer of grey matter 2–4 mm thick, forming a highly folded *cerebral cortex*. Beneath the cortex is the white matter. There is a deep *longitudinal fissure* dividing the cerebrum into right and left *hemispheres*, which are connected by a bundle of transverse nerve fibres, the *corpus callosum*.

The cerebral cortex is divided up into areas of three main types:
(a) *Motor areas* towards the anterior end control the main pathways for muscular movement;
(b) *Sensory areas* posterior to the motor areas interpret sensory impulses;
(c) *Association areas* at the posterior end of the cortex and in the anterior frontal lobes are concerned with intellectual processes of thought and memory, emotions, and personality traits.

Figure 6.8
Areas of the cerebral cortex (side view)

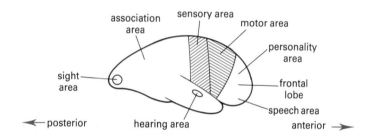

In the cerebral cortex activity of the neurons making up the grey matter generates *brain waves*. These can be detected and recorded to produce an *electroencephalogram* (EEG). Abnormal brain activity, as in epilepsy, shows up on an EEG.

The peripheral nervous system

Nerves are bundles of axons (nerve fibres) surrounded by a connective tissue sheath, which carry impulses to and from the central nervous system. The peripheral nervous system includes mainly those nerves involved in voluntary actions. The 12 pairs of *cranial nerves* originate from the brain inside the skull which they leave via foramina. The 31 pairs of *spinal nerves* originate from the spinal cord, and leave between the vertebrae.

Cranial nerves

Some of these nerves are *mixed*, containing both motor and sensory axons, while others are either *sensory* or *motor*. Most cranial nerves are confined to the head and neck, but the tenth pair have branches in the trunk. Details of the cranial nerves are given in Table 6.1.

Spinal nerves

Each spinal nerve has two points of attachment, or roots, to the spinal cord. These are the *dorsal root* carrying *sensory* axons whose impulses are passing inwards, and the *ventral root* carrying

Table 6.1
Cranial nerves

No	Name	Branches	Type	Role
I	Olfactory		sensory	Takes impulses giving the sense of smell from the nose to the brain
II	Optic	Some fibres from each nerve cross over at the optic chiasma	sensory	Takes impulses related to vision from both eyes to the brain
III	Oculo-motor		motor	Takes impulses from the brain to most of the muscles moving the eyeball, and to the muscle of the upper eyelid
IV	Pathetic (trochlear)		motor	Takes impulses from the brain to the superior oblique eyeball muscle
V	Trigeminal		mixed	
		Ophthalmic	sensory	Receives impulses from skin of front of scalp, forehead, upper eyelid, eyeball, and upper part of the nose
		Maxillary	sensory	Receives impulses from the upper jaw, palate, lower part of the nose, lower eyelid and cheek
		Mandibular	mixed	Receives sensory impulses from the lower jaw, floor of the mouth, and skin in front of the ear; takes motor impulses to the muscles of mastication (masseter temporalis and pterygoid)
VI	Abducens		mixed	Takes motor impulses to the lateral rectus muscle of the eyeball; receives sensory impulses from the proprioceptors in this muscle
VII	Facial		mixed	Receives sensory impulses of taste; supplies the muscles of facial expression
		Temporal	motor	Takes motor impulses to auricular, frontalis, orbicularis oculi, and corrugator muscles

Table 6.1 (cont)

No	Name	Branches	Type	Role
VII	Facial	Zygomatic	motor	Takes motor impulses to the orbicularis oculi muscles
		Buccal	motor	Takes motor impulses to the procerus, buccinator, orbicularis oris, zygomaticus, and levator muscles of mouth
		Mandibular	motor	Takes motor impulses to the lower lip and chin supplying risorius, mentalis, and triangularis muscles
		Cerivcal	motor	Takes motor impulses to the platysma muscle
VIII	Auditory		sensory	Receives impulses relating to hearing and balance
IX	Glosso-pharyngeal		mixed	Takes motor impulses to the muscles used in swallowing and to the salivary glands; receives sensory impulses from the taste buds on the back of the tongue
X	Vagus		mixed	Takes motor impulses to muscles of the pharynx, thorax, and food canal; receives sensory impulses from the same organs; carries parasympathetic fibres to slow heart rate
XI	Accessory	Originate from the brain stem and spinal cord	mixed	Cranial part supplies muscles of the pharynx and larynx; spinal part supplies trapezius and sternocleidomastoid muscles of the neck; receives sensory impulses from proprioceptors in the muscles
XII	Hypoglossal		mixed	Takes motor impulses to tongue muscles; receives sensory impulses from proprioceptors in the tongue muscles

motor axons whose impulses are passing outwards. A short distance from the spinal cord the two roots combine to form a *mixed* spinal nerve, which is surrounded by a fibrous sheath. The dorsal root has a swelling, or *ganglion,* containing the cell bodies of the sensory neurons (see Fig. 6.5).

Figure 6.9
Distribution of fifth and seventh
cranial nerves to the face (side view)

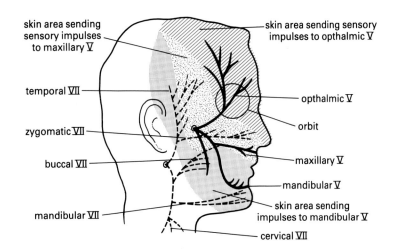

skin area sending
sensory impulses
to maxillary V

skin area sending sensory
impulses to opthalmic V

temporal VII

zygomatic VII

buccal VII

mandibular VII

opthalmic V

orbit

maxillary V

mandibular V

skin area sending
impulses to mandibular V

cervical VII

The thirty-one pairs of spinal nerves are named according to the region of the spinal cord from which they emerge. There are:

- eight pairs of *cervical* nerves;
- twelve pairs of *thoracic* nerves;
- five pairs of *lumbar* nerves;
- five pairs of *sacral* nerves;
- one pair of *coccygeal* nerves.

Each spinal nerve divides into several *rami* (branches) just beyond the point where its two roots join. The posterior rami supply the muscles and skin of the back. Some of the anterior rami join up with those of adjacent nerves to form *plexuses* (networks). There are four main plexuses on each side of the body.

- The *cervical plexuses* of the neck supply the skin and muscles of the head, neck, and upper region of the shoulders. The *phrenic* nerves to the diaphragm come from the cervical plexus;
- The *brachial plexuses* at the top of the shoulders supply the skin and muscles of the arms, shoulders, and upper chest;
- The *lumbar plexuses* occur between the waist and hip bone and supply the front and sides of the abdomen wall, and part of the leg. The *femoral* nerves, passing down the front of the thighs to the flexor muscles of the thigh and extensor muscles of the leg, are the largest nerves from the lumbar plexuses;
- The *sacral plexuses* at the base of the abdomen supply the buttocks and some leg muscles. The *sciatic nerves* from these plexuses are the largest nerves in the body, and supply muscles of the legs and feet. The sciatic nerves pass from the buttocks down the back of the thighs, and give branches to the lower legs and feet. (For the nerve supply to individual muscles see Chapter 5.)

Most thoracic nerves pass directly to the structures they supply in the chest wall. Each spinal nerve has two thin branches, the *rami communicans*, which link it with the autonomic nervous system.

The autonomic nervous system

The autonomic nervous system controls the involuntary activities of smooth and cardiac muscle, and of glands. It is largely concerned with motor reflexes, and is regulated by centres in the medulla oblongata, hypothalamus, and cerebral cortex of the brain, to which it sends sensory impulses. It has two divisions, or sets of nerves, known as *sympathetic* and *parasympathetic*, which usually have opposite effects. The opposite effects result from the different *chemical transmitters* secreted at the nerve/effector synapse. Parasympathetic nerve endings produce *acetylcholine*. Sympathetic nerve endings produce *nor-adrenalin*, which has similar effects to those of the hormone adrenalin.

In general, the effects of the sympathetic division are to increase the body's use of energy, eg during exercise or stress. The effects of the parasympathetic division are concerned with energy conservation. Together they maintain *homeostasis*, as one division counteracts the effects of the other; one acting as an 'accelerator' and the other as a 'brake' for example. The autonomic nervous system acts with the endocrine system to maintain homeostasis by regulating the body's physiology.

Some of the *functions* of the autonomic nervous system are shown in Table 6.2.

Substances that affect the nervous system

Drugs

- *Sedatives* are drugs that reduce nervousness and excitement by their action on the central nervous system. One group are the *tranquillizers*, used to treat anxiety;

- *Hypnotics* are drugs which induce sleep. One group are the *barbiturates*, although these have been largely replaced by tranquillizers. Both barbiturates and tranquillizers are addictive if prescribed for long periods of time;

- *Narcotics* are drugs producing a condition of stupor. *Opium* drugs such as morphine and heroin have this effect. These drugs too, are addictive;

Table 6.2
Functions of the autonomic nervous system

Organ (effector)	Parasympathetic division	Sympathetic division
Heart	Slows the rate	Accelerates the rate
Bronchioles	Constricts	Dilates
Arteries supplying the skeletal muscles	Dilates	Constricts
Sphincters of the food canal	Relaxes (opens)	Contracts (closes)
Bladder	Relaxes the wall	Contracts the wall
Pupil of the eye	Constricts	Dilates
Arrector pili muscles of the hairs		Contracts (gooseflesh)
Sweat glands		Increases secretion of sweat

- *Analgesics* act by inhibiting impulses of pain. *Aspirin* and *paracetamol* are commonly used to treat minor pains. Too frequent use of aspirin can damage the lining of the food canal, and too frequent use of paracetamol can cause liver damage;

- *Stimulants* act by stimulating the sympathetic nervous system. *Amphetamines,* which are drugs related to the hormone adrenalin, are stimulants and also cause weight loss. As they are addictive, they should not be used as slimming aids. *Caffeine* from coffee is a brain stimulant, as it speeds up transmission across synapses.

Nerve poisons

These are substances which have adverse effects on the nervous system.

- *Alcohol* (ethanol) is a depressant, having a narcotic and sedative action. It affects the intellectual faculties of the brain, reducing self-control. Larger amounts of alcohol dull sense perception and slow the transmission of nerve impulses. Co-ordination of muscular movements is affected, causing clumsiness and slurring of speech. High alcohol consumption has dangerous social consequences by inducing violent behaviour and seriously reducing driving ability. Excess consumption finally results in heavy sleep or stupor, prolonged until the alcohol absorbed has been oxidized;

- *Methanol* (methyl alcohol) is present in methylated spirit, and has effects on the body similar to those of ethanol. It is however even more toxic, having a pronounced adverse effect on the nervous system. In large quantities it causes *neuritis,* affecting the optic nerves particularly, and resulting in blindness;

- *Lead* is a nerve poison. The general sources of the lead absorbed by the nervous system are *tetraethyl lead* from petrol exhaust gases, and *lead salts* in soft drinking water that has been standing in lead pipes. Lead poisoning causes mental and behavioural impairment. It causes tremors and paralysis due to nerve damage, usually starting in the muscles on the back of the wrist, and causing 'wrist drop' as an early symptom.

Self-assessment questions

1   List **eight** structural components of a mulitpolar motor neuron.

2   Where in the body would you expect to find:

(a) a motor end plate;
(b) a myelin sheath;
(c) nor-adrenalin;
(d) a proprioceptor?

3   What is the function of a synapse?

4   Give one example of:

(a) a mineral salt;
(b) a chemical transmitter;

(c) a cutaneous receptor;

each of which have a role in the functioning of the nervous system.

5   List the structures forming the brain stem.

6   Give examples of reflex actions associated with:

(a) the eye;
(b) the digestive system
(c) the blood vessels.

7   Explain the functions of the hypothalamus in controlling the body's activities.

8   Explain what is meant by the terms:

(a) sensory nerve;
(b) analgesic;
(c) pia mater;
(d) hyperaesthesia.

9   Give the position and functions of the following:

(a) the sciatic nerve;
(b) the temporal branch of the facial nerve.

10   Describe the functions of:

(a) the cerebro-spinal fluid;
(b) the cerebellum.

CHAPTER 7

The Digestive System

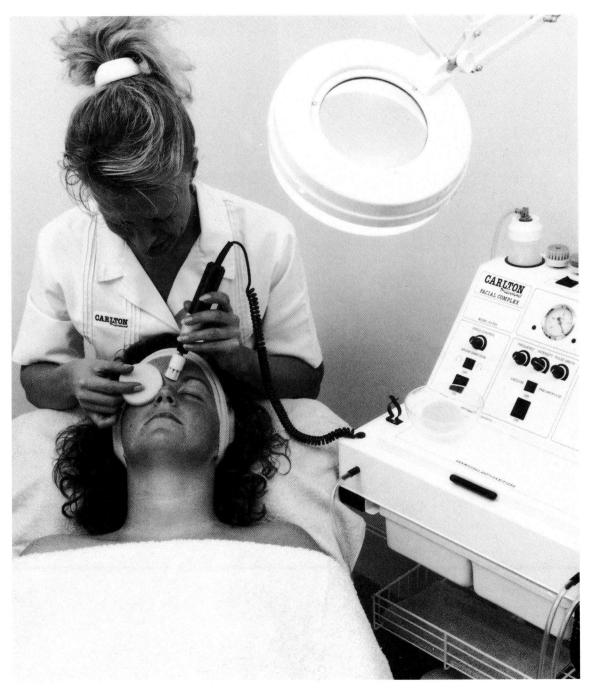

Brush cleanser

The digestive system is involved in obtaining the chemicals required to sustain life. The chemicals required by the body for energy and warmth, growth and repair, and protection against disease, are called *nutrients*. There are six groups of nutrients which must be supplied in our food and drink. Carbohydrates and fats are the nutrients required for *energy*, proteins, water and mineral salts are used in *tissue building*, while vitamins are *protective* in function.

Nutrients

Carbohydrates

The main *function* of carbohydrates is to provide *energy*. They are also a source of body fat. Carbohydrates are compounds of the elements carbon, hydrogen, and oxygen. *Sugars, starches*, and *celluloses* are the three groups of carbohydrates which occur in food.

- **Sugars** are white crystalline solids which dissolve in water, and usually taste sweet:
  (a) *Monosaccharides* such as glucose and fructose are simple sugars. *Glucose* is the sugar present in blood, and other carbohydrates are converted into glucose during digestion and metabolism. Glucose also occurs in some fruits, eg grapes and figs. *Fructose* is the sweetest of the sugars and occurs in honey and fruits;
  (b) *Disaccharide* sugars such as sucrose, maltose, and lactose, consist of two monosaccharides linked together by the removal of a water molecule. *Sucrose* is present in sugar cane, sugar beet, carrots, and fruits. It is formed by linking a glucose with a fructose molecule. *Maltose* is malt sugar from barley grains, and is not very sweet. It is formed by linking two glucose molecules. *Lactose* is the sugar present in milk;

- **Starches** are *polysaccharides*, being composed of large numbers of glucose units linked together by the removal of water molecules. The compact bush-like starch molecules contain straight chain *amylose* units, and branched chain *amylopectin* units, and are *storage* products. Starches occur in granules inside the cells of cereals, potatoes, and root vegetables. The starch granules are enclosed by a membrane which is destroyed by cooking. Starch is insoluble in water but cooked starch forms a colloidal suspension. *Glycogen* is the starch formed in the body from glucose, and stored in liver cells as star-shaped granules. It is also stored in muscles;

- **Celluloses** are fibrous *polysaccharides* built up from glucose units. Together with pecten, they form the cell walls of plants, and are present in cereal bran, root vegetables, and hard fruits. Cellulose is not broken down by human digestive juices but forms roughage, or *dietary fibre*.

Figure 7.1
Structure of carbohydrate molecules
(a) Monosaccharide: glucose
(b) Disaccharide: maltose
(c) Polysaccharide: starch

(a) formula $C_6H_{12}O_6$
the molecule has a 6-membered ring structure

simplified to

(b) formula $C_{12}H_{22}O_{11}$
the molecule has two 6-membered rings joined through an oxygen atom by the removal of water

(c) chains of linked glucose units form a bush-shaped molecule

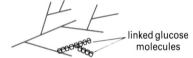

linked glucose molecules

Lipids

Lipids are *fatty* materials which *function* as an *energy* source. They have a higher energy value than carbohydrates as they contain less oxygen in their molecules. Fats can be stored in the body, the subcutaneous fat insulating the body against heat loss as well as providing an energy reserve. *Phospholipids* and *cholesterol* have the important function of forming cell membranes.

Lipids contain carbon and hydrogen as well as oxygen, and are organic substances which are insoluble in water. The lipids include *triglycerides* (fats and oils), *phospholipids, sterols* (cholesterol) and *steroid* hormones and vitamins.

● **Triglycerides** are built up from three fatty acid molecules combined with glycerol. Many different fats occur in food, varying in the particular fatty acids they contain.
(a) *Polyunsaturated* fats have two or more double bonds in their fatty acids, and are oily. They are not very stable as they gradually oxidize in the air, becoming rancid;
(b) *Saturated* fats contain fatty acids lacking double bonds, and are more stable solid fats. Examples of unsaturated fatty acids are *oleic* acid (in olive oil), *linoleic* acid (in corn and soya oils), and *arachidonic* acid. All three of these unsaturated

fatty acids occur in sunflower oil, and are essential for life. As they cannot be synthesised by the liver, they must be obtained from food. Examples of saturated fatty acids are *palmitic* acid (cocoa butter), *stearic* acid (in lard and suet), and *butyric* acid (in butter).

Triglycerides form the neutral fat deposits in the body. The waxes forming sebum and ear wax are formed from triglycerides. *Animal fats* contain mainly saturated fatty acids, and occur in dairy produce, egg yolk, oily fish, red meat, and bacon. *Plant seed oils* contain a higher percentage of unsaturated fatty acids. Soft margarine contains around 60% of polyunsaturates;

- **Phospholipids** form the middle layer of cell membranes and the myelin sheath round nerve fibres. The phospholipid molecule is similar to that of a triglyceride, but one of the fatty acid molecules is replaced by phosphoric acid. They are present in fish oils;

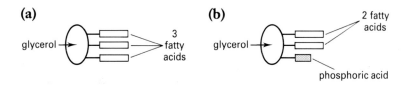

Figure 7.2
Structure of lipid molecules
(a) Triglyceride (fat or oil)
(b) Phospholipid

- **Cholesterol** is a complex lipid formed from saturated fats. It is present in the blood, and is a component of cell membranes. It is needed for the synthesis of several hormones (eg sex hormones) and the bile salts.

Proteins

Proteins *function* as *tissue building materials* and are active components of *biochemical reactions*. They can be oxidized as an energy source if carbohydrate or fat is not available, but this results in tissue loss as protein is not stored in the body.

Fibrous proteins have long chain molecules. Examples of fibrous proteins are *collagen* (in connective tissue), *myosin* and *actin* (in muscle fibres), *keratin* (in skin, hair, and nails), and *fibrin* (in blood clots). Other types of proteins act as enzymes and antibodies, and as hormones (insulin and adrenalin). Protein forms part of the haemoglobin molecule which carries oxygen in the blood.

Proteins contain *nitrogen* in addition to carbon, hydrogen, and oxygen, and may also contain sulphur and/or phosphorus. They are built up from smaller molecules called *amino-acids* which are linked by *peptide bonds* to form polypeptide chains. Several polypeptide chains may be linked together, or the chains may be

Figure 7.3
Structure of protein molecules
(a) General formula for an amino-acid
(b) Polypeptide or protein

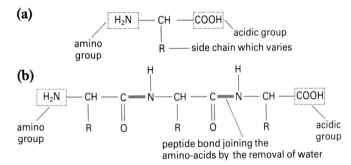

coiled into complex shapes. Heat causes proteins to '*denature*' by altering the shape of the molecules.

There are around twenty different amino-acids divided into two types, **essential amino-acids** which cannot be made by the body, and **inessential** ones made by converting other amino-acids. The eight amino-acids essential for adults are lysine, tryptophan, phenylalanine, methionine, valine, threonine, leucine, and isoleucine. Among the inessential amino-acids are glycine, tyrosine and alanine.

Animal proteins contain more of the essential amino-acids than *plant proteins*, as the proteins of animals are more like those of man. Wheat protein is low in lysine, and maize protein is low in tryptophan. Plant proteins are described as being of *low biological value* because they do not contain the complete range of essential amino-acids. A wide variety of vegetable foods in large quantities is needed to obtain all the essential amino-acids from plant protein alone (vegan diet). If milk, cheese, and eggs are also included all the essential amino-acids will be obtained. *Plant proteins* occur in cereal products, legumes, pulses and nuts. Texturized vegetable protein (meat substitute) is also available. *Animal proteins* occur in meat, fish, cheese, milk and egg white.

Minerals

The *functions* of minerals are (a) to form components of body tissue (bone and blood); (b) to take part in biochemical reactions involving enzymes, and (c) to maintain the osmotic (salt/water) balance of the body fluids. Some eight major minerals are required in relatively large amounts, while only traces of several other minerals are necessary.

The *major minerals* include calcium, iron, phosphorus, sulphur, sodium, potassium, chlorine, and magnesium:

- **Calcium** is essential for the ossification of bones and teeth, for blood coagulation, and for muscle contraction. It is also required for the normal functioning of cell membranes, transmitter release at nerve endings, and glandular secretion. In an adult there is approximately 1 kg of calcium of which 99% occurs in bone tissue, from which it is constantly being withdrawn and replaced. The food sources of calcium include milk, cheese, bread, pilchards, and green vegetables. It is also present in hard drinking water;

- **Iron** forms part of the blood pigment haemoglobin, and the muscle pigment myoglobin. It is needed for the production of ATP in cells (see chapter 8). Iron is stored in the liver. Foods containing iron are liver, red meat, egg yolk, nuts, beans and dried fruits;

- **Phosphorus** occurs as the calcium salt (calcium phosphate) in bones and teeth. Phosphates are involved in the release of energy from glucose, and form part of biologically active substances such as ATP and DNA. Phosphorus is present in most foods and good sources are yeast extract, cheese, eggs, white fish, peanuts and wholemeal bread;

- **Sulphur** is a component of many structural proteins including the keratin of skin and hair. It occurs in egg yolk, fish, red meat, and liver;

- **Sodium** and **chlorine** occur as sodium chloride (common salt) in all the body fluids. Salt is needed to maintain the body's osmotic balance. It is essential for the conduction of nerve impulses, and prevention of muscle cramps. A high salt intake may be associated with high blood pressure which may result in strokes. All processed foods contain salt, particularly bacon and kippers;

- **Magnesium** occurs in bones as magnesium phosphate and is involved in ossification. It is also needed for the activity of enzymes which release energy in the cell. It occurs in green vegetables and salads;

- **Trace minerals** required by the body are shown in Table 7.1.

Vitamins

The *function* of vitamins is to *maintain good health*. They are organic substances required in very small amounts which the body is (in most cases) unable to synthesize. Vitamins are involved in enzyme reactions forming part of the body's physiological processes. Many act as co-enzymes (enzyme activators).

Vitamins are divided into two groups according to their solubility. The **fat-soluble** vitamins are A, D, E, and K, while the **water-soluble** ones include the B group and C. A large unnecessary intake of vitamin pills has little useful effect, and results in their being excreted.

Fat-soluble vitamins can only be absorbed from the food canal in the presence of fatty foods, in which they usually occur. Surpluses are stored in the liver and if taken in excess reach toxic levels, causing liver damage:

Table 7.1
Trace minerals required by the body

Mineral	Food source	Role in the body
Boron	Fruit, nuts, leafy vegetables	Reduces calcium loss from the bones and increases the level of blood oestrogen, protecting against osteoporosis
Cobalt	Liver	Forms part of the Vitamin B12 molecule
Copper	Eggs, cereals, fish and spinach	Required for the formation of haemoglobin; it is part of an enzyme involved in melanin synthesis also
Fluorine	Some drinking water	Makes tooth enamel more resistant to dental caries (decay)
Iodine	Fish	Forms part of the hormone thyroxin
Manganese	Tea, nuts, and cereals	Required for the formation of haemoglobin, and for enzymes concerned with growth, reproduction and lactation
Zinc	Protein foods	It is an activator of several enzymes and is necessary for growth; it is required for the synthesis of insulin; larger amounts are required by women taking the oral contraceptive pill

- **Vitamin A** (Retinol) is essential for dim-light vision, and the health of epithelia such as mucous membranes and skin epidermis. Vitamin A can be produced in the intestine from dietary carotene, an orange pigment in carrots and tomatoes. Other sources of the vitamin are fish liver oils, liver and kidney, eggs, and dairy products;

- **Vitamin D** (Calciferol) is essential for maintaining the blood calcium level by increasing calcium absorption from food. It regulates the interchange of blood and bone calcium, and thus affects the hardening of bones and teeth. Children and pregnant or lactating women require larger amounts of Vitamin D. Its dietary sources are fish liver oils, fatty fish, margarine and eggs. It is also formed in the skin by the action of ultra-violet rays in sunlight on a cholesterol derivative;

- **Vitamin E** (Tocopherol) inhibits the oxidation of polyunsaturated fatty acids that form part of cell membranes. It also protects the liver from damage by some toxic chemicals (eg carbon tetrachloride). It is present in most foods;

- **Vitamin K** (Phylloquinone) is necessary for the production of prothrombin, which aids normal blood clotting. This vitamin occurs in leafy vegetables and cereals. It is also produced by bacteria in the intestine.

Water-soluble vitamins are absorbed along with water in the food canal:

- **Vitamin B** is a group of chemically varied substances which act as co-enzymes in the enzyme reactions of metabolism. All members of the group tend to occur in the same foods, and cannot be stored by the body. Not all the B vitamins are numbered;

- **Thiamin (B1)** is necessary for the steady release of energy from glucose. It is rapidly destroyed by heat. Sources are wholegrain cereals, yeast extract, eggs, liver, milk, vegetables and fruit;

- **Riboflavin (B2)** is essential for using the energy released from food. Its main source is milk, but riboflavin is destroyed if milk is exposed to the ultra-violet rays of sunlight;

- **Nicotinic acid** or **niacin (B5)** is also involved in the breakdown of glucose to release energy. It inhibits the production of cholesterol and assists in fat breakdown. Its source is wholegrain cereals, yeast extract, meat, liver, beans and nuts;

- **Pyridoxine (B6)** is an essential co-enzyme in protein metabolism, including the repair of body tissues. It also acts in fat metabolism. It is destroyed by heat. It is required in larger amounts by women taking the contraceptive pill. It occurs in wholegrain cereals, yeast extract, liver, meat, nuts, bananas, salmon, and tomatoes;

- **Cyanocobalamin (B12)** is a co-enzyme needed for the formation of red blood cells in the red bone marrow. It is also involved in amino-acid metabolism. It is unusual in containing the mineral *cobalt*. Its source is liver, kidney, milk, eggs and cheese. Because it is not present in vegetable foods, a *vegan* diet will be deficient in this vitamin;

- **Folic acid** is essential for the normal formation of red and white blood cells, and for the synthesis of DNA. It is required in larger amounts by women taking the contraceptive pill, and during pregnancy. It occurs in liver, raw leafy vegetables, oranges and bananas. It is also synthesized by bacteria in the food canal;

- **Pantothenic acid** is necessary for the release of energy from glucose, and the conversion of fats and amino-acids to glucose. It is also needed for the synthesis of cholesterol and adrenal hormones. It occurs in kidney, liver, yeast extract, cereals and green vegetables;

- **Biotin** is necessary for the release of energy from glucose, and for the synthesis of fatty acids. It occurs in liver, kidney, yeast extract and egg yolk. It is synthesized by bacteria in the food canal;

- **Vitamin C** (Ascorbic acid) is needed to maintain healthy connective tissue by its involvement in collagen formation. It prevents bleeding from small blood vessels particularly those in the gums. It helps wound to heal. It is rapidly destroyed by heat and by cooking food in water containing bicarbonate of soda. However, potatoes and green vegetables retain much of their Vitamin C if they are placed into boiling water, to which no bicarbonate of soda has been added, and cooked for the minimum time. Fresh fruits, particularly citrus fruits and blackcurrants, are good sources of Vitamin C;

Water

Water forms about two-thirds of the body weight, and is a major structural component. It is the solvent in which all the biochemical reactions of metabolism take place. Water acts as the suspending fluid for blood and lymph cells, and lubricates the tissues.

The evaporation of water in sweat cools the body, but excessive water loss can result from vomiting or diarrhoea, causing *dehydration*. At least one litre of water should be swallowed daily in a temperate climate. In addition to drinks, water is obtained from fruit and vegetables in the diet.

Diet

A *balanced diet* contains all six main nutrients in adequate amounts for energy, growth, reproduction, and protection of the body. The precise amount of each nutrient needed will vary for each individual, but *recommended amounts* for various groups of people have been proposed. The current recommended daily allowances for women and girls are shown in Table 7.3.

Factors to take into account when advising on a balanced diet relate to *individual* nutritional requirements. The energy requirement varies with the age, sex, and occupation of the person. Men require more energy foods than women, while young children require less. An active occupation has a heavier energy demand than a sedentary one. Girls and women require

Table 7.2
Nutrients present in selected foods

Food	Sugar	Starch	Fat	Protein	Calcium	Iron	Vitamin A	Vitamin D	Vitamin E
Baked beans	●	●	●	●					
Bread white		●	●	●		●			
Bread wholemeal	●	●	●	●		●			●
Carrots (raw)	●	●			●		●		
Cheese			●	●	●		●	●	
Chicken			●	●					
Cornflakes	●	●		●					
Cream			●		●		●	●	
Eggs				●	●	●	●	●	●
Fish (white)				●	●				
Honey	●								
Liver			●	●	●	●	●	●	
Meat (lean)			●	●	●	●			
Milk	●			●	●		●	●	
Oranges	●				●				
Pilchards			●	●	●	●		●	
Potatoes		●							
Yeast extract					●	●			

Key F = dietary fibre present   ▓ major source   ▒ minor source   ☐ absent

present

Vitamin K	Thiamin	Ribo-flavin	Niacin	Pyridox-ine	Cyanocob-alamin	Folic acid	Pantoth-enic acid	Biotin	Vitamin C	
										F
										F
										F
										F

Table 7.3
Recommended daily allowances in
the diet for women and girls

Nutrient	Weight (in grams)
Protein	50.0
Total fat ($\frac{1}{3}$ saturated fat) ($\frac{2}{3}$ polyunsaturates)	75.0
Carbohydrates	275.0
Fibre	25.0–30.0
Calcium	0.5
Iron	0.012
Salt	not exceeding 9.0

additional iron in their diet to compensate for losses resulting from menstruation. During pregnancy and lactation extra protein, iron, calcium, folic acid, and Vitamins C and D are required. Children need extra protein for growth.

The *energy-value* of a nutrient is obtained by burning a known weight of it in a bomb calorimeter. The heat given out on burning the nutrient increases the temperature of a known weight of water. From this data, the amount of heat energy can be calculated, and is measured either in **kilocalories** (kcal) or in **kilojoules** (kJ). A *kilocalorie* is the amount of heat needed to raise the temperature of 1 kilogram of water by 1 °C. 1 kcal is equivalent to 4.2 kJ, so 4.2 kJ raise the temperature of 1 kg of water by 1 °C. *Glucose, protein, fat* and *alcohol* all produce energy when taken into the body, but fats have the highest energy (calorific) value.

Table 7.4
Energy values of nutrients

Weight (in g)	Nutrient	Energy value	
		kcals	kJ
1	Glucose	3.75	16
1	Protein	4.00	17
1	Fat	9.00	37
1	Alcohol	7.00	29

The recommended daily energy intake from foods for women and girls is 2000 kcals or 8400 kJ. Women who are pregnant or lactating require a higher energy intake, 2400 and 2750 kcals respectively.

Malnutrition is the result of having a diet which is inadequate or not balanced. If all the nutrients are present in

Table 7.5
Deficiency diseases

Deficient nutrient	Name of disease	Symptoms of the disease
Calcium	Rickets	Soft bones which become deformed in children
	Osteomalacia	Soft bones, with bowing of the legs
	Osteoporosis	Decrease in bone mass causing bones to break easily
Iron	Anaemia	The haemoglobin content of the blood is too low; it results in tiredness, breathlessness, depression
Fluorine	Dental caries	Tooth decay due to weakened tooth enamel
Iodine	Cretinism	Dwarfism and mental retardation in children
	Goitre	Enlargement of the thyroid gland in the neck
Vitamin A	Night blindness	Inability to see in dim light
	Epithelial atrophy	Scaly skin
Thiamin	Beri-beri	Muscle paralysis affecting limbs and digestive system
	Polyneuritis	Reflexes related to the senses of kinesthesia and touch are impaired
Riboflavin	Dermatitis	Skin cracking, and sores in the corners of the mouth
	Cataract	Impaired sight due to clouding of the lens of the eye
Niacin	Pellagra	Skin becomes dark and scaly; chronic diarrhoea
Pyridoxine	Dermatitis	Inflamed skin round eyes, nose and mouth
Cyanocobalamin	Pernicious anaemia	Red bone marrow is unable to form new red blood cells
	Nerve cell degeneration	The axons of the nerve cells in the spinal cord degenerate
Folic acid	Macrocytic anaemia	Abnormally large red blood cells are produced
Vitamin C	Scurvy	Tender swollen gums which bleed; teeth become loose and fall out
Vitamin D	Rickets Osteomalacia	(see Calcium)

inadequate amounts, then **undernutrition**, leading to eventual *starvation*, results. If one particular nutrient is absent or in short supply, a *deficiency disease* may occur (see Table 7.5).

Equally, if too much of any one nutrient is present in the diet, malnutrition occurs. **Obesity** (overweight) is the result of taking in more energy-providing nutrients than can be used up by the body's activities. The excess nutrients will then be converted into *fat* and deposited under the skin and round internal organs such as the heart and kidneys. Even moderate obesity is a *health-hazard*, predisposing the person to coronary heart disease, diabetes, gall-stones, gout, high blood pressure or varicose veins. *Life expectancy* is also reduced by obesity.

Obesity can be treated by adopting a *slimming diet* and increasing *physical activity,* provided the obesity has a dietary cause. *Carbohydrates* can be greatly reduced in the diet with no observable ill effects. The blood/glucose level will remain normal due to the action of the hormones *insulin, adrenalin* and *glucagon* (see Chapter 13). A small amount of glucose is required for the complete oxidation of the fats used as the alternative energy source.

Fats must not be completely excluded from the diet as polyunsaturated fatty acids are essential for life. *Arachidonic* acid is converted into *prostaglandins,* lipids which regulate a variety of body processes, including blood pressure and peristalsis (movement of food along the food canal). *Proteins* cannot be excluded from a slimming diet as they are not stored by the body, and have a short life-span in many cases, so tissue deterioration sets in rapidly unless some protein is included in each meal.

A fibre-rich diet of unrefined foods, having a reduced fat and salt content, little alcohol, and a daily energy value between 1000 and 1500 kcals, should be suitable as a slimming diet.

Anorexia nervosa is a condition involving severe appetite loss and aversion to food, resulting in serious weight loss. It occurs mainly in young women who believe themselves to be overweight and carry dieting to excess. Anorexia is frequently accompanied by *amenorrhoea* (absence of menstruation). Emotional conflicts are often involved, and the condition can develop into a serious nervous disorder requiring medical treatment, often over several years. **Bulimia nervosa** is a condition where the patient eats enormous meals, then induces vomiting or takes laxatives. Acid vomit damages tooth enamel, and retching may rupture the oesophagus.

The digestive process

Some of the nutrients contained in food are not in a suitable form for **absorption** by the body, as they do not *dissolve* in

simpler soluble substances. Most carbohydrates, fats, and proteins need digesting. Minerals and some vitamins are already water-soluble, and do not need digesting.

The digestion and absorption of food occurs in the *alimentary canal* (food canal). Food is pushed along this long tubular structure by the squeezing movements of its walls, which are known as *peristalsis*. **Ingestion** is the act of taking food into the alimentary canal through the mouth. **Elimination** (defaecation) is the expulsion from the alimentary canal of the undigested food remains. It occurs through the *anus*.

During the process of digestion food is broken down *mechanically* by the teeth and peristaltic churning movements. Food is also *chemically* broken down by a series of *digestive juices*. Most of these juices contain *enzymes*, biological catalysts which speed up chemical reactions in the body without being destroyed themselves. Enzymes are proteins synthesized by living glandular cells. They are most active at body temperature (37 °C) and at a specific pH value.

The digestive organs

The digestive organs consist of the **alimentary canal** and the **accessory organs**, which include the teeth, tongue, salivary glands, liver, gallbladder, and pancreas.

The alimentary canal

The wall of the alimentary canal has the same basic structure along its length, having four layers or *tunics*. On the outside is the *serosa* tunic, a serous membrane which is part of the *peritoneum* which attaches the alimentary canal to the wall of the abdominal cavity. Below the serosa is the thick *muscularis* tunic

Figure 7.4
Structure of wall of alimentary canal (small intestine region)

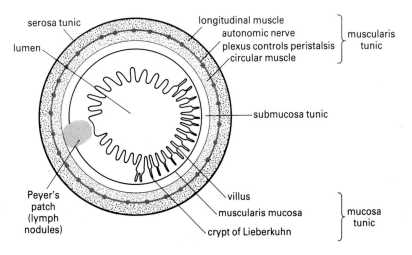

consisting of smooth muscle as a *longitudinal* layer outside and a *circular* layer inside. An *autonomic nerve plexus* controlling peristalsis occurs betwen the two muscle layers. Below the muscle layer is the *submucosa*, a layer of connective tissue which contains many blood vessels. On the inside, lining the lumen or food cavity, is the *mucosa* consisting of a thin layer of smooth muscle, the *muscularis mucosa*, attached to a mucous membrane. The mucous membrane is *stratified* in regions needing protection against friction from the food, or *simple* in regions where absorption of nutrients occurs.

The alimentary canal is divided into several regions of varying length and width:

- The **buccal cavity** is the space inside the mouth, and is bounded by the cheeks, hard and soft palates and the tongue. It is lined by stratified squamous epithelium. Hanging below the soft palate is the *uvula* on each side of which are the *palatine tonsils*. The *lingual tonsils* are at the base of the tongue. The tonsils are part of the lymphatic system (see Chapter 12);

- The **pharynx** (throat) links the buccal cavity to the oesophagus (gullet), and is lined with stratified squamous epithelium. Although it is both an air and a food passage, when food is being swallowed breathing is temporarily stopped as the larynx (air passage) is closed by the *epiglottis*. Swallowing begins as a voluntary action, aided by the tongue, but further movement of the food is involuntary by peristalsis;

- The **oesophagus** is a long narrow tube passing through the thorax, which it leaves through a hole in the diaphragm called the *hiatus*. *Hiatus hernia* is the protrusion of the lower end of the oesophagus and the upper part of the stomach into the thoracic cavity through an enlargement of the hiatus. It occurs mainly in women over 50 years of age, as a result of previous pregnancy, obesity, or continual lifting of heavy weights. The oesophagus is lined by a stratified squamous epithelium, and secretes *mucus* as a lubricant to aid peristalsis. Just below the diaphragm it opens into the stomach;

- The **stomach** occurs in the upper left region of the abdominal cavity. It is a curved enlargement of the alimentary canal, divided into four regions, the *cardia, fundus, body* and *pylorus*.
  (a) The upper region, or *cardia*, is separated from the oesophagus by the *cardiac sphincter*, a ring-shaped muscle which, on contracting, narrows the opening between the oesophagus and the stomach. It relaxes during swallowing

so that food can pass into the stomach. It contracts to retain food in the stomach, but relaxes when the reflex action of *vomiting* occurs;

(b) Above and to the left of the cardia is the *fundus* of the stomach;

(c) Below is the large central region or *body* of the stomach, where the mucosa lies in large folds (rugae) which smooth out as the stomach fills;

(d) The stomach then narrows at the *pylorus* region where it opens into the small intestine. The *pyloric sphincter* is a ring of muscle controlling this opening. It contracts to retain food in the stomach for around three to four hours, by which time the food has been converted into a creamy suspension called *chyme*.

The stomach mucosa contains *gastric glands* with three types of cells:

(a) *Peptic* cells at the base of the glands which secrete pepsinogen;

(b) *Oxyntic* cells which secrete hydrochloric acid that activates pepsinogen to form the enzyme pepsin;

Figure 7.5
Digestive organs (transverse colon removed)

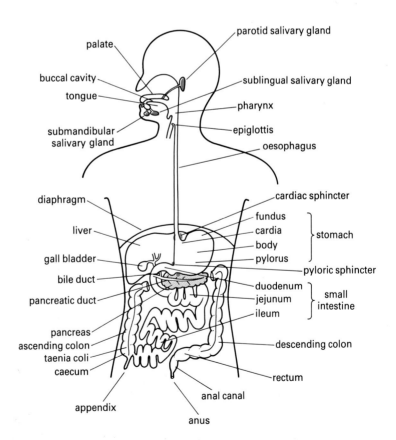

(c) *Goblet* cells at the top of the glands which secrete a thick mucus to protect the stomach wall from damage by the acid and enzyme in the *gastric juice*. Very vigorous peristaltic movements in the stomach churn the food and mix it with the gastric juice;

- The **small intestine** is divided into three parts:
  (a) the duodenum;
  (b) the jejunum;
  (c) the ileum.

  The *duodenum* begins at the pyloric sphincter and is 25 cm long. It merges with the narrower *jejunum* which is 2.5 m long and leads into the *ileum* whose length is 3.6 m. The coils of the small intestine are bound together and to the abdominal wall by a membrane, the *mesentery*, which is part of the peritoneum. The walls of the small intestine contain glands which secrete a digestive juice from deep pits in the mucosa called *crypts of Lieberkuhn*. In the duodenum only, the submucosa contains *Brunner's* glands which secrete an alkaline mucus to neutralize stomach acids and protect the wall of the duodenum from ulceration.

  The mucosa of the small intestine has small finger-like projections called *villi*, which increase the internal surface area enormously to aid the absorption of digested nutrients. The villi are covered by a simple columnar epithelium so that nutrients can pass through easily. The epithelial cells have tiny *microvilli* projecting from their free surface which further increase the absorptive area. Goblet cells occur amongst the epithelial cells to secrete mucus. Each villus contains a central *lymphatic duct* surrounded by a network of *blood capillaries*. Lymph nodules in groups called *Peyer's patches* occur in the mucosa and submucosa of the ileum. They act as a defense against harmful bacteria in the alimentary canal;

Figure 7.6
Villus in small intestine

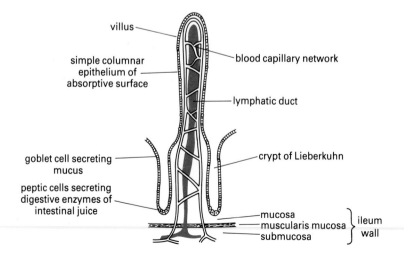

- The **large intestine** is 1.5 m long and is twice as wide as the small intestine. It extends from the ileum to its opening at the anus. It is divided into four regions:
  (a) the caecum;
  (b) the colon;
  (c) the rectum;
  (d) the anal canal.

  The opening into the *caecum* from the ileum is guarded by a fold of membrane called the *ileocaecal valve*. The caecum is 6 cm long and ends in a narrow closed tube 8 cm long called the *vermiform appendix*. At the other end the caecum leads into the colon. The caecum and appendix have no known function in human digestion;

  The *colon* has ascending, transverse, and descending portions, ending in the pelvic colon which leads into the rectum. It is 1.3 m long. The longitudinal muscle of its wall consists of three strips only, the *taenia coli*, which are shorter than the colon in length and pucker its wall. There are no villi in the mucosa which is bounded by a simple columnar epithelium containing goblet cells to secrete mucus;

  The *rectum* is the continuation of the colon, and lies anterior to the sacrum in the pelvic cavity. It is 20 cm long and its last few centimetres form the anal canal;

  The *anal canal* has longitudinal folds in its highly vascular lining. Inflammation of the anal veins results in *haemorrhoids* (piles). At the external end of the anal canal is the *anal sphincter* which contracts to close the anus. The sphincter consists of an internal ring of *smooth* muscle and an external ring of *skeletal* (voluntary) muscle. The anus normally remains closed except during the elimination of the undigested food remains (faeces).

The accessory organs

- The **teeth** of the permanent dentition occupy sockets in the maxillae and mandible. Teeth are composed of bone-like *dentine* and consist of a *crown* above the gum, and a *root* embedded in the socket. The crown has a thin covering of very hard *enamel*, while the root is covered by a layer of *cement*. The tooth socket is lined by a fibrous *periodontal membrane* attached to the cement, which anchors the tooth in the jaw, and acts as a shock absorber. In the centre of the dentine is a *pulp cavity*. Pulp is a connective tissue containing nerves and blood vessels which enter the tooth through the root.

  The 32 teeth vary in shape and function, and can be represented by a dental formula viz: $i\frac{2}{2} \, c\frac{1}{1} \, p\frac{2}{2} \, m\frac{3}{3}$, giving the numbers of teeth of each type on one side of the jaws. *Incisors* (i) are chisel-shaped teeth used to cut food. *Canines*

(c) are pointed and tear food. *Premolars* (p) and *molars* (m) have flattened surfaces with small projections called cusps, and grind or crush food;

- The **tongue** forms the floor of the buccal cavity. A fold of mucous membrane called the *lingual frenulum* is attached to the underside of the tongue to anchor it in the buccal cavity. The surface of the tongue is roughened by small projections called *papillae,* and it carries *taste buds* which respond to chemical stimuli (sour, salt, bitter, and sweet);

- Three pairs of **salivary glands** open into the buccal cavity:
  (a) The *parotid* pair lie below and in front of the ears, on top of the masseter muscle. Their ducts open opposite the upper second molar teeth;
  (b) The *submandibular* pair occur posteriorly below the tongue, and their ducts open behind the middle lower incisors;
  (c) The *sublingual* pair occur anteriorly below the tongue and they have several ducts opening into the floor of the buccal cavity.
     The parotids are compound tubuloacinar glands, while the other two pairs are of the compound acinar type. The glands produce a digestive juice called *saliva,* but the secretions of the individual glands vary. The parotids secrete a thin watery liquid containing the enzyme *salivary amylase* (pytalin). The submandibulars also secrete this enzyme, but as they produce *mucus* the secretion is thicker. The sublingual secretion contains mainly mucus. Saliva contains 99.5% water, and provides the solvent for food. It is slightly *acidic* due to the action of mouth bacteria on food debris, with a pH between 6.5 and 6.9. The mucus in saliva lubricates the food so that it is easily swallowed. The secretion of saliva is a *reflex action* in response to taste stimuli from the tongue. The smell and sight of food also stimulate saliva secretion;

- The **liver** occurs on the right side of the abdominal cavity under the diaphragm, to which it is attached by the *falciform ligament.* It is a large red glandular organ covered by a fibrous capsule, and composed of several lobes. It has a small left lobe and a larger right lobe which is subdivided into *caudate* and *quadrate* lobes.
     The liver consists of a large number of *lobules* which are hexagonal blocks of *hepatic cells.* The vertical plates of hepatic cells radiate from a central *hepatic vein* branch in each lobule. The hepatic veins return blood to the heart from the liver. The blood supply to each lobule comes from two vessels. The *hepatic artery* brings oxygen-containing blood from the heart, while the *hepatic portal vein* brings

Figure 7.7
Blood supply of liver lobule
(a) Side view
(b) Cross-section

(a)

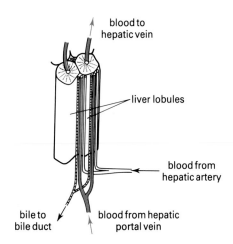

(b)

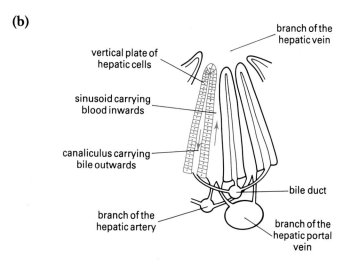

digested food from the small intestine. Branches of these vessels occur in spaces between the liver lobules.

Between the plates of hepatic cells in the lobules are narrow channels called *canaliculi*. The hepatic cells secrete the digestive juice *bile* into the canaliculi, which carry it to the bile ducts between the lobules. Bile is a greenish alkaline fluid containing *bile salts* (sodium bicarbonate, glycocholate, and taurate), and the *bile pigments* bilirubin and biliverdin produced from worn out red blood cells. Alternating with the canaliculi are similar spaces called *sinusoids*, in which blood passes from the hepatic artery and hepatic portal vein branches to the central hepatic vein branches;

● The **gall bladder** is a sac on the underside of the liver. Its inner wall is thrown into folds which allow it to expand as it fills with bile from the liver. Contraction of its muscular wall forces the stored bile into the main *bile duct* which opens into the duodenum;

- The **pancreas** is a compound tubuloacinar gland lying below the stomach. It contains small clusters of glandular epithelial cells of two types. One type, the *islets of Langerhans*, are endocrine glands secreting the hormones *insulin* and *glucagon* into the blood stream. The other type, the *acini*, are exocrine glands secreting *pancreatic digestive juice* which passes down the *pancreatic duct* to the duodenum. Just before reaching the duodenum the pancreatic duct joins the bile duct, both ducts opening together just below the pyloric sphincter.

Chemical digestion

The food broken down by the teeth is rolled round the buccal cavity by the tongue and mixed with saliva. Each swallowed food mass (bolus) then travels the length of the alimentary canal by peristaltic movements. The food is acted upon by a series of *digestive juices* which chemically break it down into simpler soluble nutrients. The smell and sight of food, and its presence in the alimentary canal, stimulate the autonomic nervous system and the secretion of certain hormones, which regulate the ordered secretion of the digestive juices.

The *end-products* of this chemical digestion are simple sugars from carbohydrates, amino-acids from proteins, and fatty acids and glycerol from fats. The actions of the digestive juices are shown in Table 7.6.

Absorption

The soluble nutrients from food are able to diffuse through the mucosa of the alimentary canal wall, and enter the body's transport systems, the blood or lymph vessels.

The *stomach* absorbs *alcohol*, which enters the blood capillaries in the stomach wall. Absorption of alcohol occurs very rapidly once it has been consumed, particularly when the stomach is empty.

The *small intestine* absorbs most of the nutrients through the villi, which contain smooth muscle and are able to move about gently, to bring them into close contact with the digested food. *Glucose* and *amino-acids* are absorbed by a combination of diffusion and active transport, and pass into the capillary networks of the villi which drain into the hepatic portal vein.

Table 7.6
Chemical digestion in the
alimentary canal

Region where digestion occurs	Digestive glands	Digestive juice	Enzymes present	Food acted on	Nutrients produced
Buccal cavity (continuing in oesophagus)	Salivary (three pairs)	Saliva (slightly acid)	Salivary amylase	Cooked starch	Maltose sugar
Stomach	Gastric (in stomach wall)	Gastric (acid)	Pepsin (activated by acid)	Protein	Peptides
Duodenum	Pancreas	Pancreatic (alkaline)	Trypsin (activated by enterokinase)	Protein and peptides	Dipeptides and amino-acids
			Pancreatic amylase	Starch	Maltose sugar
			Lipase	Fats	Fatty acids and glycerol
	Brunner's (in duodenal wall)	Intestinal (alkaline)	Protease	Protein and peptides	Amino-acids
	Liver	Bile (alkaline)	None	Bile salts act on fats	Emulsified fat
Jejunum and Ileum	Crypts of Lieberkuhn (in intestine wall)	Intestinal (slightly alkaline)	Erepsin Lipase Maltase Amylase Lactase (Enterokinase)	Peptides Fats Maltose Starch Lactose (Trypsinogen)	Amino-acids Fatty acids and glycerol Glucose Maltose Simple sugars (Trypsin)

Fatty acids and *glycerol* pass into the columnar epithelial cells of the villi by *pinocytosis*. Here they are converted back into *fat* droplets and enter the lymph vessels as a white emulsion. The fat is carried by the lymphatic system to the blood in the main veins. *Fat-soluble vitamins* are also absorbed in this way. Inorganic *salts* and *water-soluble vitamins* are absorved into the blood capillary networks of the villi.

The colon absorbs much of the water from the undigested food remains. If this material contains large amounts of *dietary fibre*, less water is removed from it and it remains much softer. The water-holding properties of fibre allow the soft undigested food remains to pass quickly through the intestine and be easily eliminated. This prevents *constipation*, and the build-up of toxic materials in the bowel which can cause *diverticulitis* and *cancer*. Adequate dietary fibre may also prevent *haemorrhoids* (piles) or *appendicitis*.

Fibre (cellulose) can be broken down by *bacteria* in the large intestine, and some of the by-products are the gases carbon dioxide and methane, leading to some flatulence. Other by-products are some of the vitamins, eg folic acid and biotin. Such bateria are described as *symbiotic* because both they, and their human carrier, obtain benefit from the association. The bacteria obtain food and a protected environment, while the person obtains extra nutrients. By the time the food remains reach the rectum they have become *faeces*.

Metabolism

Metabolism involves all the chemical activities of the body and the use or production of energy. Once nutrients have been absorbed from the alimentary canal and enter the blood, they are taken to the living cells of all the body's tissues, and become involved in cell metabolism. This is known as nutrient *assimilation*.

Carbohydrate metabolism

Glucose is the end product of carbohydrate digestion, and it is used by living cells as the preferred source of *energy*. The level of glucose in the blood is kept constant by the activity of the hepatic cells of the liver, regulated by the pancreatic hormones and adrenalin. Excess glucose is either converted into *glycogen* and stored in the hepatic cells, or converted into *fatty acids* and carried by the blood to the body's *fat deposits* for storage.

If the diet contains insufficient carbohydrate for the body's needs, stored glycogen and fat are converted back to glucose by the liver to maintain the *blood glucose* level. Thus the liver has a *homeostatic* function in keeping the blood glucose level constant.

Fat metabolism

The end products of fat digestion are **fatty acids** and **glycerol** which are used as an energy source in addition to glucose. In a normal balanced diet 35% of the body's energy would come from fat. The liver cells can convert glycerol to glucose, which is then used as described above. Fatty acids cannot be converted into glucose, but are broken down by a series of chemical changes called *beta-oxidation*.

Incomplete breakdown of fatty acids (*ketosis*) produces an increased level of blood ketones (eg acetone) which are harmful. Ketones may escape from the blood into the lungs and appear in the breath. This commonly happens in diabetics. Excess fat in the diet is stored in the body's *fat deposits.*

Protein metabolism

The end products of protein digestion are **amino-acids**. In the body cells they are built up into new protein molecules required for building new tissues and for enzyme synthesis. If there is no other energy nutrient available, protein can be broken down by the liver and used to produce energy.

The first stage in protein breakdown is called *deamination*, during which the nitrogen-containing amino group is removed, and converted into *urea* to be excreted in the urine. The rest of the amino-acid molecule is used to provide energy. Surplus amino-acids from the dietary proteins cannot be stored by the body, so they too are deaminated and used for energy. Proteins extracted from worn out cells are broken down into their constituent amino-acids in the liver, and used similarly.

Functions of the liver in metabolism

As a result of its functions in carbohydrate, fat, and protein metabolism, the liver produces a lot of *heat* from chemical reactions. This heat is transferred to the blood which distributes it to cooler parts of the body.

The liver also synthesizes *cholesterol*. Excess cholesterol from dietary fats is excreted in the bile, where a high concentration may produce *gall-stones* during storage. The liver secretes a chemical which stimulates the *red bone marrow* to produce new red blood cells. This chemical can only be secreted if *Vitamin B12* is available. The liver also breaks down worn out red blood cells forming the *bile pigments* in the process. The veins in the liver act as a blood *reservoir*, so the liver stores blood. The liver synthesizes the *plasma proteins* of the blood.

Sex hormones are broken down in the liver once they are no longer required. The liver stores *minerals* such as iron, potassium and copper, and *Vitamins* A, D, E, K and B12. It can also deal with some *poisons*, converting them into less toxic substances, or storing them to prevent harm to more sensitive tissues.

Self-assessment questions

1 Define the following terms:

(a) vitamin;   (b) enzyme;
(c) peristalsis.

2 Compare the chemical structure of a starch molecule with that of a triglyceride.

3 List the advantages of a high-fibre diet.

4 Explain the functions of:

(a) the pyloric sphincter;
(b) the mesentery;
(c) villi.

5 Which nutrient is associated with the following diseases:

(a) goitre;   (b) osteoporosis;
(c) scurvy;   (d) polyneuritis;
(e) dental caries?

6 Describe the composition and functions of bile.

7 Describe the structure of the ileum wall.

8 In which foods do the majority of the B group vitamins occur?

9 List **six** major functions of the liver.

10 In which digestive juices do the following occur:

(a) amylase;
(b) lipase;
(c) mucus;
(d) hydrochloric acid;
(e) sodium glycocholate?

CHAPTER 8

The Respiratory System

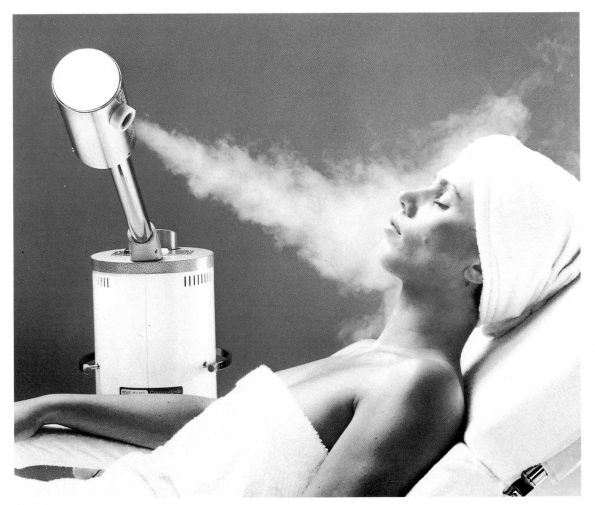

Facial steamer

Respiration

Respiration is the process by which the body obtains a supply of *energy* by breaking down nutrients. This process occurs in every living cell of the body tissues, and is part of *cell metabolism*. The chemical reactions involved in cell respiration may be *aerobic*, if oxygen is required, or *anaerobic* if they occur in the absence of oxygen. Anaerobic respiration occurs in the cells of actively

Table 8.1
Composition of air

Gases in the air	Composition in volumes %	
	Air breathed in (inspired)	Air breathed out (expired)
Oxygen	21	17
Carbon dioxide	0.03	4
Water vapour	variable	increased
Nitrogen	78	78
Rare gases	0.9	0.9

contracting muscle, while *resting* muscle cells respire aerobically. The cells of other tissues respire aerobically all the time. The *complete* chemical breakdown of glucose molecules to supply energy occurs in the presence of *oxygen*. Anaerobic respiration results in the partial or *incomplete* breakdown of glucose molecules, and releases less energy. *Respiratory enzymes* act as catalysts during the chemical breakdown of energy foods in all the living body cells.

During aerobic cell respiration *carbon dioxide* is liberated and *oxygen* is used up. The tissues therefore require a continuous supply of oxygen from the blood. As carbon dioxide is acidic and toxic to living cells, the blood must continuously remove it from the tissues, together with other toxic waste products. The oxygen supply is obtained from the air, and the carbon dioxide is expelled into the air. Table 8.1 shows the way the *composition* of the *air* is changed by human respiration.

The process by which air enters and leaves the body is known as *breathing* or *ventilation*. *External* respiration is the exchange of gases between the lungs and the blood. *Internal* respiration is the exchange of gases between the blood and the living cells of the body tissues.

Respiratory organs

The air must be brought into contact with a vascular *respiratory surface* where the *exchange* of oxygen and carbon dioxide gases can occur during external respiration. Substantial amounts of *water* will evaporate from such a surface. To prevent dehydration by reducing evaporation, the respiratory surface occurs *inside* the lungs. A system of tubes connects the lungs to the outside air. The **nose, nasopharynx, pharynx, larynx, bronchi,** and the **bronchioles** and **alveoli** of the lungs, form the *respiratory organs.*

The nose

The nose consists of two *nasal cavities* opening to the outside at the *nostrils* (external nares). Internally the nasal cavities connect with the nasopharynx by two *internal nares.* A vertical partition, the *nasal septum,* separates the nasal cavities which are roofed by the nasal bones and nasal cartilage. The floor of the nasal cavities is formed by the palate.

The ethmoid *conchi* and *turbinate* bones subdivide each nasal cavity into three groove-like air passages lined with a *mucous membrane* containing ciliated and goblet cells. These scroll-shaped bones provide a large surface area for the membrane. The *mucus* secreted traps dust and bacteria entering with the air, and the outward beating of the cilia keeps dirt out of the lungs.

The functions of the nose are to moisten, warm and filter the air breathed in. It acts as the organ of smell, and as a resonating chamber for the voice.

The nasopharynx

The nasopharynx is the upper part of the cavity behind the nose, and is lined with mucous membrane. The two *Eustachian* tubes from the middle ears open into it so that air pressure inside the ear can be adjusted to prevent damage to the ear drum. The posterior wall of the nasopharynx carries the *pharyngeal tonsil* composed of lymphoid tissue. When enlarged it is known as the adenoids, and can block the internal nares and cause *mouth-breathing,* with the loss of the protective function of nose-breathing.

The pharynx

The pharynx (throat) is a continuation of the nasopharynx extending to the larynx (voice box) in the neck. It is lined with a protective stratified squamous epithelium. The *palatine* and *lingual tonsils* occur on its lateral walls.

The functions of the pharynx are to act as both an air and a food passage, and as a resonating chamber for the voice.

The larynx

The larynx is a short passage connecting the pharynx to the trachea (windpipe). It opens from the pharynx at a slit-like *glottis.* Its walls are supported by nine pieces of cartilage, one of which is the *thyroid cartilage* or Adam's apple. These cartilages hold the air passage permanently open. The *epiglottis* is a leaf-shaped piece of cartilage lying on top of the larynx, and closes the glottis when food is swallowed. This prevents food going down the wrong way and blocking the air passage.

Figure 8.1
Section through head to show
respiratory organs (side view)

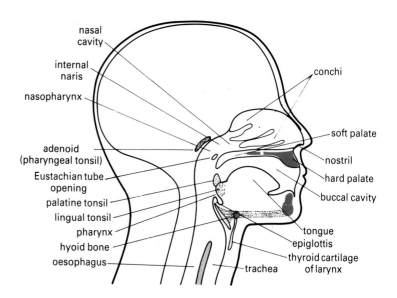

nasal cavity

internal naris

nasopharynx

conchi

adenoid (pharyngeal tonsil)

soft palate

nostril

Eustachian tube opening

hard palate

palatine tonsil

buccal cavity

lingual tonsil

pharynx

tongue

hyoid bone

epiglottis

oesophagus

thyroid cartilage of larynx

trachea

Two pairs of folds in the larynx wall form the *vocal cords* on each side of the glottis. When the muscles attached to these cords contract, the space between them is narrowed. When air passes the vocal cords, they vibrate and cause sound waves in the air in the pharynx, nose and buccal cavity.

The trachea

The trachea extends into the thorax from the larynx, and is a narrow tube 11 cm long. Its wall is composed of three layers. On the inside is a pseudostratified ciliated epithelium which secretes mucus. The middle layer is composed of elastic connective tissue. The outer layer contains approximately 20 C–shaped bands of hyaline *cartilage* to keep the trachea permanently open. The open ends of the cartilages are posterior, so that where the trachea touches the oesophagus, food boluses in the oesophagus can bulge slightly into the trachea as they are swallowed.

The bronchi

The two bronchi are formed by forking of the lower end of the trachea. They carry the air into the lungs. The right bronchus is only half as long as the left bronchus and is nearly vertical. The walls of the bronchi are lined by a ciliated columnar epithelium, and, like the trachea, contain C–shaped cartilages to hold them open.

The lungs

The lungs lie on each side of the thoracic cavity, extending from the clavicles to the diaphragm. They are roughly conical in shape, and both are lobed. The right lung has three lobes, and the left lung has two. Each lung is enclosed in a *pleural membrane* and another pleural membrane lines the thoracic cavity.

Figure 8.2
Respiratory organs of the thorax
(anterior view)

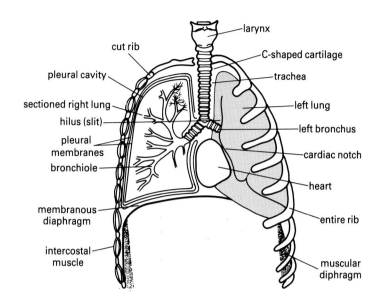

Between the pleura there is a cavity containing a *lubricating fluid*, allowing the lungs to slide freely over the thoracic wall during breathing. The medial surface of each lung contains a vertical slit called the *hilus*. The pulmonary blood vessels, nerves and bronchi enter or leave the lung at the hilus. The left lung has a *cardial notch*, a medial depression into which the heart fits.

The bronchioles

Within the lungs each bronchus subdivides forming a tree-like system of bronchioles, which become progressively narrower. The walls of the wider bronchioles are supported by small plates of *cartilage*, while those of the narrower *terminal* bronchioles contain smooth muscle but no cartilage supports. The columnar ciliated epithelium lining the walls of the wider bronchioles changes to a squamous epithelium in the terminal bronchioles, where no goblet cells secreting mucus are present.

The alveoli

Alveoli are cup-shaped cavities within the lungs. They are lined by a thin film of water, essential for dissolving oxygen from the alveolar air. The alveoli are grouped round an air space, the *alveolar duct*, which leads from a terminal bronchiole.

The alveolar wall consists of two types of epithelial cells. It is a simple *squamous* epithelium with interspersed *septal* cells, which are cuboid and secrete a *detergent-like* chemical to lower the surface tension of the water film, and allow the alveoli to expand so that air can enter. *Phagocytes* (dust cells) also occur in the alveolar wall to remove foreign particles which have entered the lungs.

On the outer side of the alveolar wall is a network of *blood capillaries* linking branches of the pulmonary arteries with

Figure 8.3
Functional unit of the lung

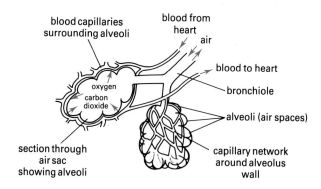

branches of the pulmonary veins. The lungs contain around 300 million alveoli, and provide an enormous respiratory surface for the exchange of gases.

Breathing or ventilation

Breathing or ventilation is the passage of air into and out of the lungs, known as **inspiration** and **expiration** respectively. The *pressure* inside the thoracic cavity is increased to cause expiration, and decreased to cause inspiration. The pressure changes are brought about by *volume* changes of the thoracic cavity. Reducing the volume of the thorax increases the pressure on the lungs, leading to expiration. Increasing the volume of the thorax reduces the pressure on the lungs by causing a partial *vacuum* which draws air into the lungs during inspiration.

These volume changes are caused by the **external intercostal** muscles between the ribs, and the **diaphragm** muscle. The muscles contract to cause inspiration, and relax to cause expiration. *Contraction* of the external *intercostal* muscles lifts the ribs and pushes the sternum forward. This increases the dimensions of the thorax from back to front, and increases its circumference. *Contraction* of the radiating *diaphragm* muscles flattens the diaphragm by decreasing its surface area, and increases the dimensions of the thorax from top to bottom.

Both sets of muscles *relax* to decrease the volume of the thorax. The ribs then slope downwards and the sternum moves inwards, reducing the circumference of the thorax. The stomach and liver push the relaxed diaphragm upwards so that it bulges up into the thoracic cavity. The respiratory muscles contract and relax *alternately*, so inspiration and expiration alternate.

A *respiratory centre* in the medulla oblongata of the brain controls these *reflex* breathing movements. A person at rest takes in and gives out only 0.5 litre of air with each breath. This is

Figure 8.4
Changes in volume of the thorax
(a) Due to intercostal muscles
(b) Due to diaphragm muscle

(a)

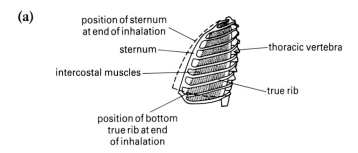

(b)

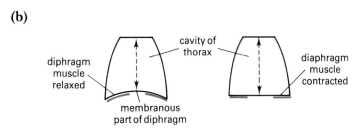

known as the *tidal volume*. The tidal volume multiplied by the rate of respiration per minute is called the *minute volume*. The number of breaths per minute varies between 12 and 20, so the minute volume varies between 6 litres (0.5 × 12) and 10 litres (0.5 × 20). The *total lung capacity* is about 5 litres of air while the tidal volume is only 0.5 litre, so only one-tenth of the air is exchanged during each *quiet* breath.

By taking a *deep* breath an extra 3 litres of air will enter the lungs and be expelled when breathing out. The 3.5 litres of air entering and leaving the lungs during deep breathing is the *vital capacity*. It is the maximum volume of air that can be exchanged during breathing. The remaining 1.5 litres of air which is not expelled is the *residual volume*. The lungs therefore never collapse completely during ventilation. The *functional residual capacity* is the air remaining in the lungs throughout normal quiet breathing. These volumes are measured by an instrument called a recording spirometer which produces a tracing similar to that in Fig 8.5.

External respiration

This is the exchange of the gases oxygen and carbon dioxide between the blood in the capillaries covering the alveoli walls, and the air in the alveolar cavities. The *deoxygenated* blood entering the lungs in the pulmonary arteries becomes *oxygenated* as it flows through the capillaries, then returns to the heart in the pulmonary veins. This movement of the blood from the

Figure 8.5
Recording spirometer tracing

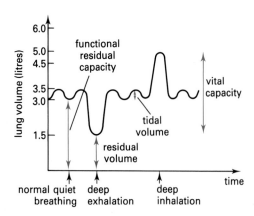

heart to the lungs and back again, is known as the *pulmonary circulation*.

The enormous surface area of the alveoli and the narrowness of the blood capillaries gives the maximum surface exposure for gaseous exchange. The thinness of the alveolar and blood capillary walls allow the dissolved gases to diffuse across very readily. *Diffusion* of the oxygen and carbon dioxide depends on the difference in the amount of each gas present in the alveolar air and in the blood. As there is more oxygen in the alveolar air and less in the blood, oxygen will diffuse into the blood. The higher concentration of carbon dioxide in the deoxygenated blood in the pulmonary capillaries causes it to diffuse into the alveolar air spaces.

Figure 8.6
External respiration

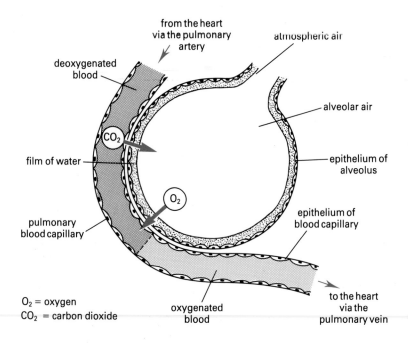

Internal respiration

This is the exchange of *oxygen* and *carbon dioxide* between the blood and the living cells of the body tissues. During this process the oxygenated blood in the tissue capillaries becomes deoxygenated. The different concentrations of oxygen and carbon dioxide in the blood and body cells results in gaseous exchange by *diffusion*. Oxygen diffuses from the blood into the body cells, and carbon dioxide formed in the body cells diffuses into the blood.

Oxygen is carried by *haemoglobin*, inside the red blood cells, as bright red *oxyhaemoglobin*. Where living tissue cells are using up oxygen rapidly so the oxygen concentration in the cells remains low, oxyhaemglobin readily releases its oxygen. The oxygen dissolves in the blood plasma, and diffuses into the tissue cells. The deoxygenated haemoglobin is purple in colour.

Figure 8.7
Internal respiration

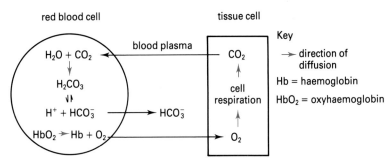

Carbon dioxide diffuses in solution from the living tissue cells into the blood in the tissue capillaries. The red blood cells contain an *enzyme* which speeds up the reaction between carbon dioxide and water to form *carbonic acid*.

$$CO_2 + H_2O \xrightarrow{\text{enzyme}} H_2CO_3$$

The carbonic acid splits up into *ions*, forming positive hydrogen ions (H^+) and negative hydrogen carbonate ions (HCO_3^-).

$$H_2CO_3 \rightleftharpoons H^+ + HCO_3^-$$

The hydrogen carbonate ions can readily pass through the wall of red blood cells so they diffuse out into the blood plasma because of the concentration gradient between the red cells (high) and the plasma (low).

Metabolic rate

The body requires a certain amount of energy daily just to keep alive, ie to maintain its *basal metabolism*. *Basal metabolic rate* (BMR) is a measure of how fast the body cells break down energy nutrients to release enough energy just to stay alive. The rate of oxygen consumption and carbon dioxide production are convenient ways of measuring BMR, which accounts for around 60% of the daily energy expenditure. The volume of carbon dioxide produced divided by the volume of oxygen used up in a definite time is called the *respiratory quotient* (RQ).

$$RQ = \frac{\text{volume of CO}_2 \text{ produced}}{\text{volume of O}_2 \text{ used}}$$

During *aerobic* respiration, if the energy nutrient is solely *glucose*, equal volumes of oxygen and carbon dioxide are exchanged, and the RQ = 6/6 = 1.

$$C_6H_{12}O_6 + 6\ O_2 \rightarrow 6\ CO_2 + 6\ H_2O$$
(glucose)
(equal volumes)

When *triglyceride* (fat) alone is the energy source, as more oxygen is used up than carbon dioxide produced, the fraction is less than one, and the RQ = 0.7. When *protein* alone is the energy source, the RQ = 0.99. Using a *mixture* of these three energy sources gives an RQ of between 0.8 and 0.9. A *balanced diet* gives an RQ of 0.85, showing that both carbohydrates and fats are used as energy sources.

In most body cells *aerobic* respiration occurs. *Glucose* is first broken down to *pyruvic acid* by a series of *anaerobic* reactions called *glycolysis*. The further breakdown of pyruvic acid into carbon dioxide and water cannot occur unless *oxygen* is present, and is the aerobic phase of the process. The energy released from the glucose molecules is stored in *ATP molecules*.

In all the living body cells *ADP molecules* and *phosphate ions* are present. The energy released from the breakdown of glucose is used to join a phosphate ion to an ADP molecule by a *high energy bond*. This forms an ATP molecule, which stores the energy temporarily. When the cell requires energy for its metabolism, ATP molecules release it by breaking their high energy bonds, and reforming ADP molecules and phosphate ions.

(i) ADP + phosphate +   energy   → ATP
(from glucose)

(ii) ATP → ADP + phosphate +   energy
(for cell's use)

During *anaerobic* respiration, which occurs in vigorously contracting muscle cells, glucose is incompletely broken down, as the blood is unable to supply oxygen fast enough for aerobic respiration to occur. The glucose is first converted to pyruvic acid, which is then partially broken down into *lactic acid*. About 80% of the lactic acid is carried to the *liver* by the blood. In the liver it is converted back into glucose which can be used again as an energy source. Some of the lactic acid accumulates in the muscle tissue causing *muscle fatigue*. This toxic lactic acid must eventually be removed by breaking it down into carbon dioxide and water by reactions requiring additional oxygen, known as the *oxygen debt*. After vigorous exercise *deep breathing* occurs to obtain this extra oxygen to pay back the oxygen debt. When a muscle is *not contracting*, the breakdown of glucose occurs only slowly, as very little energy is required by the muscle. The blood supplying the muscle is able to bring sufficient oxygen for the complete breakdown of glucose to carbon dioxide and water to occur by aerobic respiration.

Disorders of the respiratory system

All the following disorders contra-indicate facial massage and electrical muscle stimulation.

* *Rhinitis* is inflammation of the mucous membrane lining the nasal cavities and covering the conchi. The membrane swells and blocks the free flow of air through the nose. There is increased secretion of a watery mucus;

* *Hay fever* is an allergic reaction to foreign proteins, usually those in pollen. The respiratory membranes become inflamed, and a watery fluid exudes from the eyes and nose. The allergy has a genetic cause. It runs in families, and is related to asthma and eczema;

* *Bronchial asthma* is an allergic reaction to foreign proteins, either eaten or breathed in, such as wheat products or house dust. It is characterized by attacks of wheezing and difficulty in breathing. It is caused by spasms of the smooth muscle in the walls of the bronchioles, which partly closes their air passageway. The bronchi often become clogged with mucus. Breathing out is especially difficult during these spasms;

* *A common cold* is a *rhino-viral* infection of the mucous membrane lining the nasal cavities. This predisposes the membrane to further attack by *bacteria*, which cause the secretion of thick mucus in place of the clear nasal discharge of the viral infection. Sore throat, sneezing, slight fever and headache commonly occur. It is most readily *transmitted* by

touching with contaminated fingers, rather than by droplet infection from sneezing and coughing. Frequent hand washing, and not touching the face, particularly the eyes and nose, are the best preventive measures against transmitting the virus to others;

- *Influenza* is a viral infection of the respiratory system causing a feverish illness. It is readily *transmitted* by droplet infection, particularly during the first few days of the illness. The symptoms are a raised temperature, shivering, sore throat, cough and eye pain. Viral pneumonia can be a serious complication. Antibiotics are ineffective in destroying the virus. Flu injections will protect vulnerable people during epidemics.

Smoking and health

If tobacco smoke is inhaled, *solid particles* and *tar droplets* enter the trachea and bronchi. The irritant chemicals from the smoke kill the *cilia* of the epithelial cells lining the upper respiratory passages, and cause the goblet cells to secrete excessive *mucus*. As the cilia become ineffective, mucus impregnated with solid particles and tar droplets remains in the bronchial tubes instead of being carried upwards towards the pharynx. Attempts to clear this mucus result in 'smoker's cough'.

The irritant chemicals trapped in the lungs slowly destroy the alveoli, greatly reducing the surface for gaseous exchange, and *emphysema* results. The loss of elasticity in the lungs causes them to be permanently inflated as the alveoli are replaced by fibrous connective tissue. The lungs then tend to succumb to other respiratory infections such as *bronchitis* or *pneumonia*. Prolonged contact with the irritant chemicals may finally cause *lung cancer*. Giving up smoking at any time reduces the chance of dying from lung cancer.

Women who smoke during *pregnancy* produce babies up to 0.23 kg lighter than average, and are more likely to miscarry or have a still-born child.

The raised level of *carbon monoxide* in tobacco smoke reaches the blood and is irreversibly combined with haemoglobin to form *carboxyhaemoglobin*. This means that the blood has less haemoglobin for carrying oxygen, which reduces the supply to the extremities. This can make limb amputations necessary. The *permeability* of the blood vessels is increased, leading to a higher rate of fatty deposition in the arteries (atherosclerosis) with an increased risk of *coronary heart disease*. Carbon monoxide may be one of the factors involved in *hypertension* (high blood pressure).

Self-assessment questions

1 Distinguish between external and internal respiration.

2 Describe the structure of the tracheal wall. How is the structure of the wall related to the function of the trachea.

3 What is the function of:

(a) pleural membranes;
(b) septal cells;
(c) intercostal muscles?

4 State the value of each of the following:

(a) %, by volume, of oxygen in expired air;
(b) %, by volume, of carbon dioxide in atmospheric air;
(c) the RQ of a dietary fat;
(d) the tidal volume of the lungs.

5 Explain the function of the film of water lining the alveolar air spaces.

6 Describe the process of respiration in a vigorously contracting muscle cell.

7 What is the molecule which temporarily stores energy for use in the cell? From what components is this molecule formed?

8 Name **two** respiratory disorders which are allergic reactions, and **two** which are viral infections.

9 Define:

(a) basal metabolism;
(b) minute volume;
(c) pulmonary circulation.

10 Describe the structure and functions of the nose.

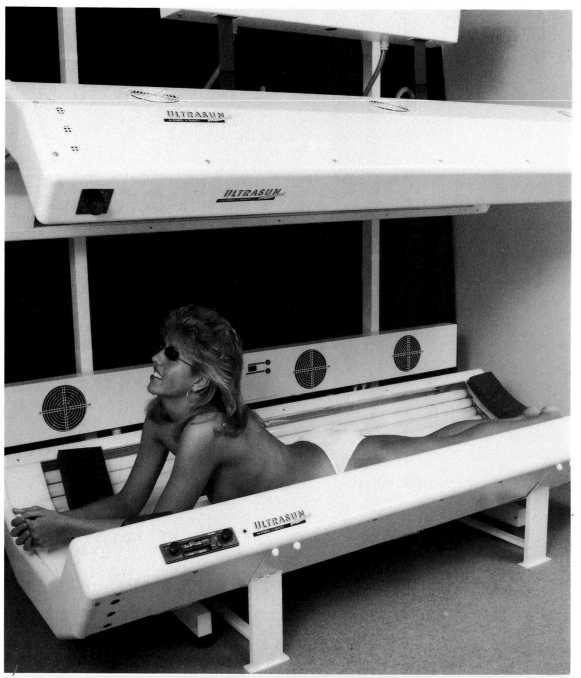

Sunbed

Excretion

The metabolism of nutrients results in the production of *waste products* in the living cells of the body tissues. If these waste products accumulated in the tissues and organs they would become *toxic*, preventing the body from functioning efficiently. Ill-health, and finally death, would occur.

The toxic waste materials which must be removed are *carbon dioxide, urea* and *uric acid.* Carbon dioxide is a waste product of glucose metabolism, and is removed by the lungs. Urea is formed from the nitrogen waste of protein deamination, while uric acid is a waste product of DNA breakdown. These two waste products are mainly removed by the urinary system, but small amounts are also removed by the skin in the sweat. *Gout* is a hereditary condition where there is an abnormally high level of uric acid in the blood which the kidneys are unable to remove. Crystals of uric acid are deposited in the joints, particularly the big toe joints, causing considerable pain.

The removal of these toxic waste products of metabolism is known as *excretion.*

Osmoregulation

Excess of some essential materials such as *water* and *mineral salts* must also be removed if the body is to maintain an exact *balance* between its water and salt content. Maintaining the salt/water balance is known as *osmoregulation,* and involves the urinary system. The *osmotic* (salt/water) balance is also affected by water loss through the skin (in sweat), lungs (in expired air) and alimentary canal (in faeces).

The primary function of the urinary system is the regulation of the *composition* and *volume* of the *blood,* and involves both excretion and osmoregulation. Thus the urinary system maintains a stable internal environment for the body tissues by regulating the composition of the blood. The urinary system therefore carries out *homeostasis.*

Organs of the urinary system

The organs of the urinary system are the two **kidneys**, connected by the two **ureters** to the urinary **bladder**. A single **urethra** connects the bladder with the exterior urinary opening. In addition, there are the *renal arteries* and *veins* which carry blood to and from the kidneys.

Figure 9.1
Organs of the urinary system

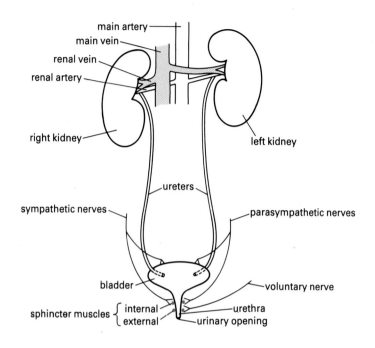

main artery
main vein
renal vein
renal artery
right kidney
left kidney
ureters
sympathetic nerves
parasympathetic nerves
bladder
voluntary nerve
sphincter muscles { internal / external
urethra
urinary opening

The kidneys

The two kidneys are attached to the posterior body wall on either side of the vertebral column between the twelfth thoracic and third lumbar vertebrae, ie. just above the waist. They lie outside the *peritoneum*, the membrane lining the abdominal cavity. The *right* kidney is placed slightly *lower* than the left kidney to provide space for the liver, which lies on the right side of the abdominal cavity and superior to the kidney. The kidneys are protected by the eleventh and twelfth pairs of ribs.

Externally, the kidneys are two bean-shaped dark red organs, which are approximately 11 cm long, 6 cm wide and 2.5 cm thick. Their medial surface is concave, and contains a notch called the **hilum**. A ureter leaves each kidney at the hilum and the renal blood vessels, lymph vessels and nerves connect with the kidney there. Each kidney is surrounded by a transparent fibrous membrane, the *renal capsule*. *Adipose* tissue is deposited on the outside of this membrane, so the kidneys are embedded in a fatty layer for cushioning and heat insulation. The kidneys are *anchored* to the body wall by an outer thin layer of fibrous connective tissue.

Internally, the kidney is divided into two regions, the **cortex** and the **medulla**. The outer cortex is dark red in colour, while the inner medulla is reddish-brown. Within the medulla are a number of triangular *pyramids* with their apices directed towards the hilum. A large cavity called the **renal pelvis** occurs in the region of the hilum. The *ureter* is a continuation of the renal pelvis.

Each kidney is composed of around one million functional units called *nephrons*. Each nephron is associated with networks

Figure 9.2
Internal structure of the kidney

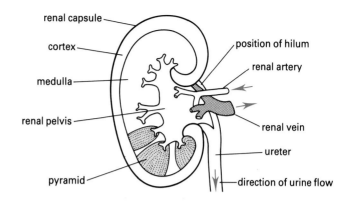

of blood capillaries and branches from the renal arteries (arterioles) and renal veins.

Nephrons are very small thin-walled tubes with a cup-shaped *Bowman's capsule* at one end, which encloses a knot of blood capillaries called a *glomerulus*. Blood enters the glomerulus from a branch of the renal artery called an *afferent arteriole* and leaves by an *efferent arteriole*. Below the capsule the nephron tubule has three distinct regions. A coiled *proximal convoluted tubule* is followed by a U-shaped *loop of Henle* and a coiled *distal convoluted tubule*. Each nephron opens into a *common collecting duct*.

The capsules and convoluted tubules of the nephrons lie in the cortex of the kidney. The loops of Henle and the collecting ducts lie in the medulla. The common collecting ducts open into the renal pelvis at the apex of a pyramid.

Figure 9.3
Nephron and its blood supply

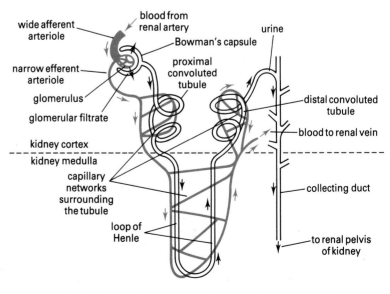

The *wall* of the Bowman's capsule is composed of a single layer of *podocyte* cells which have foot-like projections wrapped around the capillaries of the glomerulus and resting on their basement membrane. The wall of the proximal convoluted tubule is lined by a simple cubical epithelium, the cells having *microvilli* on their free surface. The wall of the descending limb of the loop of Henle is lined by a simple squamous epithelium, while the wall of the ascending limb has a simple cubical epithelium. The cubical epithelium lining the distal convoluted tubule is without microvilli. A simple cubical epithelium also forms the wall of the collecting ducts.

Capillary networks surround each region of the nephron tubule. These capillaries originate from the efferent arteriole leaving the glomerulus, and drain into a branch of the renal vein.

The ureters

Each ureter is a narrow tubular extension of the renal pelvis. Like the kidneys, the ureters lie outside the peritoneum. They enter the posterior surface of the *bladder* at separate openings. Their *function* is to carry the waste product or urine from the kidney to the bladder.

The bladder

The bladder is a hollow muscular organ situated in the pelvic cavity. Its muscular wall is highly extensible, and is lined on the inside by *transitional* epithelium which is able to stretch. The bladder opens at its base into a tube, the *urethra*. This opening is surrounded by *internal* and *external sphincter* muscles.

The **internal sphincter** is controlled by the *autonomic* nervous system. As the bladder fills with urine its wall stretches and eventually stimulates a parasympathetic reflex which relaxes the internal sphincter muscle and contracts the bladder. The **external sphincter** is controlled by the *conscious* part of the brain, so its relaxation is a voluntary action not an involuntary reflex. The external sphincter normally relaxes following the relaxation of the internal sphincter. *Urination* (micturition) then occurs. Thus emptying the bladder is brought about by a combination of involuntary and voluntary nerve impulses.

The urethra

The urethra is a narrow tube leading from the floor of the bladder, and opening at the body surface. It opens close to the vaginal opening and anus in the female, and at the tip of the penis in the male. It carries *urine* to the exterior in both sexes, and in the male it carries the reproductive fluid (semen) also.

Cystitis is an inflammation of the wall of the bladder. It causes frequent and painful urination, producing a burning pain in the urethra. It is caused by a bacterial infection, usually *E coli bacteria* from the intestine. These bacteria are present on the skin round the anus, and in women can easily enter the urethra and reach the bladder. Careful hygiene in the anal region is important in preventing this infection.

Formation of urine

The two processes occurring in the kidney which are responsible for the formation of urine are **ultra-filtration** and **reabsorption.**

Ultra-filtration

Ultra-filtration occurs in the *Bowman's capsules* of the nephrons. It occurs because the *efferent arteriole* taking blood from the glomerulus is *narrower* than the afferent arteriole bringing blood to it. As blood is held back in the glomerular capillaries, the *blood pressure* there becomes much higher than normal. The increased pressure forces the fluid part of the blood (plasma) through the capillary wall pores, and into the space within the capsule wall. This fluid is then called the *glomerular filtrate*. Blood cells and plasma proteins remain in the glomerulus, as they are too large to pass through the walls of the capillaries and Bowman's capsule.

The glomerular filtrate contains a number of substances which are *useful* to the body, as well as the toxic waste materials which were being carried by the blood.

Reabsorption

Reabsorption of the useful constituents of the glomerular filtrate occurs through the wall of the nephron *tubule.* The reabsorbed substances pass into the blood contained in the capillary networks surrounding the nephron tubule.

In the proximal convoluted tubule *glucose, water* and some *sodium ions* are reabsorbed. In the loop of Henle more *sodium ions* are reabsorbed, greatly increasing the *osmotic pressure* of the blood in the capillaries surrounding the tubule. The higher osmotic pressure increases the blood's ability to absorb *water* from the glomerular filtrate passing through the distal convoluted tubule and collecting ducts. Water passes back into the blood by *osmosis.* Altogether, all the glucose and 99% of the water in the glomerular filtrate is reabsorbed by the blood. In *diabetics*, not all the glucose is reabsorbed so some occurs in the urine. Osmoregulation, the control of the relative amounts of sodium salts and water in the blood, is thus carried out by the nephron tubule.

This osmoregulatory activity of the nephron is controlled by *hormones*, and is homeostatic in nature. *Aldosterone*, a hormone secreted by the adrenal glands, stimulates increased *sodium reabsorption* from the tubule into the blood. ADH (anti-diuretic hormone) secreted by the posterior lobe of the pituitary gland, stimulates increased *reabsorption of water* from the tubule into the blood, and therefore reduces the volume of urine and the frequency of urination.

Urine

Urine has an average pH of 6, so it is slightly *acid*. It contains 95% water by weight, 2% urea, 0.05% uric acid, 0.05% ammonia, 0.35% sodium ions and small amounts of other salts. Its *yellow* colour is due to a pigment formed from the breakdown of haemoglobin.

The *factors* influencing the volume of urine produced are the salt/water (osmotic) balance, the blood pressure, high external temperature or feverish illnesses, diet and emotional state:

- The *salt/water balance* in the blood is controlled by aldosterone and ADH, and affects the volume of urine produced as explained above;
- When *blood pressure* falls the homeostatic control mechanism causes more water to be reabsorbed into the blood, increasing its volume and raising the blood pressure. The volume of urine will therefore be reduced;
- When the *body temperature* increases more water is lost from the body by sweating. The volume of urine is therefore reduced to compensate for the extra water loss;
- A *diet* with a high salt content results in more water being reabsorbed in the kidney, as the blood has a higher osmotic pressure. This reduces the volume of urine produced. Where large amounts of liquid are swallowed the volume of urine will obviously be increased. Some chemicals known as *diuretics* (present in tea, coffee and alcoholic drinks) increase urine volume by partially inhibiting the reabsorption of water from the nephron tubule;
- *Emotional states* such as nervousness result in increased production of urine.

Self-assessment questions

1   List **three** toxic waste products, and explain how each one originates during cell metabolism.

2   Define:

(a) ultra-filtration;
(b) excretion;
(c) osmoregulation.

3   List the major components of urine in order of decreasing percentage by weight.

4   Name the **two** hormones which bring about the homeostatic control of the salt/water balance in the blood. Explain the role of each hormone in this regulatory process.

5   List the parts of a nephron.

6   Describe the position of the two kidneys in the body.

7   What is the role of each of the following in the formation of urine:

(a) glomerulus;
(b) loop of Henle;
(c) efferent arteriole;
(d) distal convoluted tubule?

8   List **five** factors which influence the volume of urine produced.

9   Explain the mechanism by which urination is controlled.

10   Where, in the urinary system, would you find the following:

(a) microvilli;
(b) podocytes;
(c) simple squamous epithelium;
(d) transitional epithelium?

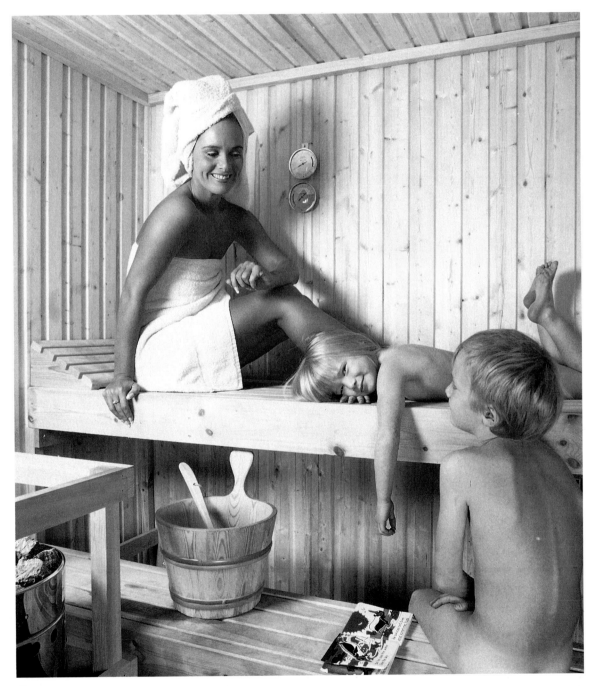

Sauna

The body fluids form between half and three-quarters of the body weight. About two-thirds of the body fluid is *intracellular*, occurring inside the body cells. The remaining one third lies outside the cells in vessels, ducts and body spaces, and is *extracellular*. It includes the blood and lymph, cerebrospinal fluid, urine, glomerular filtrate (in the kidney tubules), synovial fluid (in the joints), tears, saliva and other digestive juices, the fluid in the pleural cavity surrounding the lungs, and tissue fluid bathing the cells.

The body fluids are separated from one another to form distinct *fluid compartments* of variable size. A fluid compartment may be as small as the inside of a single cell, where it is bounded by the cell membrane. The spaces inside the heart and blood vessels form a very large compartment.

Homeostasis

Homeostatic mechanisms keep the volume of fluid in each compartment constant, in spite of the fact that water can readily move from one compartment to another.

Fluid balance

When the body is in fluid balance it contains the *correct volume* of water in each of its fluid compartments to allow normal functioning of the body. The fluid balance in the various compartments is maintained by *osmosis*, ie the transfer of water through the *semi-permeable* membranes separating each fluid compartment. As the body must contain a constant volume of water to maintain fluid balance, water intake must be equal to water loss.

Water is *obtained* from food and drink, and also from cell metabolism, as water is formed during many of the chemical reactions which occur. Water is *lost* from the kidneys in urine, from the skin in sweat, from the lungs in the water-saturated expired air, and from the rectum in the faeces.

In the *hypothalamus* of the brain there is an *osmoregulation centre* which is sensitive to the *osmotic pressure* of the blood. The osmotic pressure of the blood increases if the volume of water in the blood plasma falls. This increase in osmotic pressure of the blood leads to a sensation of *thirst*, so the person will take more water into the body by drinking. Water loss is reduced by the production of less urine due to the action of ADH (antidiuretic hormone) on the kidneys. If large quantities of liquid are drunk, the osmotic pressure of the blood will decrease, and water loss by the production of large volumes of urine will restore the fluid balance.

Some *diseases* result in considerable water loss leading to marked *dehydration* of the body tissues. *Vomiting* and *diarrhoea* cause abnormally large water loss from the alimentary canal. *Feverish* illnesses which cause considerable sweating result in great water loss from the skin. Severe dehydration is corrected by drinking water containing sugar and a little salt. Water containing sugar is more readily absorbed by the alimentary canal than pure water. The salt is required to replace the sodium ions lost in sweat, faeces and vomit.

Salt balance

The *osmotic pressure* of the body fluids is also determined by some of the solutes present in them. Some of these solutes are *electrolytes,* chemicals which split up or ionize in water, to form electrically charged *ions.* Salts, acids, bases and some proteins are electrolytes. Many essential minerals are present as salts such as calcium phosphate and sodium and potassium chlorides, and occur as ions in the body fluids. These salts help to maintain the osmotic pressure of the blood and other body fluids. *Sodium ions* are particularly important in this respect. The amount of sodium excreted in the urine is controlled by the hormone *aldosterone.* If the sodium concentration of the blood falls, less sodium is removed by the kidney tubules due to the action of aldosterone.

Acid/base balance

Some electrolytes help to regulate the *acid/base balance*, or pH, of the body fluids. A stable pH is required for normal cell metabolism. The *enzymes* which speed up the chemical reactions of metabolism will only function effectively at a particular pH. The majority of enzymes are most *active* at a slightly alkaline pH between 7.35 and 7.45, known as the *optimum* pH. Some of the digestive enzymes, which do not act inside cells, function best at a lower or higher pH.

To keep the pH approximately constant, substances called *buffers* occur in the body fluids. *Hydrogen carbonate* (bicarbonate) and *phosphate ions* are two important buffers in the blood. Because the presence of large amounts of carbon dioxide from cell respiration makes the blood increasingly *acidic*, the blood pH is lowered to below 7. The carbonic acid produced when carbon dioxide reacts with water in the blood plasma is taken up by the buffers, so the pH rises again.

An increased rate of *breathing* will remove carbon dioxide from the blood more rapidly, and help to increase its pH. The *respiratory centre* in the medulla oblongata of the brain is stimulated by a drop in blood pH, and triggers the increased rate of breathing which restores the acid/base balance.

Blood

Structure

Blood is a red viscous body fluid composed of a liquid **plasma** in which several types of *cells* are suspended. *Plasma* is a pale yellow liquid 91% of which is water. The remaining 9% consists of dissolved solids, of which 7% are plasma proteins and the remaining 2% are salts, glucose, amino-acids, waste products, hormones and antibodies.

The **plasma proteins** are of three main types, *clotting agents*, *albumins* and *globulins:*

- The **clotting agent** *fibrinogen* is converted into insoluble threads of fibrin when blood clots, and is produced in the liver. *Prothrombin* is another plasma protein which acts as a clotting agent;
- **Albumins** form over half of the plasma proteins and are largely responsible for the *viscosity* of the blood. Together with electrolytes, albumins help to regulate blood volume by determining the *osmotic pressure* of the blood, which maintains the fluid balance. By their effect on blood volume, they have an important function in maintaining *blood pressure*. Albumins are formed by the liver;
- The third type of plasma proteins are the **globulins**, and all antibodies are globulins. *Antibodies* can locate and destroy the foreign proteins present in disease-producing organisms (pathogens). *Gamma globulins*, for example, destroy the measles and hepatitis viruses. Other globulins are used to *transport* other materials in the blood. Iron is carried in the blood to the bone marrow combined with a globulin called *transferrin*. Globulins are formed either in the liver or by white blood cells.

Blood cells of three types are suspended in the plasma. These are the *erythrocytes* or red cells, the *leucocytes* or white cells, and the *thrombocytes* or blood platelets:

- **Erythrocytes** are the most numerous cells in the blood. Five million or so occur in every mm^3 of blood. They give the blood its colour and increase its viscosity. Each cell is a biconcave disc 8 μm in diameter, and is without a nucleus. The outer cell membrane encloses a solution of the oxygen-carrying pigment *haemoglobin*, a purple iron-containing compound which becomes bright red oxyhaemoglobin when it absorbs oxygen. The biconcave shape of the erythrocyte provides a large surface area for absorbing *oxygen*.

    Erythrocytes are formed in red bone marrow, and survive for about three months. They then break down and are destroyed in the liver, where their haemoglobin is converted into bile pigments, and the iron retained and recycled;

Figure 10.1
Three types of cell found in human blood (not to scale). From left to right: erythrocyte (8μm diam), leucocyte (10μm diam) and thrombocyte (2μm diam)

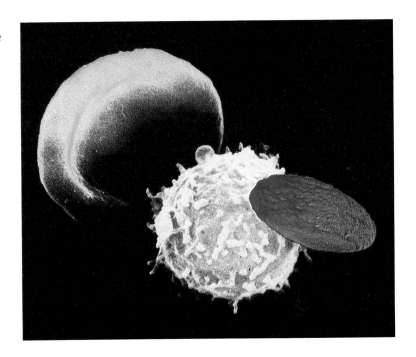

- **Leucocytes** are white blood cells, and are fewer in number than red blood cells. Their diameter is around 10 μm so they are slightly larger than red blood cells. They have an irregular spherical shape and contain a nucleus. Some types carry out amoeboid movement and engulf bacteria by *phagocytosis.* They then secrete *lysozymes* (enzymes) into vacuoles which are formed, to destroy the engulfed bacteria. Other types of leucocytes secrete *antibodies* which react with foreign proteins (antigens). These antigens may be chemicals released by bacteria (toxins), or may be attached to the outside of the cell membrane of bacteria, viruses, or foreign red blood cells etc.

    There are two main groups of leucocytes called polymorpho- and mono-nuclear types, which have differently shaped nuclei:

    (a) *Polymorphonuclear* leucocytes (polymorphs) have a lobed nucleus and granular cytoplasm. They form around three quarters of all leucocytes. They can migrate through the walls of small blood vessels to reach sites of infection. They carry out phagocytosis, engulfing and destroying bacteria until their lysozyme granules are used up. When loaded with killed bacteria, they die, forming *pus.* Their life span is approximately three weeks, but in the event of a bacterial infection it is much shorter. New polymorphs form in the red bone marrow;

    (b) *Mononuclear* leucocytes have a spherical nucleus and

their cytoplasm is without granules. One type, the *lymphocytes*, form antibodies to destroy antigens. Another type, the *monocytes*, are phagocytic producing lysozymes continuously. In the tissues monocytes develop into *macrophages* and destroy invading bacteria. Mononuclear leucocytes are produced in lymphoid tissues, eg the lymph nodes and spleen;

Figure 10.2
Leucocytes
(a) Polymorph
(b) Lymphocyte
(c) Monocyte

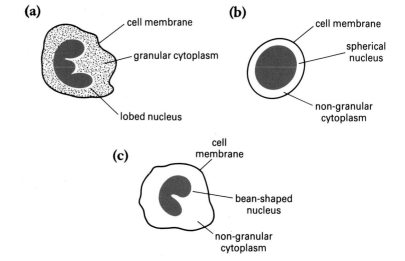

- **Thrombocytes** are small disc-shaped cell fragments shed from large cells in the red bone marrow. They are surrounded by membrane but have no nucleus, and are about 2 μm in diameter. They prevent fluid loss by aiding the clotting of blood. They will also adhere to form plugs at small wounds such as pinpricks. They have a short life span of one or two weeks.

Functions

Between 4 and 5 litres of blood occur in the female body, and an additional litre is present in males.

Blood has the *major function* of moving substances round the body, providing a **transport system**:

- **Oxygen** is carried in the erythrocytes, loosely attached to the haemoglobin pigment they contain to form oxyhaemoglobin. In *tissues* where the oxygen content is low oxygen is released, and diffuses out of the erythrocytes into the blood plasma, and then into the tissues. A low concentration of haemoglobin in the blood causes *anaemia*. In the *lungs*, where the concentration of oxygen in the alveolar air is much higher than in the blood, oxygen gas, dissolved in the water film lining the alveoli, diffuses into the blood. Oxygen is then absorbed by the haemoglobin in the erythrocytes;

- **Carbon dioxide** is carried partly by the erythrocytes and partly in the plasma, either as dissolved gas or as hydrogen carbonate ions. Carbon dioxide is formed in the tissues as a result of cellular respiration, and diffuses into the blood. In the lungs, the carbon dioxide diffuses out of the blood into the alveolar air spaces, where its concentration is lower. Some *nitrogen* gas also diffuses in solution from the alveolar air spaces into the blood plasma, especially when the body is subjected to high pressures as in sub-aqua sports;

- **Absorbed nutrients** are transported in the blood from the small intestine to the liver, and then to the body cells. Normally the blood contains a regulated amount of *glucose* to ensure that all tissues, particularly the brain tissue, have enough glucose to survive. The normal level of blood glucose (before meals) is between 810 and 990 mg/litre of blood. An abnormally high level of blood glucose is known as *hyperglycaemia*, and causes cell damage. The constant level of blood glucose is *homeostatically* controlled by the hormones insulin, adrenalin and glucagon. Other nutrients required for cell metabolism and tissue building are transported to the tissues by the blood;

- **Nitrogen waste** from protein metabolism is carried by the blood from the tissue cells to the liver. Here the nitrogen waste is converted into the less toxic *urea*, and carried to the kidneys to be excreted;

- **Hormones** produced by endocrine glands are transported by the blood to their target organs, in which they induce a response;

- **Heat** is also distributed round the body in the blood. As the blood passes through actively working organs such as contracting muscles or the liver, it is warmed. The blood travels on to the colder parts of the body which absorb some of the heat. Surplus heat is lost from the blood via the skin blood vessels.

Another *major function* of the blood is to **protect** the body against pathogens. The leucocytes carry out this function by means of phagocytosis and antibody production. *Antibodies* destroy pathogens by attaching themselves to the cell membrane of the pathogen and causing it to burst (lysis), or by making the pathogens clump together (agglutinate). This protective method is known as the *immune reaction*.

Immunity is the ability to resist disease, and *innate* immunity is present at birth. *Adaptive* immunity against specific pathogens can be *acquired*. An attack on the body by the pathogen results in the formation of the specific antibody by the lymphocytes. This antibody destroys the pathogen and its toxins, and may then remain in the blood for a considerable time. Any further attack by the same pathogen will be dealt with by the existing antibodies, so the person has acquired immunity to that particular disease. New antibodies against the pathogen can also be produced very rapidly.

Active artificial immunity can be conferred by injecting a small amount of material from a pathogen. This material is called a *vaccine*. The lymphocytes are stimulated to form the relevant antibody by the vaccine. Immunity to *influenza* is obtained by this method.

An **allergy** is an exaggerated immune response to a type of antigen called an *allergen*, to which most people show no reaction. The antibodies to allergens such as pollen, house dust, fur, food components etc are made in the lymph nodes and circulate in the blood. The antibodies become attached to cells in the skin, and mucous membranes of the buccal cavity and respiratory ducts, making these tissues *hypersensitive*. On contact with an allergen, the hypersensitive cells release *histamine* causing an inflammatory *allergic reaction*.

Clotting

Clotting, or coagulation, of the blood prevents fluid loss from damaged blood vessels and blocks the entry of pathogens. When the blood *thrombocytes* are exposed to air at the site of a wound, a complex sequence of chemical reactions begins. It results in the conversion of the soluble plasma protein *fibrinogen* into a network of insoluble fibres of *fibrin*. Erythrocytes become entangled in the fibrin network to form a *blood clot*.

Clotting requires three *blood components* (thrombocytes and the two plasma proteins fibrinogen and prothrombin), and two *nutrients* (Vitamin K and calcium). Fig 10.3 shows the main stages in blood clotting.

Figure 10.3
Main stages in blood clotting

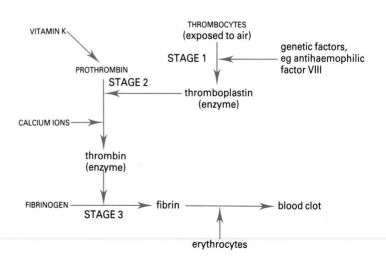

There are *genetic* factors involved also. One of these is *antihaemophilic factor VIII* produced in the liver, which affects the thrombocytes. In the absence of this factor the blood does not clot, and the disease of *haemophilia* occurs.

The clotting of blood occurs faster at higher *temperatures*, which speed up the rate of chemical changes.

After a clot forms, the remains of the blood plasma without its clotting proteins is called *serum*. Normally clotting does not occur inside undamaged blood vessels as *antithrombic* substances are present in the blood. These substances are enzymes which can dissolve fibrin if it forms unnecessarily. However, if the inside of a blood vessel becomes rough by the occurrence of *atherosclerosis*, clotting can occur inside an intact vessel. Such a clot is known as a *thrombosis*, and it may block a narrow blood vessel and prevent blood reaching an organ. Where this happens in the coronary artery to the heart, a *coronary thrombosis* is said to occur and a heart attack may result.

Blood groups

In human blood the red cells carry *antigens* on their cell membranes. These antigens vary from person to person and their occurrence is due to *inherited* genes. An individual's blood can be *classified* as belonging to a particular blood group, depending on the antigens present. About 20 such blood groups occur, of which the ABO and Rhesus groups are the best known.

In the **ABO system** the red cells in an individual's blood carry one, both or neither of two antigens A and B. Where A is present but B is absent the blood belongs to group A. Where B is present but A is absent the blood belongs to group B. Where both antigens occur the blood is of the AB type, and where neither antigen occurs the blood belongs to group O.

In blood plasma, *antibodies* to the two antigens occur, but an individual never carries the antibody to any antigen present on their own red cells. Group A blood plasma therefore carries anti-B but not anti-A antibodies. Group O blood plasma carries both anti-A and anti-B antibodies.

A and O are the *commonest* blood groups in the UK. AB is a very rare blood group. If, during a blood *transfusion*, group A or group AB blood (with red cells carrying the A antigen) are given to a patient with group B or group O blood (who has anti-A antibodies in his/her plasma), the transfused red cells will be damaged and agglutinate, as the two types of blood are *incompatible*.

In the **Rhesus system** about 85% of white people and 99% of black people have an antigen called the *Rhesus factor* (or D-antigen), on their red blood cells and are said to be *Rhesus positive*. The rest of the population do not carry the antigen and are *Rhesus negative*. If the tissues of a Rhesus negative person

Blood group	Antigens present on red cells	Antibodies present in plasma
A	A	anti-B
B	B	anti-A
AB	A and B	
O		anti-A and anti-B

come in contact with the Rhesus antigen, they will form an antibody against it which will be carried in their blood. If Rhesus positive blood is given to a Rhesus negative patient during a blood transfusion, the patient will form the antibody to destroy the Rhesus positive red cells, with often fatal results.

During *pregnancy*, when a Rhesus negative woman bears a Rhesus positive foetus, problems may occur. In the last month of pregnancy, or at the birth, small amounts of foetal blood may get into the mother's circulation, and cause her to form the antibody to the Rhesus antigen on the foetal red cells. At this late stage the current foetus may not be greatly harmed, but subsequent Rhesus positive babies will develop *haemolytic disease* (blue babies) due to the destruction of their red cells. This can be prevented by injecting the mother with an *anti-Rhesus factor globulin* (anti-D antiserum) immediately after the birth of each Rhesus positive baby. This globulin coats any escaped Rhesus positive foetal red cells, blocking the Rhesus positive antigen, and preventing the mother from forming the antibody which will damage the foetus' blood.

Lymph

Lymph is a clear colourless watery fluid resembling blood plasma. It contains all the components of blood plasma (salts, nutrients, waste products, hormones and antibodies) in similar concentrations except for the *plasma proteins*, which occur in lower concentrations in lymph (4% instead of 7%). The large size of the molecules of some plasma proteins prevent them from filtering through the cells forming the capillary walls, so they remain in the blood plasma. Lymph contains *fibrinogen* and can therefore clot to form a whitish coagulation.

Floating in the lymph are leucocytes of the *lymphocyte* type.

After a meal the lymph leaving the small intestine contains droplets of *fat* absorbed through the villi. The fat droplets produce a white *emulsion* instead of a colourless solution, so the lymph appears milky. One of the *functions* of lymph is to transport absorbed fat to the liver. Another function is to prevent water-logging of the tissues.

Tissue fluid

Tissue fluid, like lymph, contains all the components of blood plasma except the plasma proteins of large molecular size. It is a clear colourless watery fluid containing nutrients (glucose, fatty acids, amino-acids and mineral ions), dissolved oxygen and hormones which it supplies to the living cells of the tissues for their metabolism. It also contains dissolved carbon dioxide and nitrogen waste which it removes from the tissue cells where these waste products of metabolism are produced.

The tissue fluid permeates the spaces between the cells in all the body tissues and is in contact with their cell membranes. It *functions* as the link between the blood and the living cells of the body tissues.

The relationship between blood, lymph and tissue fluid

The pumping action of the heart forces the blood against the walls of the arteries creating a *hydrostatic pressure* (water pressure) known as the blood pressure. As the blood enters the much narrower blood capillaries, the hydrostatic pressure rises forcing water through the thin capillary walls from the blood plasma. This reduces the blood volume so the hydrostatic pressure of the blood in the capillaries falls. At the same time, smaller molecules dissolved in the water (glucose and hormones) are carried through the blood capillary walls to the surrounding tissues. The blood cells and plasma proteins with very large molecules are unable to pass through the capillary walls, and remain in the blood.

The fluid leaving the blood capillaries is the tissue fluid, which comes into close contact with the living cells of the tissues, allowing *exchange of materials* to occur between them.

The blood remaining inside the capillaries has an increased osmotic pressure due to the loss of water and retention of plasma proteins. It therefore absorbs back some of the tissue fluid until the osmotic pressure bringing water into the blood capillaries is equalled by the hydrostatic pressure of the blood which forces plasma out of the capillaries.

Any tissue fluid which is not reabsorbed into the blood capillaries enters the *lymphatic capillaries* through their *selectively permeable* walls, and becomes the lymph. On average, 100 ml of lymph is formed per hour. The lymphatic vessels eventually drain into a main vein at the base of the neck, and the lymph is returned to the blood.

Figure 10.4
Relationship between blood, lymph and tissue fluid

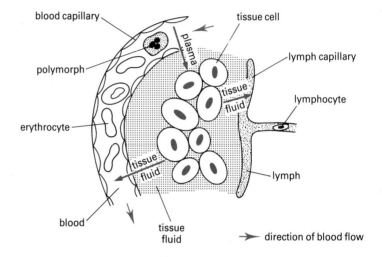

Since the lymph transport back to the blood is not very efficient, *standing* for long periods causes *swollen* feet and ankles. The plasma proteins of large molecular size do gradually leak out of the blood vessels into the tissue fluid of the feet, thus reducing the osmotic pressure of the blood. Tissue fluid return is then slowed, causing it to accumulate in the tissues of the feet. Lymph return to the blood can be aided by *gravity* on 'putting one's feet up'.

Oedema is the excessive accumulation of fluid in the tissues, leading to puffy local swellings. It is an example of *fluid-imbalance*, and has a number of possible causes. *Standing* for long periods is one cause. There may be an *obstruction* in the lymphatic drainage pathway such as an infected swollen lymph node. An increased *permeability* of the blood capillary walls may occur due to *histamine* release from damaged cells. The escape of tissue fluid from the blood capillaries will then be too rapid for its removal by the lymphatic system, where the rate of flow is slow. Cell damage may be due to a *sprain* or an *insect sting*, when considerable oedema can occur in the region of the injury. The delivery of *nutrients* to the tissue cells from the blood via the tissue fluid occurs much more slowly in oedematous tissue, as the nutrients have to diffuse greater distances to reach the cells.

Self-assessment questions

1 Define:

(a) an electrolyte;
(b) a buffer;
(c) a globulin.

Give **one** named example of each.

2 Distinguish between thrombocytes and prothrombin. In which process are they both involved?

3 List **five** functions of blood.

4 State **four** characteristics of:

(a) erythrocytes;
(b) lymphocytes.

5 What is the function of:

(a) fibrin;   (b) albumins;
(c) Anti-Rhesus factor?

6 What is meant by 'fluid balance'? What is the physical process which maintains this balance? Name a condition which is the result of fluid-imbalance.

7 Describe the process of tissue fluid formation.

8 List the antigens and antibodies present in the blood of a person belonging to:

(a) group A;   (b) group O.

Which ABO types of blood could each accept should a blood transfusion be necessary?

9 What is lymph? How does its composition differ from that of blood?

10 What is meant by:

(a) immunity;
(b) hyperglycaemia;
(c) allergen?

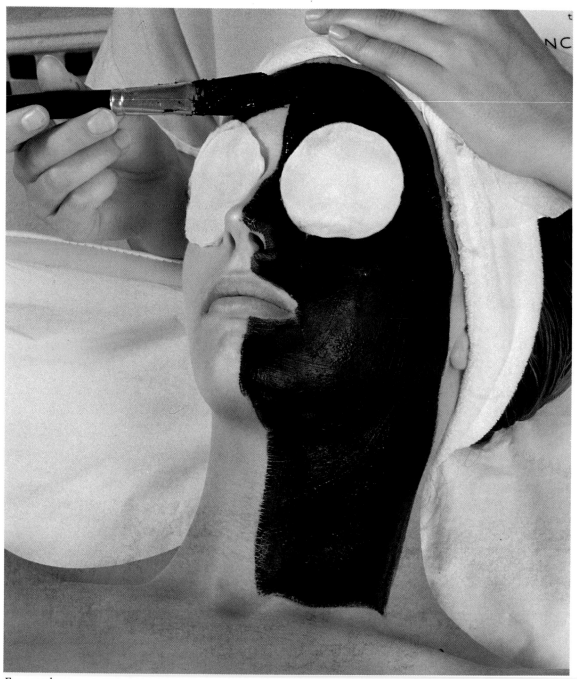

Face mask

A rapid *transport* system is needed to supply body cells with oxygen and nutrients and to remove toxic waste materials. A continuous closed system of *blood vessels* carry the transport medium, the blood, which flows in one direction round the body. The circulation of blood through the blood vessels is maintained by the *heart*, a muscular pump.

The heart

Position

The heart occurs in the *thorax* between the lungs. It is set obliquely, two-thirds of the heart lying to the left of the mid-thoracic line, fitting into the *cardiac notch* of the left lung. The heart is enclosed in a membranous *pericardium* so that it lies in a pericardial cavity which contains a watery fluid to prevent friction as the heart moves.

Structure

The heart is a hollow conical organ 12 cm long, and composed of *cardiac muscle* (see Chapter 5). It is divided into right and left halves by a vertical *septum*. Each half consists of an upper **atrium** (auricle) and a lower **ventricle**. Over the outside of the heart there is a network of blood vessels which are branches of the right and left *coronary* arteries and veins, and which supply the heart muscle. The blood in the main *veins* enters the two *atria* of the heart, and leaves in the main *arteries* from the two *ventricles*. The ventricles have much thicker walls than the atria to generate the *pressure* forcing the blood through the arteries.

Internally there are a number of *valves* in the heart to ensure that blood always flows in one direction. There are valves between the atria and ventricles on each side. These valves are flaps of tough tissue attached to the muscle of the ventricle walls by *chordae tendineae* which prevent the valves being forced up into the atria by the pressure of blood in the ventricles. The valve on the left side of the heart has two flaps and is known as the **bicuspid** (mitral) **valve**. That on the right side has three flaps and is the **tricuspid valve**. There are valves between the ventricles and main arteries called **semilunar valves**. They consist of groups of three pockets projecting internally round the inside of the artery wall. If they fill with blood trying to return to the heart, they bulge into the lumen and close the artery.

Circulation of blood through the heart

There is a double circulation of blood through the heart. In the *pulmonary* circulation between the heart and lungs, blood travels from the *right ventricle* to the lungs in the **pulmonary artery**. It returns to the *left atrium* of the heart in the **pulmonary vein**.

In the *systemic* circulation between the heart and all other

Figure 11.1
Structure of the heart

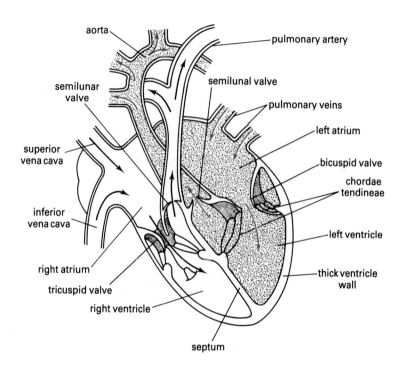

aorta

pulmonary artery

semilunar valve

semilunal valve

pulmonary veins

left atrium

superior vena cava

bicuspid valve

chordae tendineae

inferior vena cava

left ventricle

right atrium

thick ventricle wall

tricuspid valve

right ventricle

septum

oxygenated blood

deoxygenated blood

body systems except the lungs, blood travels from the *left ventricle* through the **aorta** and returns from the body tissues to the *right atrium* of the heart in the **venae cavae** (caval veins). The left side of the heart contains *oxygenated* blood which has been brought to the heart from the lungs in the pulmonary circulation. The right side of the heart contains *deoxygenated* blood which has been brought to the heart from the body tissues in the systemic circulation.

As the heart beats, contraction or *systole* of the *atria* increases the pressure of blood inside the atria and forces open the *bicuspid* and *tricuspid* valves. The blood is sucked into the relaxed ventricles as the atrial systole forces blood through the valves. The atria relax once the blood has entered the ventricles, undergoing *atrial diastole.*

Contraction or *systole* of the *ventricles* then occurs, increasing the blood pressure inside the ventricles. The pressure rises to 120 mm of mercury in the left ventricle, but is lower in the right ventricle. The pumping action of the left ventricle is so strong that it can be felt as the *pulse* in arteries a considerable distance from the heart. The normal *pulse rate* varies between 60 and 80 beats per minute, with 72 beats as the *average* pulse rate. The pressure of the blood during ventricular systole forces open the *semilunar* valves so that blood can enter the arteries. The ventricles relax once the blood has entered the arteries, and *ventricular diastole* occurs until the next contraction. During diastole the pressure of blood in the ventricles falls to zero.

Blood pressure

Blood pressure is always maintained in the *arteries* however, and does not fall to zero, due to contraction of their muscular walls. The blood pressure in the aorta at ventricular diastole is 80 mm of mercury, although that in the pulmonary artery is much lower. Less pressure is required in the pulmonary artery as the pulmonary circulation *pathway* is much shorter than that of the systemic circulation. In the systemic circulation normal blood pressure is 120 mm of mercury at systole and 80 mm of mercury at diastole, usually expressed as 120/80. Blood pressures above these values indicate *hypertension,* and above 140/95 may result in a stroke or heart attack. Blood pressure is measured in the upper arm by an instrument called a *sphygmomanometer.*

Control of the heart beat

The cardiac muscle of the heart contracts and relaxes with an *inherent* rhythm known as the *cardiac cycle.* It beats without any direct stimulus from the nerves, and can continue to beat when removed from the body if it is in a suitable supporting fluid. A single cardiac cycle lasts 0.75 seconds. During a cardiac cycle *electrical* changes occur in the heart which can be measured and displayed as an *electrocardiogram* (ECG).

Figure 11.2
The cardiac cycle

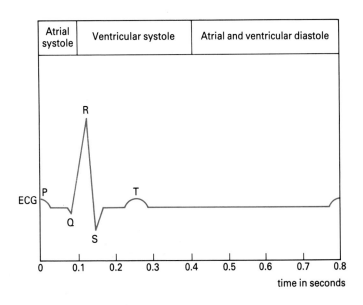

Figure 11.3
Heart showing nodes and autonomic control

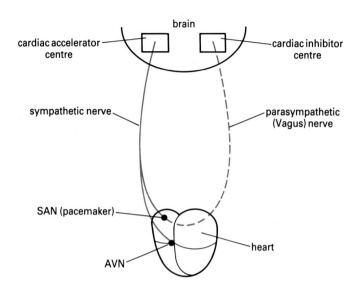

Peaks of electrical activity occur when heart muscle is contracting during systole. The QRS wave occurs at ventricular systole, and the P wave at atrial systole. Electrical activity is low when the heart muscle is relaxed during diastole. There is a short *pause* at the end of each cycle before the next cycle begins.

There are two regions in the heart where the electrical activity causing contraction starts. These regions are two small patches of tissue called *nodes*. The *sinu-auricular* node (SAN), called the *pacemaker*, is in the wall of the right atrium. The *auriculo-ventricular* node (AVN) occurs near the tricuspid valve. From the nodes electrical activity spreads through the rest of the heart muscle causing contractions. The pacemaker causes the heart to beat automatically at a regular rate.

Nerve impulses from the *autonomic* nervous system can alter this regular rate. They can act as a 'brake' or *inhibitor* slowing down the heart, or as an *accelerator* speeding up the heart rate. These nerve impulses come from *cardiac* inhibitor and accelerator *centres* in the medulla oblongata of the brain.

A *parasympathetic* (Vagus) nerve passes from the inhibitor centre to the pacemaker (SAN), and its impulses *slow* down the heart rate. A *sympathetic* nerve passes from the accelerator centre to both the nodes and its impulses *speed up* the heart rate. These autonomic nerves provide a *homeostatic* mechanism for controlling heart rate. They allow the heart rate to be adjusted to the most suitable level for the body's activity at any one time.

The hormone *adrenalin* can also speed up the heart rate. This hormone is secreted as a response to a temporarily stressful situation resulting in fear or anger, and requiring a 'flight or fight' response (see Chapter 13) but it does not provide homeostatic control.

Blood vessels

The blood vessels are tubular organs in which the blood is transported round the body. There are three types of blood vessels, **arteries, veins** and **capillaries.**

Arteries

Arteries are vessels that carry blood *away from* the heart to the body tissues. The main arteries close to the heart are wider, while the branches of the main arteries which lie close to the body tissues are narrower and are known as *arterioles.*

Arteries have a narrow *lumen* (central space for the blood) and a thick muscular wall, which is very elastic and is composed of three layers:

- The *inner* layer of the arterial wall is called the *tunica intima.* On the inside, in contact with the blood, is the smooth *endothelium* composed of simple squamous epithelium. The rest of the intima consists of connective tissue and an *internal elastic membrane,* which gives the intima a convoluted outline;
- The *middle* layer or *tunica media* is the thickest layer of the artery wall. It contains smooth *muscle* fibres which allow the artery to contract in diameter, *collagen* fibres which strengthen the artery wall, and *elastin* fibres giving elasticity. Nerves from the *sympathetic* division of the autonomic nervous system supply this muscle layer;
- The *outer* layer or *tunica adventitia* is thinner than the middle layer and is composed of connective tissue. There are many elastin fibres and some collagen and smooth muscle fibres in this connective tissue, which also contains small blood vessels.

Arterioles have thinner walls, but they always have an endothelium and a layer of smooth muscle in them.

Figure 11.4
Cross-section of an artery

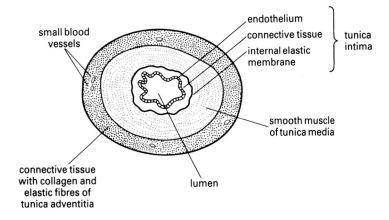

small blood vessels

endothelium
connective tissue } tunica intima
internal elastic membrane

smooth muscle of tunica media

connective tissue with collagen and elastic fibres of tunica adventitia

lumen

The *blood* in the lumen of the artery moves in a series of spurts or *pulses* due to the heart beat. The contractile muscular walls also aid the circulation of blood between the pulses. The blood in an artery, therefore, is always under *pressure*. The arteries to the lungs (pulmonary arteries) carry *deoxygenated* blood, while the rest of the arteries carry *oxygenated* blood.

Veins

Veins are vessels which carry blood away from the body tissues and *back to* the *heart*, except in the case of *portal* veins. The *hepatic portal vein* carries blood away from the small intestine to the liver, before the blood returns to the heart in the hepatic vein (see Chapter 7). The small veins leaving the tissues are called *venules*. They merge to form the larger veins.

Veins have a larger diameter and a wider lumen than arteries, and their wall are much thinner and less muscular. Their *walls* have the same three layers as the walls of the arteries:

- The inner *tunica intima* is bounded by an endothelium which is unconvoluted, and there is less elastic tissue present;
- The middle *tunica media* is a thinner less muscular layer, containing collagen and elastin fibres;
- The outer *tunica adventitia* is a thick connective tissue layer with many collagen but few elastin fibres. It contains small blood vessels.

Figure 11.5
Structure of a vein
(a) Cross-section
(b) Vertical section showing a valve

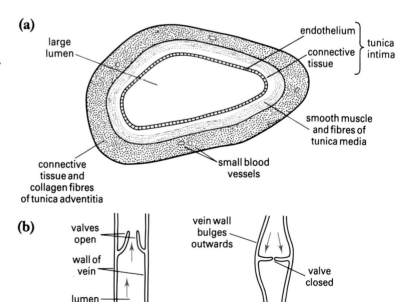

direction of blood flow

The *lumen* of the veins is subdivided by groups of two or three *semilunar valves* which prevent *backflow* of blood. If backflow starts to occur the pocket-shaped valves fill with blood, and bulge into the lumen obstructing it. The blood in veins flows smoothly; there is no pulse and the blood pressure is low. The low pressure in the veins is not sufficient to counteract the force of gravity dragging the blood downwards in the veins of the legs, when it needs to be travelling upwards. The upward movement of blood through the veins of the legs is due to the *massaging* effect of contractions of the skeletal muscles around them. *Exercise* thus aids venous return from the legs. The low blood pressure in the veins means that their walls do not need to be as strong as those of arteries.

In people whose venous valves have become weak, often as a result of standing for long periods, the thin walls of the veins become pushed outwards and lose their elasticity through over-stretching. A vein damaged in this way is said to be *varicose*. Superficial veins in the leg often become varicosed, and so do those of the anal canal when the condition is known as *haemorrhoids* (piles). Exercise is an important factor in preventing varicose veins.

Capillaries

Capillaries are very narrow blood vessels which form *networks* in the tissues linking arterioles to venules. The thin capillary walls consist of an *endothelium* only, and the small lumen allows erythrocytes to pass only in single file. The capillary network is very well developed in very active tissues and organs, which are said to be *highly vascular* (eg liver, kidney, skin).

The capillary network is very close to the living tissue cells, and exchange of substances between the blood and body cells takes place readily via the tissue fluid. Capillary blood pressure is less than that in the arterioles, but greater than that in the venules.

Figure 11.6
Cross-section of a blood capillary

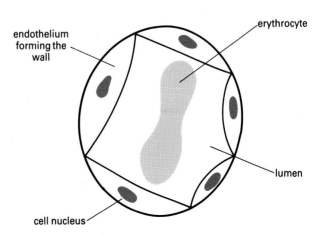

endothelium
forming the
wall

erythrocyte

lumen

cell nucleus

Vasomotor control

This is the *nervous* control of the *diameter* of blood vessels, especially the arterioles. In the walls of the *carotid* arteries taking blood to the brain, are small sense organs called *baroreceptors* which are sensitive to increased blood pressure. Nerve impulses pass from these baroreceptors to a *vasomotor centre* in the medulla oblongata of the brain. The vasomotor centre sends impulses to the smooth muscle in the tunica media of the arteriole wall via *sympathetic* nerves of the *autonomic* nervous system. These impulses are sent continuously and cause some contraction of the smooth muscle, giving a moderate amount of *vasoconstriction* (narrowing) of the arterioles at all times, which produces normal blood pressure. If the baroreceptors are stimulated by an increase in blood pressure in the carotid arteries, they send *inhibitory* impulses to the vasomotor centre. The centre then decreases the number of sympathetic impulses to the smooth muscle of the arteriole walls to below normal. More of the smooth muscle then relaxes which allows the diameter of the vessel to increase, and reduces blood pressure due to the *vasodilation*.

Figure 11.7
Vasomotor control

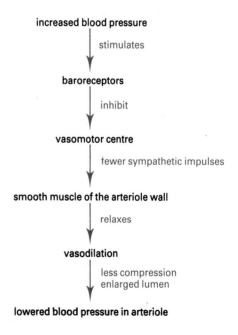

increased blood pressure

stimulates

baroreceptors

inhibit

vasomotor centre

fewer sympathetic impulses

smooth muscle of the arteriole wall

relaxes

vasodilation

less compression
enlarged lumen

lowered blood pressure in arteriole

When the blood pressure in the carotid arteries is *low* the baroreceptors are not stimulated, so inhibitory impulses are not sent to the vasomotor centre. The centre then increases the number of sympathetic impulses to the smooth muscle of the arteriole walls causing *vasoconstriction*, which increases blood pressure to its normal value.

This method of controlling blood pressure is a *homeostatic* mechanism, as it helps to restore the blood pressure to its normal level if it increases or decreases. *Another* method for controlling blood pressure involves the *heart*. Any increase in heart rate or force of contraction of the cardiac muscle will increase blood pressure. Any decrease in heart rate and force of contraction of the muscle will decrease blood pressure.

The arterial system

Pulmonary circulation

The *pulmonary artery* leaving the right ventricle of the heart emerges from the top of the heart, and immediately divides into right and left pulmonary arteries taking *deoxygenated* blood to each lung.

Figure 11.8
Pulmonary, systemic and portal circulations

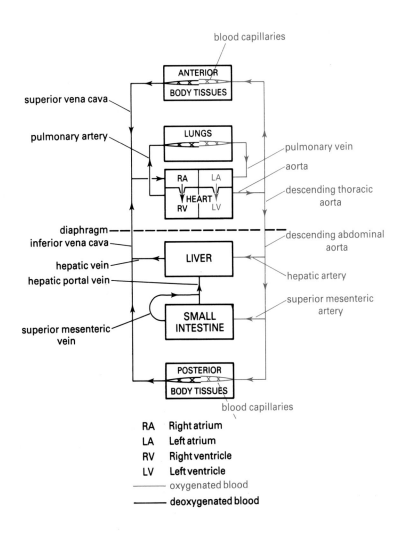

Systemic circulation

The main artery or *aorta* carries *oxygenated* blood to the body tissues. On leaving the left ventricle, the aorta emerges from the top of the heart. The right and left *coronary* arteries to the heart muscle arise from the aorta just above the point where it leaves the left ventricle. It continues anteriorly as the *ascending aorta*. It then curves to the left forming the *aortic arch*, then passes posteriorly through the thorax and abdomen as a *descending aorta*. Each of these regions of the aorta gives off branches to the various body organs as shown in Table 11.1.

Figure 11.9
Aorta and its branches

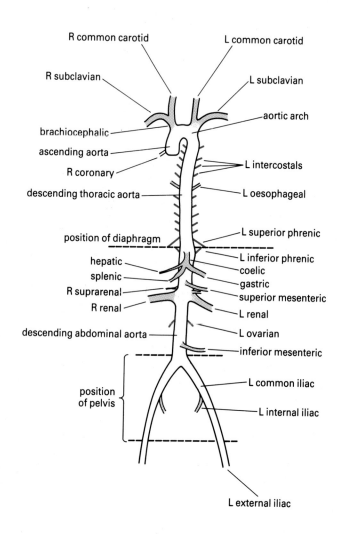

Arteries of the head

The *common carotid* artery on each side of the neck divides at the level of the larynx into two branches. An *internal carotid* artery passes through the temporal bone of the skull behind the ear, and takes blood to the brain. An *external carotid* artery remains

Table 11.1
Aorta and its branches

Region of the aorta	Names of arteries branching from aorta	Region and organs supplied
Ascending	Right and left coronary	Heart muscle
Arch	Brachiocephalic, dividing into right common carotid and right subclavian	Right side of head and neck and top of arm
	Left common carotid	Left side of head and neck
	Left subclavian	Top of left arm
Descending thoracic	Series of L and R intercostals	Intercostal and chest muscles
	L and R superior phrenics	Upper surface of diaphragm
	L and R bronchials	Bronchi of the lungs
	L and R oesophageals	Oesophagus
Descending abdominal	L and R inferior phrenics	Lower surface of diaphragm
	Coeliac dividing into hepatic	Liver
	splenic	Spleen and pancreas
	gastric	Stomach and oesophagus
	Superior mesenteric	Small intestine, caecum and upper parts of colon
	L and R suprarenals	Adrenal glands
	L and R renals	Kidneys
	L and R spermatic or ovarian	Testes or ovaries
	Inferior mesenteric	Lower part of colon and rectum
	L and R common iliacs dividing into	
	external iliacs	Legs
	internal iliacs	Buttocks, urinary bladder and reproductive ducts

outside the skull, and divides into *facial, temporal* and *occipital* arteries. These three arteries supply the skin and muscles of the face, side, and back of the head respectively.

Arteries of the arm and hand

The *brachial* artery of the upper arm is a continuation of the *subclavian* artery. Just below the elbow it divides into the *radial* and *ulnar* arteries which pass down the lateral and medial sides of the forearm respectively, and cross the wrist. The *pulse* can be felt in the radial artery in the wrist proximally to the thumb. The radial and ulnar arteries are connected across the palm of the hand by a *deep* and a *superficial palmar arch.* Three *palmar metacarpal* arteries, and a *digital* artery to the thumb, arise from the deep palmar arch. Three *digital* arteries to the fingers arise from the superficial palmar arch.

Figure 11.10
Main arteries of the head (side view)

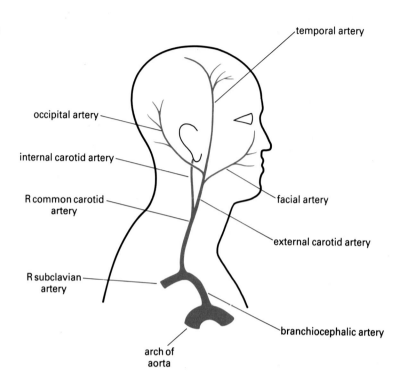

temporal artery

occipital artery

internal carotid artery

R common carotid artery

facial artery

external carotid artery

R subclavian artery

branchiocephalic artery

arch of aorta

Figure 11.11
Arteries of the arm and hand (anterior view)

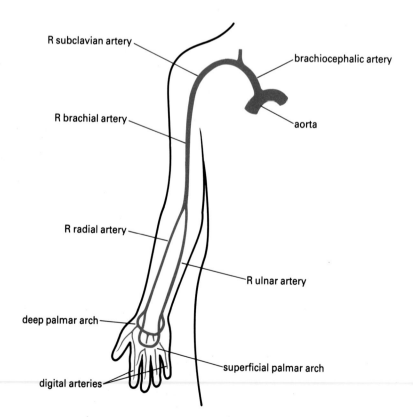

R subclavian artery

brachiocephalic artery

R brachial artery

aorta

R radial artery

R ulnar artery

deep palmar arch

superficial palmar arch

digital arteries

Arteries of the leg and foot

Two *external iliac* arteries pass into the two thighs from the descending abdominal aorta and continue down the front of the thighs as the *femoral* arteries. Just below the knee each femoral artery branches to form the anterior and posterior *tibial* arteries. A *peroneal* artery branches off each posterior tibial artery in the upper region of the calf. At the ankle the anterior tibial artery becomes the *dorsalis pedis* artery on the dorsum of the foot. The posterior tibial artery divides at the ankle into *medial* and *lateral plantar* arteries on the plantar surface of the foot. These plantar arteries link up with the dorsalis pedis artery, and give off *digital* arteries supplying the toes.

Figure 11.12
Arteries of the leg and foot (anterior view)

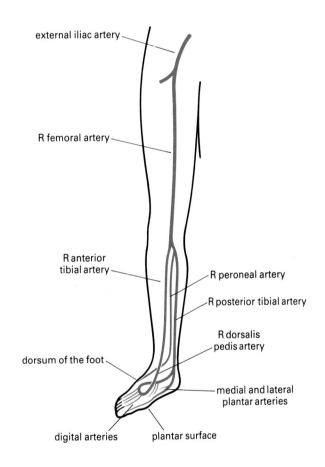

The venous system

Pulmonary circulation

The pulmonary veins which contain *oxygenated* blood from the alveolar capillaries of the lungs return blood to the left atrium of the heart.

Systemic circulation

The systemic veins return *deoxygenated* blood to the right atrium of the heart through one of three large vessels. The veins of the arms, head, neck and thorax open into the *superior vena cava* (caval vein), the veins of the legs, pelvis and abdomen open into the *inferior vena cava*, and the coronary veins from the heart muscle open into the *coronary sinus*.

The *deep* veins supplying internal organs usually run parallel to the arteries and have the same names, eg renal vein and renal artery supplying the kidneys. *Superficial* veins occur just below the skin and are often visible, the purple colour of the deoxygenated haemoglobin showing through the thin walls.

Veins of the head

Blood is collected up from the scalp capillaries by the *facial, temporal, occipital* and *posterior auricular* veins which run alongside similarly named arteries. These veins join to form an

Figure 11.13
Veins of the head (side view)

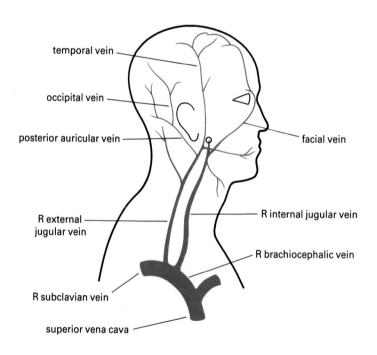

external jugular vein on each side behind and below the ear. The external jugular veins continue laterally down the neck and enter the *subclavian* veins. An *internal jugular* vein bringing blood from the brain descends on either side of the neck, and enters the subclavian vein. The subclavian veins continue towards the heart as the *brachiocephalic* veins after joining with the jugular veins. The brachiocephalic veins enter the superior vena cava.

Veins of the arm and hand

Blood in the *digital* veins from the fingers drains into the *dorsal arch*, leading to a dorsal venous network on the back of the hand. This venous network drains into superficial *cephalic* (lateral) and *basilic* (medial) veins in the forearm. There is another venous network on the palmar surface of the hand extending over the thenar and hypothenar eminences. This palmar network links up with the dorsal network into a *median antibrachial* vein, which passes up the anterior side of the forearm and joins the basilic vein at the elbow. The basilic vein is joined by a *brachial* vein in the upper arm to form the *axillary* vein. The axillary and cephalic veins join to form the *subclavian* vein at the top of each arm.

Figure 11.14
Veins of the arm and hand (anterior view)

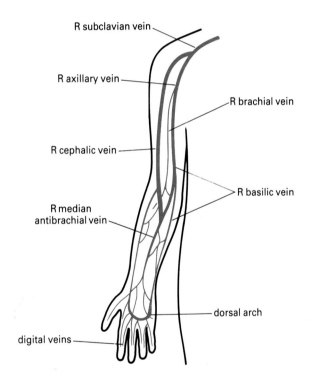

R subclavian vein

R axillary vein

R brachial vein

R cephalic vein

R basilic vein

R median antibrachial vein

dorsal arch

digital veins

Veins of the leg and foot

The *digital* veins from the toes drain into a *plantar arch* on the sole of the foot, and into a *dorsal venous arch* on the dorsum, from which *dorsalis pedis* veins pass medially and laterally to the ankle. The main *superficial* veins of the leg are the *saphenous* veins which pass from the ankle medially up each leg to join with the *external iliac* veins. The saphenous veins frequently become *varicosed*.

The *deep* veins of the leg are the *posterior tibial* vein passing up the back of the leg and joined by the *peroneal* vein, and the *anterior tibial* vein passing up the front of the leg. These two deep tibial veins join below the knee to form the *popliteal* vein. Above the knee the popliteal vein continues up the back of the thigh as the *femoral* vein, which enters the *external iliac* vein. The blood from the leg is then returned to the heart in the *inferior vena cava*.

Figure 11.15
Veins of the leg and foot (anterior view)

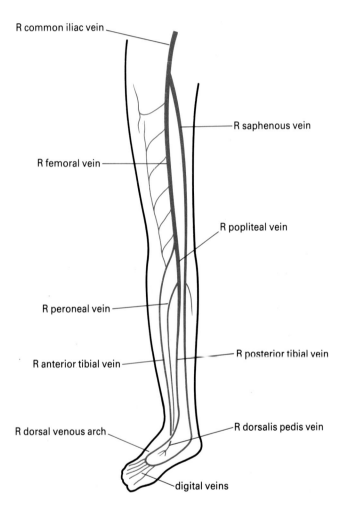

R common iliac vein

R saphenous vein

R femoral vein

R popliteal vein

R peroneal vein

R posterior tibial vein

R anterior tibial vein

R dorsal venous arch

R dorsalis pedis vein

digital veins

Portal circulation

The *hepatic portal* vein contains blood which has absorbed nutrients from the intestine, and which it transports to the liver. The liver controls the amount of each nutrient remaining in the blood. The hepatic portal vein is formed by the fusion of the *superior mesenteric* vein from the small intestine, the *inferior mesenteric* vein from the large intestine and the *splenic* vein from the spleen, stomach and pancreas. The hepatic portal is the only vein in the body which does not return blood directly to the heart.

Contra-indications

Disorders of the cardiovascular system which contra-indicate beauty therapy treatments such as massage and faradism are abnormal pulse rates, high blood pressure (hypertension), highly vascular skin conditions, varicose veins, angina pectoris (insufficient oxygen supply to the heart muscle) or the presence of an artificial pacemaker in the heart.

Self-assessment questions

1 Describe the nature and function of an artery in blood transport.

2 What is meant by the pulmonary circulation?
Name the blood vessels involved, and state whether they carry oxygenated or deoxygenated blood.

3 Distinguish between systole and diastole in relation to the heart.

4 What is the function of:

(a) the tricuspid valve;
(b) the pericardium;
(c) the pacemaker (SAN)?

5 List **four** points of difference between the wall of the aorta and the wall of a large vein.

6 Why does backflow of blood often occur in the veins of the leg?
How does the body reduce backflow in these veins?
Name **one** disorder of the veins that can result from backflow.

7 Give the names of the following blood vessels:

(a) that taking blood to the left side of the head and neck;
(b) that bringing blood away from the kidneys;
(c) the superficial medial vessel returning blood from the right foot and leg;
(d) that in which the pulse rate is commonly timed.

8 What is meant by vasomotor control?
Name the sense organs involved in this process, and the position of the vasomotor centre.

9 Where in the body would you expect to find:

(a) an atrium;
(b) a dorsal venous arch;
(c) a semilunar valve;
(d) a portal vein?

10 Name the regions of the aorta. Give the name of **one** artery which arises from each region of the aorta.

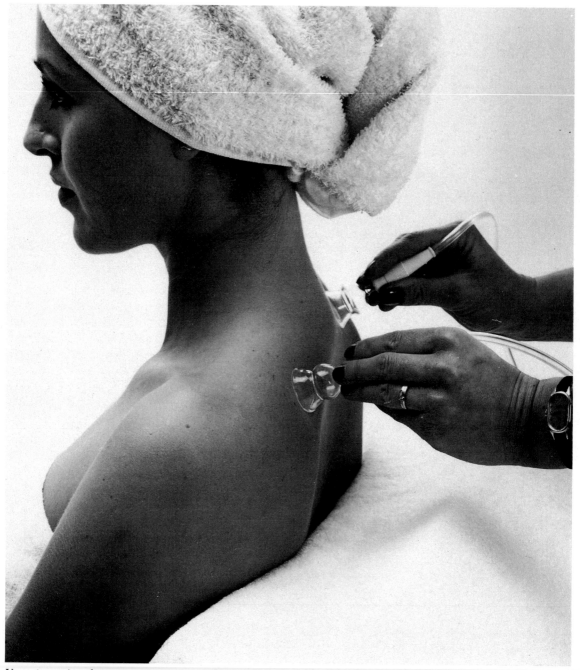

Vacuum suction therapy

The lymphatic system comprises the **lymph** and the vessels in which it is transported, including **lymph capillaries, lymphatics** and the lymph **ducts**. Chains of small lymph glands or *nodes* occur along the lymphatics. The *spleen, tonsils* and *thymus gland* are three organs that form part of the lymphatic system. The *lymphoid* tissue of these structures is a specialized type of connective tissue.

The *functions* of the lymphatic system are to *drain* tissue fluid from the organs and *prevent* oedema, and to *return* to the blood protein molecules which are unable to pass back through the blood capillary walls because of their large size. The lymphatic system also transports fats from the ileum, where they are absorbed by the villi, to the liver. Lymphocytes, which are part of the body's immune system, are produced by the lymphatic system.

Lymph

See Chapter 10.

Lymph capillaries

Lymph capillaries occur in the spaces between the cells of all vascular body tissues, but are absent from the nervous tissue of the brain and spinal cord. They are narrow closed vessels which may form extensive networks. Lymph capillaries are slightly larger in diameter than blood capillaries, and are surrounded by *collagen* fibres on the outside. The lymph capillary wall is composed of simple squamous epithelium forming an *endothelium* which is more permeable than that of a blood capillary wall. Some larger molecules such as proteins are able to pass into the lymph capillaries, although they cannot normally pass through the blood capillary walls.

The lymph capillaries drain into an extensive system of larger lymph vessels, the lymphatics. The lymph capillaries remove tissue fluid and prevent oedema.

Lymphatics

Lymphatics resemble veins in structure. Their walls, though thinner, are composed of the same three layers that occur in veins. Lymphatic also contain internal *valves* to prevent backflow. The flow of lymph through the lymphatics is aided by skeletal muscle contractions which have a massaging effect, and by respiratory movements. *Exercise* is therefore of great importance in maintaining lymph circulation. The rate of flow of lymph is very much slower than the rate of flow of blood in the blood capillaries. Lymphatics in the skin usually occur alongside veins. Lymphatics of the internal organs usually occur alongside arteries, and form networks round them. Lymph nodes occur along the length of the lymphatics.

Lymph nodes

Lymph nodes occur in *groups*, often concentrated in particular regions of the body, eg. the neck and axillae. The groups of nodes are arranged in two sets, *deep* and *superficial*.

Lymph nodes are small oval structures varying between 1 mm and 25 mm in length. On one side of each node there is a slight depression called the *hilum*. Each node is surrounded by an external *capsule* of collagen fibres. Projecting inwards from the capsule are septa or *trabeculae*. The lymphoid tissue inside the node is divided into two regions, an outer *cortex* and an inner *medulla*. The outer cortex contains blocks of lymphocytes called *lymph nodules* which are separated from one another by the trabeculae. In the medulla the lymphoctes are arranged on collagen strands forming *cords*.

Lymph nodes occur at the junctions of several lymphatics, and *afferent lymphatics* enter one lymph node at several points on its surface. The valves of the afferent lymphatics allow lymph to enter the series of irregular channels inside the cortex called the *cortical sinuses*. From here the lymph diffuses into the *medullary sinuses* in the centre of the node between the cords. The sinuses are lined with phagocytic cells called *macrophages* which *filter* the lymph by ingesting bacteria, damaged cell material and unwanted proteins. The *lymphocytes* on the medullary cords produce *antibodies*. Some lymphocytes become detached and carried out of the node by the lymph into the blood circulation. They will then destroy bacteria and their toxins in the tissues. If the lymph carries large numbers of bacteria due to an infection, some of the lymph nodes may enlarge and become *painful*. Infected lymph nodes may become blocked so that lymph is unable to drain away, causing local oedema.

A smaller number of *efferent lymphatics* leave the lymph node from the region of the hilum. These vessels are a little wider than the afferent lymphatics, and their valves allow lymph to pass out of the node. The efferent vessels leaving a lymph node then enter another node in the chain, becoming afferent vessels.

Figure 12.1
Structure of a lymph node

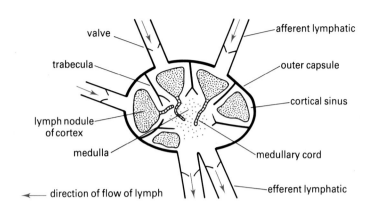

Main groups of lymph nodes

Major groups of lymph nodes occur in the head and neck, in the axillae (armpits), in the groin, in the thorax and breasts, and in the abdomen. Tables 12.1 and 12.2 show the groups of lymph nodes in the head and neck and in the shoulders and axillae.

In the *groin*, superficial and deep *inguinal* lymph nodes occur, draining the pelvic region and the legs. The lymph nodes of the *breast* are described in Chapter 14.

Figure 12.2
Lymph nodes of the head and neck

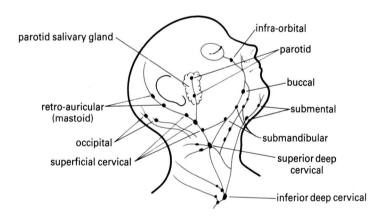

Figure 12.3
Lymph nodes of the shoulders and axillae

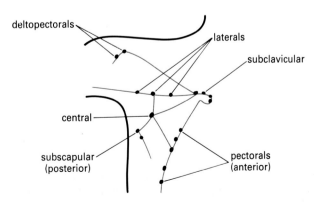

Table 12.1
Groups of lymph nodes of the head
and neck

Name of node group	Position and areas drained
Infraorbital	Face: drains eyelids and conjunctiva of the eye
Buccal	Face: drains eyelids, nose and skin of the face
Mandibular	Face: drains chin, lips, nose, cheeks and tongue
Submental	Face: drains chin, lower lip and floor of mouth
Retroauricular (mastoid)	Side of head: drains skin of ear and temporal region of the scalp
Superficial cervical	Neck below ear: drains lower part of ear and parotid area
Occipital	Back of head: drains back of scalp and upper part of neck
Parotid	Face over parotid gland: drains nose, eyelids and ear
Superior deep cervical	Neck: drains posterior region of head and neck, tongue, larynx and oesophagus
Inferior deep cervical	Neck: drains posterior region of scalp and neck, superficial region of chest, and arm

Table 12.2
Groups of lymph nodes of the
shoulders and axillae

Name of node group	Position and areas drained
Deltopectorals	Shoulder below clavicle: drain the upper arm
Laterals	Axilla: drain the upper arm
Pectorals	Axilla: drain the skin and muscles of the thoracic wall and breast
Subscapular	Axilla: drain skin and muscles of the posterior region of the neck and thoracic wall
Central	Axilla: drains lateral, pectoral and subscapular nodes
Subclavicular	Axilla: drain deltopectoral nodes

Lymph ducts

From each chain of lymph nodes the efferent lymphatics combine to form lymph trunks which empty into two main lymph ducts, the *thoracic* duct and the *right lymphatic duct*. The *thoracic* duct is the main collecting duct of the lymphatic system. It receives lymph from the left side of the head, neck and thorax, and from the left arm and the whole of the abdomen and both legs. The lymph from the ileum containing absorbed fat also drains into the thoracic duct. The duct begins in the abdomen as a small dilatation, the *cisterna chyli*, in front of the second lumbar vertebra. It is approximately 40 cm in length, and passes up through the thorax to open into the left subclavian vein.

The *right lymphatic duct* receives lymph from the right side of the head, neck and thorax, and from the right arm. It is very short, only 1.5 cm in length, and opens into the right subclavian vein.

Through these two lymph ducts the lymph is returned to the blood circulation via the subclavian veins.

Figure 12.4
Lymph ducts

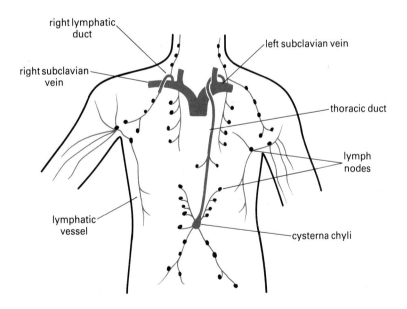

The spleen

The spleen is an oval organ 12 cm in length. It lies on the left side of the upper abdomen between the fundus of the stomach and the diaphragm. It is a dark red *highly vascular* organ, surrounded by a fibroelastic *capsule* containing some smooth muscle. On the outside of the capsule is a *serous membrane* of the peritoneum, which allows the spleen to slide over other organs without damage.

Internally its structure is similar to that of the lymph nodes. It has *trabeculae* projecting inwards from the capsule, and a *hilum* through which the splenic artery and vein and the efferent lymphatics pass. The trabeculae form a framework consisting of bands of collagen and elastin fibres. The spaces between the trabeculae are filled with cells.

These cells belong to two different kinds of tissue called *white* and *red pulp*. The *white pulp* is lymphoid tissue arranged round arterioles. The cluster of lymphocytes in this tissue are called *splenic nodules*. The *red pulp* is closely associated with the branches of the splenic vein, and consists of small spaces filled with blood and cords of phagocytic cells which contain red pigment and red blood cells.

The *functions* of the spleen are to destroy bacteria and worn out red blood cells and platelets by phagocytosis (in the red pulp), and to form lymphocytes (in the white pulp). The spleen has such a large blood supply that it 'stores' blood, and will divert some of it if extra blood is required in the circulation due to *haemorrhage*. A *sympathetic* nerve causes the smooth muscle cells in the capsule to contract and squeeze out blood into the splenic vein.

The tonsils

The tonsils are patches of lymphoid tissue embedded in mucous membrane which occur at the back of the nose and throat. The *pharyngeal* tonsil occurs in the posterior wall of the nasopharynx, and is known as the adenoids when it becomes enlarged. The *palatine* tonsils occur on each side of the uvula in the pharynx, and the *lingual* tonsils occur at the base of the tongue. The tonsils guard the opening into the respiratory passages, their lymphocytes acting as a *defense* against bacterial attack.

The thymus gland

The thymus gland is a mass of lymphoid tissue in the thoracic cavity which occurs over the trachea and underneath the sternum. It is relatively large in children, but in adults the lymphoid tissue is replaced by fat and connective tissue. The thymus gland produces special lymphocytes which are involved in the body's immune system as they attack and destroy antigens.

Peyer's patches

Peyer's patches are groups of lymph nodules in the ileum wall. They provide a defense against bacteria which have entered the alimentary canal with the food.

Self-assessment questions

1 Describe the means by which lymph flow is maintained in the lymphatics.

2 List the functions of the lymphatic system.

3 Describe the structure of a lymph node.

4 Name the **five** groups of axillary lymph nodes.

5 Describe the functions of the spleen.

6 Explain how lymph in the lymphatics is finally returned to the blood circulation.

7 What is the role of macrophages, and where do they occur in the lymphatic system?

8 Name the body regions which are drained by the following lymph nodes:

(a) buccal;
(b) superior deep cervical;
(c) deltopectoral;
(d) deep inguinal.

9 Where in the body would you find:

(a) the cisterna chyli;
(b) white pulp;
(c) Peyer's patches?

10 What are the functions of:

(a) the tonsils;
(b) lymph nodes?

CHAPTER 13

The Endocrine System

The endocrine system acts with the nervous system to *control* and *co-ordinate* the body's activities. It consists of the **endocrine glands** and the **hormones** or chemical messengers they secrete and/or store. Because the endocrine glands have no ducts and

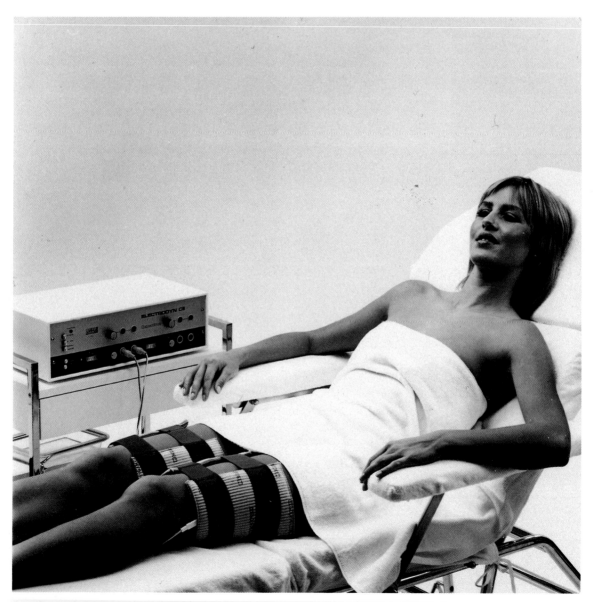

Interferential therapy

their hormones are transported by the blood, they are known as *ductless* glands. The secretory cells of the endocrine gland cluster round *blood capillaries* inside the gland, so the hormones can readily pass into the blood. In the blood the hormones become attached to plasma proteins, and are transported round the body to the *target organs* in which they produce a response. A hormone may affect a number of target organs which can be widely separated in the body.

Hormonal responses in the target organs are usually less rapid than nervous responses, and frequently continue over long periods of time. Many hormonal responses are related to growth and development which are slow and prolonged processes. Although only small amounts of hormones are present in the blood, their effects on the target organs are considerable.

Figure 13.1
Positions of the endocrine glands

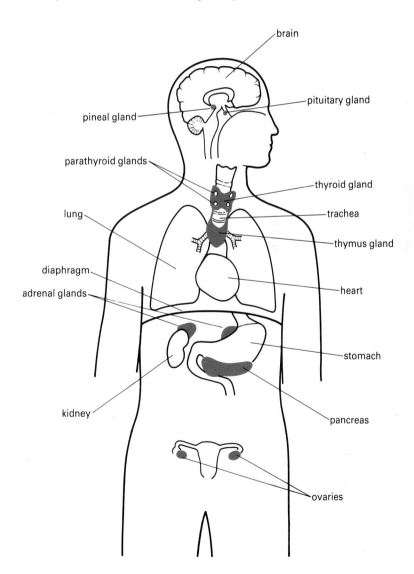

The activity of most endocrine glands is ultimately controlled by the nervous system. The *hypothalamus* links the functioning of the central nervous and endocrine systems by releasing *regulating factors* that affect hormone secretion by the endocrine glands. The hormone *adrenalin* is almost identical to the transmitter substance *nor-adrenalin* produced at the synapses at the ends of sympathetic nerves. Both chemicals produce the same responses in the body.

The main *function* of hormones is to maintain *homeostasis* by regulating the composition of the internal environment to keep it relatively constant. Some hormones produce cyclic patterns of activity (eg the sex hormones) and others control the rate of growth.

The endocrine glands are distributed throughout the body. They consist of the **pituitary** and **pineal glands** in the head, the **thyroid** and four **parathyroid** glands in the neck, the **thymus** gland in the thorax, and the two **adrenal** glands and the **pancreas** in the abdomen. In addition, the **reproductive organs** (ovary or testis) are endocrine glands.

Thyroid gland

The thyroid gland occurs in the neck close to the larynx. It is composed of hollow spherical sacs called *follicles* held together by connective tissue containing many blood capillaries. The follicle walls are composed of a simple cubical epithelium. The epithelial cells secrete hormone into the cavity of the follicle where it is stored, and later passed into the blood for transport to the target organs.

Figure 13.2
Section through part of thryoid gland

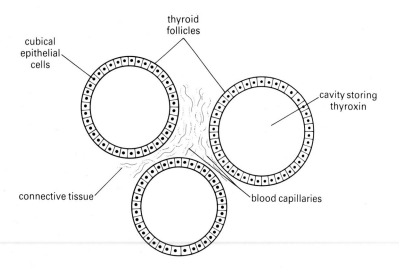

The thyroid gland removes *iodine* from the blood, the iodine being provided by food and water in the diet. In the cells of the follicles iodine is combined with the amino-acid *tyrosine* to form the hormone **thyroxin**. Thyroxin affects all the body tissues and has two main functions. It controls the *basal metabolic rate* (BMR) adjusting it to a low level just adequate for survival when the body is at rest. Its other main function is to regulate the *growth and development* of the body, especially the growth of *nervous* tissue. Thyroxin increases the rate at which carbohydrates are oxidized in the tissue cells to produce *energy*, and it stimulates cells to break down *proteins* for energy instead of using them to build new tissues.

Abnormal activity of the thyroid gland

- **Hypersecretion** (overactivity) of the thyroid gland may be caused by a *tumour* in the gland, or it may be due to malfunction of the *pituitary* gland which controls thyroid activity. Too much thyroxin in the blood increases the BMR and the heart rate, and results in considerable weight loss by using protein as an energy source. It also makes the person very excitable. A side-effect of overactivity of the thyroid gland is that the eyes bulge due to the accumulation of fluid behind the eyeball. The thyroid gland may increase in size to form a *goitre* or neck swelling. Because of its effect on the eyes and on the size of the thyroid gland this disorder is called *exophthalmic goitre*;

- **Hyposecretion** (underactivity) of the thyroid gland may be due to a deficiency of *iodine* in the diet, and also results in the formation of a goitre. In adults the effect of too little thyroxin is to cause a condition called *myxoedema*. The BMR is slow and the body weight increases. Mental activity also slows down so the person is less alert. The skin becomes dry and puffy, and the hair becomes thinned and brittle. In children too little thyroxin results in *cretinism*, a condition in which mental, physical and sexual development are retarded. Thyroid hyposecretion is now treated by giving thyroxin in carefully controlled amounts.

Control of the thyroxin level in the blood

The release of the thyroxin from the thyroid gland into the blood is stimulated by the presence of *thyroid stimulating hormone* (TSH) in the blood. TSH is secreted by the *pituitary* gland. An increase in the amount of thyroxin in the blood inhibits (supresses) the secretion of TSH by the pituitary gland, a situation described as *negative feedback control.*

The pituitary gland is stimulated to produce TSH by a *thyroxin releasing factor* (TRF) formed in the *hypothalamus* of the brain, which is close to the pituitary gland. TRF passes into small blood vessels leading from the hypothalamus directly to

Figure 13.3
Homeostatic control of thryoxin level
in the blood

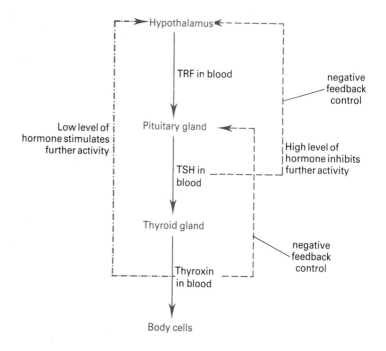

the pituitary gland. A high level of TSH in the blood will inhibit TRF secretion, while a low level of TSH will stimulate TRF secretion. As information about the hormone level is fed back to the endocrine gland this is *negative feedback* control. It prevents overproduction or underproduction of the hormone, and is an example of *homeostasis*.

Parathyroid glands

There are four small parathyroid glands embedded on the posterior surface of the thyroid gland. They produce a hormone **parathyrin** which is a *protein*. Parathyrin affects the level of *calcium ions* in the blood and other body fluids. By releasing calcium ions from bone, increasing calcium reabsorption in the kidney tubules, and increasing calcium absorption from food in the intestine, parathyrin raises the calcium level of the blood. A high level of calcium in the blood has a direct effect on the parathyroid glands, inhibiting the secretion of parathyrin. This is an example of *negative feedback* control.

Abnormal activity of the parathyroid glands

- **Hypersecretion** of the parathyroid glands increases the level of calcium in the blood by breaking down bone structure. This activity of parathyrin increases after the

menopause when parathyrin is no longer inhibited by
oestrogen hormone from the ovaries. The fragile bones of
older women, a condition called *osteoporosis,* are due to the
parathyroid overactivity resulting from oestrogen deficiency;

- **Hyposecretion** of the parathyroid glands results in a low
level of calcium ions reaching the skeletal muscles. This
affects muscle contraction resulting in *tetany,* when muscles
go into spasm producing involuntary convulsive
contractions.

Pancreas

The pancreas occurs in the abdominal cavity just below the
stomach. It is both an endocrine and an exocrine gland. Its
endocrine portion consists of clusters of hormone-secreting
cells called *islets of Langerhans.* These islets contain two types of
hormone-secreting cells: α-cells which produce **glucagon,** and
β-cells which produce **insulin.** Both these hormones are
proteins, and both affect the level of *glucose* in the blood.
Glucagon raises the blood glucose level while insulin lowers it.
Insulin also increases the rate of entry of glucose into living cells
from the blood. Insulin is dominant immediately after meals to
store glucose. Glucagon acts between meals to top up blood
glucose as fast as it is used up by the tissues. (See Chapters 10
and 7.)

Abnormal activity of the pancreas

Hyposecretion of the islets of Langerhans results in *diabetes
mellitus* (sugar diabetes) due to a shortage of *insulin.* The
glucose level in the blood rises causing *hyperglycaemia,* and
glucose is excreted in the *urine* (glycosuria). The presence of
glucose in urine disturbs the body's *fluid balance,* as it reduces
water reabsorption from the kidney tubules by increasing the
osmotic pressure of the glomerular filtrate. Feeling *thirsty* is
therefore one of the symptoms of diabetes mellitus.

The stores of glycogen in the liver are broken down rapidly
where the insulin level is low, and glucose enters the tissue cells
much more slowly. *Fats* are therefore broken down in the tissue
cells to provide enough energy, which results in **ketosis** (see
Chapter 7). *Weight loss* occurs as *proteins* are also used to supply
energy.

Diabetes mellitus is treated by regular doses of insulin and/or
a low carbohydrate diet. In the *elderly*, diabetes mellitus is often
not insulin-dependent. It can be due to raised levels of other
hormones (eg cortisol, aldosterone, adrenalin, somatotropin)
while insulin secretion is normal.

Adrenal glands

There are two adrenal glands one above each kidney. Each gland is divided into an outer adrenal *cortex* and an inner adrenal *medulla*. The cortex has a firm texture and is deep yellow in colour, while the medulla is soft and dark brown in colour. The two parts of the gland secrete different hormones.

Adrenal cortex

The adrenal cortex secretes the *steroid* hormones *cortisol* and *aldosterone*:

- **Cortisol** affects normal *metabolism* and resistance to stress. It ensures that the body cells have sufficient glucose for energy, and stimulates the use of fats and proteins as energy foods if necessary. It depresses the action of lysosomes in breaking down damaged cells, and causes wounds to heal more slowly. Cortisol also controls the body *rhythms*, providing an 'internal clock' determined by the body's cortisol level. Around midnight the level of cortisol drops, reaching its lowest level between 2 and 4 am. The cortisol level then starts to rise again until there is enough to trigger waking from sleep between 6 and 9 am. Just after lunch the cortisol level falls slightly again, inducing sleepiness, but then rises towards the evening.

- **Aldosterone** regulates the level of *sodium* and *potassium* ions in the body, and affects the osmotic pressure of the body fluids and *fluid balance*. Aldosterone increases the reabsorption of sodium ions in the kidney tubules, thus increasing the sodium level of the blood. A high sodium level in the blood inhibits further secretion of aldosterone, providing negative feedback control.

The adrenal cortex also secretes both the male and female *sex hormones*, **androgen** and **oestrogen**.

Abnormal activity of the adrenal cortex

- **Hypersecretion** of
  (a) *cortisol* results in *Cushing's syndrome*. It can be due to an adrenal tumour. In this disorder the patient gains weight and the *body fat* is redistributed in a characteristic way. It results in very thin legs, a large 'moon face', a shoulder hump and an enlarged abdomen. The *blood pressure* is raised and the skin of the face appears flushed. *Bruising* of the tissues occurs readily. There is an increased growth of hair (*hirsuitism*) in women, and the bones become soft and fragile due to *osteoporosis*. Beauty therapy treatments are contra-indicated where Cushing's syndrome is present;
  (b) *aldosterone* decreases the level of *potassium* in the body which affects nerve transmission resulting in muscular

paralysis. It also causes retention of sodium and water by the blood resulting in high *blood pressure*, and *oedema* in the tissues;

(c) the adrenal *sex hormones* may be due to a tumour in the gland. In most cases it is the male *androgens* which are increased, causing *virilism* in females who develop male sexual characteristics such as the growth of a beard and deepening of the voice.

An *adrenal tumour* will result in an abnormal increase in the number of cells in the gland, a condition known as *adrenal hyperplasia*;

- **Hyposecretion** of androgen, cortisol and aldosterone results in *Addison's disease*. The symptoms of this disease are muscular weakness, weight loss and mental lethargy, as there is insufficient *glucose* in the blood for tissue cell respiration, particularly in skeletal muscle. Increased *potassium* and decreased *sodium* in the blood lead to reduced blood pressure and dehydration through water loss. Bronzing of the skin occurs, and women may lose their axillary hair.

Adrenal medulla

The adrenal medulla secretes the hormone **adrenalin**. Larger quantities of adrenalin are secreted when the body is very *active*, or under *stress*. The hormone prepares the body to use more energy during the 'flight-or-fight' response to stress or danger. It affects a large number of target organs, and has the same effects as stimulation by the *sympathetic* nervous system.

Adrenalin increases the depth and frequency of contraction of the heart muscle, increasing the *heart rate* and blood pressure. It dilates the *bronchi* so that more air enters the lungs, increasing the oxygen supply. It causes the *arterioles* in the skin and alimentary canal to contract, and those supplying the skeletal muscles to relax, to bring more food and oxygen for greater muscular effort. Glycogen in the liver and muscles is converted into glucose to provide additional energy, so the blood glucose level is raised.

Adrenalin increases the *sensitivity* of the nervous system so that the body responds more rapidly to external stimuli. The smooth muscle of the wall of the alimentary canal relaxes, slowing *peristalsis*. In addition, the *pupil* of the eye is dilated, and the *arrector pili* muscles contract, making the hairs stand on end.

Abnormal activity of the adrenal medulla

Hypersecretion of adrenalin causes high blood pressure and an increase in the BMR. There are high levels of glucose in the blood and urine. Nervousness and sweating increase. Hypersecretion can be the result of a tumour, but can also occur where there is a continuously high stress level in an individual's lifestyle. It may be one factor in causing coronary thrombosis and early death by heart failure.

Pituitary gland

The pituitary gland projects downwards from the *hypothalamus* of the brain, and is surrounded by the *sphenoid* bone which lies below. It consists of two parts: the *anterior* and *posterior lobes*, which secrete different hormones. Some of the pituitary hormones regulate the activity of the other endocrine glands so the pituitary has been described as the '*master gland*'.

Figure 13.4
Structure of pituitary gland

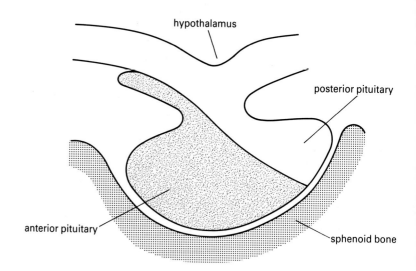

Anterior pituitary lobe

This region produces a number of hormones which act on other endocrine glands. One of these is **TSH** which acts on the thyroid gland to control the secretion of thyroxin. Another is **ACTH** (corticotropin) which controls the secretion of cortisol by the adrenal cortex. The **gonadotropins** (FSH and LH) which control the secretion of ovarian hormones, and **prolactin** which controls the milk secretion of the mammary glands, are also produced by the anterior pituitary (see Chapter 14).

The growth hormone **somatotropin** from the anterior pituitary affects the body tissues directly, increasing protein synthesis in the cells which causes tissue growth. Although secretion of somatotropin occurs throughout life, the amount secreted falls once growth is completed at maturity. The anterior pituitary secretes a *melanocyte stimulating hormone* which increases skin pigmentation.

Abnormal activity of the anterior pituitary lobe

- **Hypersecretion** of
  (a) *ACTH* causes *Cushing's syndrome* by its effect on cortisol secretion;
  (b) the growth hormone *somatotropin* in childhood leads to *giantism* as the limb bones increase in length enormously. If hypersecretion starts in adults it causes *acromegaly*, resulting in enlargement of the hands, feet, nose, jaws and ears;

- **Hyposecretion** of somatotropin in childhood leads to *dwarfism*.

Posterior pituitary lobe

This region *stores* two hormones which are secreted by the *hypothalamus* of the brain, and pass into blood capillaries supplying the posterior pituitary. The two hormones are **oxytocin** and **ADH** (antidiuretic hormone) and both are proteins.

Oxytocin affects smooth muscle and causes the contractions of the uterine wall during childbirth. It also controls the flow of milk from the mammary glands. ADH increases the reabsorption of water into the blood by the kidney tubules, and reduces the volume of urine formed, preventing excessive water loss.

Abnormal activity of the posterior pituitary lobe

Hyposecretion of *ADH* is usually caused by damage to either the hypothalamus or the posterior pituitary lobe, and causes *diabetes insipidus*. The kidney tubules reabsorb very little water due to the low level of ADH so large volumes of very dilute urine are produced. *Alcohol* inhibits the secretion of ADH, increasing the volume of urine produced, so it has a dehydrating effect on the body.

Thymus gland

The thymus gland lies in the thorax beneath the sternum. It is a bilobed gland composed of lymphoid tissue and forms part of the lymphatic system. It produces the hormone **thymosin** which stimulates antibody production by the lymphocytes.

Pineal gland

The pineal gland which is shaped like a small pine cone projects from the roof of the diencephalon of the brain. It is well developed in young children, but starts to degenerate from the age of seven. It secretes the hormone **melatonin** which affects secretion of hormones by the ovaries. Recent research shows that light entering the eyes makes the gland inactive. Secretion of melatonin occurs in darkness, and the hormone controls body rhythms.

Jet lag is thought to be due to changes in melatonin secretion, because of the altered day and night periods in other parts of the world experienced after long flights. Between Britain and the USA jet lag is noticeable for about ten days following the return flight from the USA (after travelling east). It is less noticeable after the flight out, having travelled west.

Testes

In the male, the testes are two oval organs lying outside the body cavity in the scrotum. They produce the male sex hormones or **androgens** (eg testosterone) that stimulate the development of the male organs, and maintain the male secondary sexual characteristics such as body hair patterns, a deeper voice, and skeletal and muscular development.

Ovaries

In the female, the two ovaries which lie in the pelvic cavity secrete two hormones, **oestrogen** and **progesterone** (see Chapter 14).

Table 13.1
Summary of the endocrine system

Name of gland	Hormones	Effects	Associated disorders
Thyroid	Thyroxin	Controls BMR, growth and development	Exophthalmic goitre; Simple goitre; Myxoedema; Cretinism
Parathyroid	Parathyrin	Raises blood calcium level	Osteoporosis Tetany
Pancreas islets of Langerhans	Glucagon	Raises blood glucose level	Hyperglycaemia
	Insulin	Lowers blood glucose level Increased entry of glucose into the cells	Diabetes mellitus

Table 13.1 (cont)

Name of gland	Hormones	Effects	Associated disorders
Adrenal cortex	Cortisol	Makes energy available for cell metabolism; resists stress; controls body rhythms	Cushing's syndrome Addison's disease
	Aldosterone	Controls potassium and sodium levels in the blood; affects fluid balance	Addison's disease
	Androgens	Cause male sexual characteristics to develop	Addison's disease Virilism in women
Adrenal medulla	Adrenalin	Increases BMR; prepares the body for the flight-or-fight response	High blood pressure
Anterior pituitary	TSH	Stimulates the release of thyroxin	
	ACTH	Increases the output of cortisol from the adrenal cortex	Cushing's syndrome
	Gonadotropins (FSH, LH)	Control the menstrual cycle and reproduction	Infertility
	Prolactin	Initiates and maintains lactation	
	Somatotropin	Controls growth	Giantism; Acromegaly; Dwarfism
Posterior pituitary	Stores and releases Oxytocin	Uterine contractions at childbirth; milk flow	
	ADH	Reduces urine volume	Diabetes insipidus
Thymus	Thymosin	Stimulates antibody production	
Pineal	Melatonin	Affects body rhythms and reproductive cycle	Jet lag
Testes	Testosterone	Male sexual characteristics	Infertility
Ovaries	Oestrogen Progesterone	Control the menstrual cycle and pregnancy	Breast cancer Premenstrual tension

The influence of hormone balance on external appearance

Hormones affect the size, masculinity or femininity of the body shape, the distribution of terminal hair, and the amount and distribution of subcutaneous fat. All these factors are involved in the external appearance of an individual.

As different hormones may affect one of these factors in opposite ways, the balance between the hormones can, to some extent, determine an individual's appearance. The situation is very complex however as genetic factors and diet also have marked effects on external appearance.

An individual's height is affected by *somatotropin*, the anterior pituitary growth hormone, and by *thyroxin*. A childhood deficiency in either of these hormones retards growth, resulting in small stature in the adult. Hypersecretion of somatotropin in childhood will result in very tall stature as the limb bones are likely to grow longer than average. Hypersecretion of somatotropin which begins in adult life will have a marked effect on the appearance of the face, as the nose, jaws and ears enlarge. The hands and feet also increase in size. These changes are due to the deposition of extra bone. The lips thicken and the skin coarsens at the onset of the acromegaly.

The masculinity or femininity of body shape in women is influenced by the balance between the *ovarian* hormones and the *adrenal sex* hormones. Hypersecretion of adrenal androgens and/or reduced secretion of ovarian hormones will result in the development of a more masculine body shape. Ovarian hormones will promote the increased width of the pelvis and the development of the breasts. Reduced secretion of *thyroxin* in children prevents the maturation of the body normally promoted by the ovarian sex hormones.

The masculine type of distribution of terminal hair in women (hirsuties) with hair growth in the mustache and beard region, may result from hypersecretion of adrenal androgens or cortisol counteracting the feminizing effect of ovarian hormones. After the *menopause* when the level of ovarian hormones falls, the adrenal sex hormones become dominant and facial hair may develop. A deficiency of *thyroxin* causes thinning and loss of terminal hair including that of the eyebrows.

The typical female subcutaneous fat distribution on thighs, hips, shoulders and breasts is an effect of the *ovarian* hormones. Hypersecretion of *cortisol* results in a change in the distribution of fat from the legs and thighs to the face and abdomen, with increased deposition on the shoulders. *Thyroxin* imbalance affects the amount of fat deposited. Hypersecretion results in loss of subcutaneous fat and therefore in weight loss. Hyposecretion of thyroxin causes increased deposition of fat and weight gain.

Self-assessment questions

1 What is a hormone? In what type of organs are hormones produced? What is their main function?

2 Describe the position of the thyroid gland. Name the other endocrine glands which occur close to it.

3 What effect do the following hormones have on the basal metabolic rate (BMR):

(a) thyroxin;   (b) adrenalin?

4 Distinguish between diabetes mellitus and diabetes insipidus.

5 What is the effect on the external appearance of the body of hypersecretion of:

(a) cortisol;
(b) somatotropin?

6 Name the bone conditions resulting from the increased secretion in adults of:

(a) parathyrin;
(b) somatotropin.

7 Name the hormone secreted by:

(a) the pineal gland;
(b) the adrenal medulla;
(c) the parathyroid glands;
(d) the α-cells of the islets of Langerhans.

8 Describe the effects of ADH (antidiuretic hormone) on the body.

9 Using aldosterone as an example, explain the meaning of negative feedback control in homeostasis.

10 Which hormone may be associated with jet lag? Explain why the hormone is believed to produce this condition.

CHAPTER 14   *The Reproductive System*

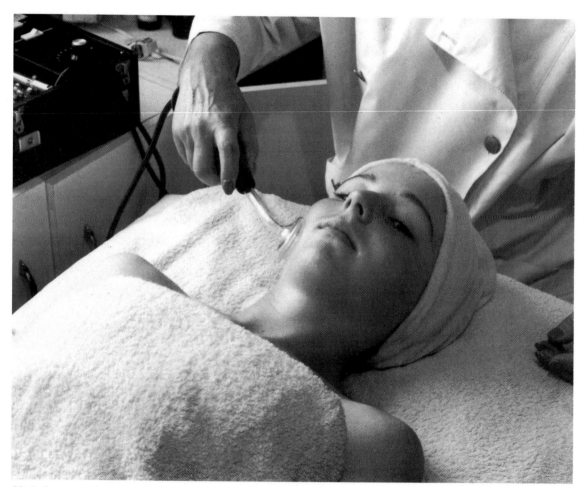

High frequency therapy – direct method

Sexual reproduction occurs in humans. The reproductive cells or *gametes* are produced separately in males and females in the sex organs or *gonads*. The *testes* are the male gonads and the *ovaries* are the female gonads. The reproductive cells or gametes are the *sperms* in the male and the *ova* or eggs in the female. The sperms gain access to the ova through sexual intercourse so that *fertilization*, the fusion of egg and sperm, can occur within the female reproductive system. This ensures that any resulting *embryo* can be protected and nourished. Sexual reproduction allows considerable *genetic variation* to occur among the offspring.

The female reproductive system

The female *organs* of reproduction occur in the pelvic cavity except the *mammary glands* (breasts) which are on the anterior wall of the chest. The **ovaries** are two organs 3 cm long and 1.5 cm wide, which produce the *ova*, and secrete *sex hormones*. They occur, one on each side, in a depression on the lateral wall of the pelvis, attached to it by a *suspensory* ligament. An *ovarian* ligament anchors each ovary to the uterus also. Two **fallopian tubes**, which are lined with ciliated epithelium and have a funnel-shaped opening close to the ovary, carry the ova to the **uterus** (womb) following *ovulation*, ie the extrusion of a ripe ovum from an ovary. It is accompanied by a small rise in body temperature.

An ovum is fertilized in the fallopian tube, and the embryo becomes attached to the lining of the uterus. The *foetus* then continues to develop in the uterus during pregnancy. The uterus connects with the **vagina** by a narrowed **cervix**. The external genital organs, known as the **vulva**, occur at the entrance to the

Figure 14.1
Female reproductive organs (anterior view)

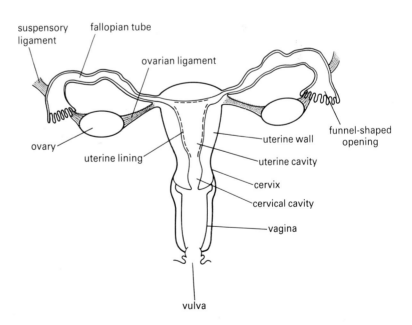

vagina. The urinary opening is just anterior to that of the vagina. The vagina serves as a passageway for the menstrual flow, and acts as the birth canal. It also holds the male penis during sexual intercourse so that the sperms can enter the uterus and reach the fallopian tubes. At the lower end of the vagina is a thin fold of mucous membrane called the **hymen** which initially partly closes the vaginal opening. The vaginal opening is enlarged during the first experience of sexual intercourse.

Puberty in the female

Puberty is the period in life at which the reproductive organs become functional and usually occurs between 10 and 14 years of age. At puberty the ovary responds to pituitary *gonadotropic* (gonadotrophic) hormones which appear in the blood, and ova are produced. The ovary then begins to produce the two hormones, *oestrogen* and *progesterone,* which travel in the blood to the body tissues. Under the influence of these hormones *bones* begin to grow, so that body height increases and the pelvis becomes broader. Extra *fat* is deposited in the subcutaneous layer on the thighs, hips and shoulders.

The ovaries and uterus enlarge and change shape, and as the *menstrual cycle* becomes established, the *uterus lining* undergoes a cycle of thickening followed by the sloughing off of the extra tissue at menstruation.

Terminal hair grows on the axillae and in the pubic region, and the *mammary glands* develop. These are known as the *secondary sexual characters.* Psychological and personality changes occur of the type associated with adolescence.

Precocious puberty occurs when females become fertile at a very young age, even as young as five years. This may be due to an ovarian tumour which is secreting oestrogen. Surgical removal of the tumour is necessary.

The menstrual cycle

The 28-day (average) menstrual cycle involves changes in the ovaries and uterus controlled by *interacting hormones.* If pregnancy occurs, the cycle is interrupted. Each cycle starts at the onset of menstruation and ovulation from one of the ovaries occurs at the midpoint of the cycle. During the first 14 days, an ovum develops inside a *follicle* in the ovary. During the second 14 days, following ovulation, the empty follicle in the ovary develops into a *corpus luteum* (yellow body) as yellow pigment accumulates there. If the relased ovum is not fertilized, the corpus luteum degenerates at the end of the cycle.

From the end of menstruation, around the fifth day of the menstrual cycle, the uterus lining thickens and becomes very vascular. This tissue is separated from the uterus at the end of the cycle and forms the *menstrual flow*. If the ovum is fertilized, the thick uterus lining remains intact and the embryo becomes attached to it, to begin pregnancy.

The stages in the menstrual cycle are regulated by *four* hormones which interact. Two are *gonadotropins* formed by the anterior lobe of the pituitary gland and known as *FSH* (follicle

Figure 14.2
Stages in the menstrual cycle

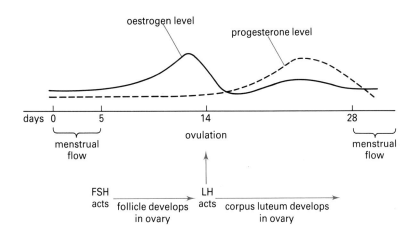

stimulating hormone) and *LH* (luteinizing hormone). The other two are the ovarian hormones *oestrogen* and *progesterone*.

At the end of menstruation **FSH** causes a follicle to develop in the ovary and stimulates the secretion of **oestrogen**. Oestrogen initiates the repair and thickening of the uterus lining. The level of oestrogen in the blood steadily increases towards the midpoint of the cycle. At its peak, oestrogen stimulates the pituitary gland to produce **LH** while inhibiting the production of FSH, so that no further follicles start to develop. LH induces ovulation followed by the conversion of the empty follicle into a corpus luteum, which then secretes **progesterone**. The oestrogen level in the blood then falls, while the progesterone level rises and continues to promote the thickening of the uterus lining. Progesterone inhibits the production of LH so the corpus luteum degenerates. Progesterone also inhibits the production of FSH so that new follicles do not start to develop in the ovary. Degeneration of the corpus luteum occurs if fertilization has not taken place and this causes a

Figure 14.3
Hormonal control of the menstrual
cycle

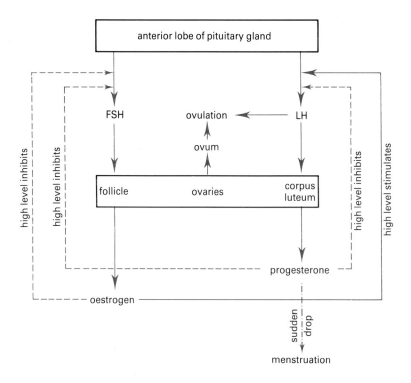

sudden drop in progesterone level which triggers menstruation thus starting the next menstrual cycle.

The interaction between the four hormones controlling the menstrual cycle is a *negative feedback* mechanism which stabilizes the reproductive cycle.

Female reproductive disorders

These may be abnormalities of the menstrual cycle, ovarian cysts, or infectious diseases of the reproductive ducts.

- *Amenorrhoea* is the absence of menstruation and is usually due to hormone imbalance. In cases where menstruation usually occurs but then stops for two or three months, a sudden weight change may be the cause. Both obesity and extreme weight loss due to Anorexia nervosa may stop menstruation.

- *Dysmenorrhoea* is painful menstruation accompanied by vomiting, diarrhoea and headache. It can be due to over-production of *tissue hormones* (prostaglandins) by the uterus, or to the presence of ovarian or uterine tumors.

- *Ovarian cysts* are tumours in the ovary which may become cancerous and must be surgically removed. The cysts are filled with a thick jelly-like material and are usually painless until their increasing size causes pressure on other organs. This may result in abdominal swelling, frequent urination, vomiting and constipation. Pressure on leg veins may cause varicose veins and swelling ankles.

  If the cyst becomes inflamed, sudden severe pain may occur in the pelvic region. Some ovarian cysts produce oestrogen causing irregular menstrual bleeding or precocious puberty. Their presence may be suspected by the beauty therapist where abdominal swelling occurs, when the client should be directed to seek medical advice.

- *Sexually transmitted diseases* are a group of infectious diseases spread primarily through sexual intercourse:

  (a) *Gonorrhoea* affects the mucous membrane of the urinogenital ducts and rectum, and is caused by a *Neisseria* bacterium. If untreated it causes sterility;

  (b) *Syphilis* causes lesions in the vagina and if untreated leads to still-births, and finally to degenerative conditions of most of the body systems. It is caused by a spirochaete *Treponema* bacterium;

  (c) *Genital herpes* is caused by the *Herpes simplex II* virus and is uncurable. It causes painful blisters on the vulva or vagina and may be associated with the later development of cervical cancer;

  (d) *Trichomoniasis* is an inflammation of the vaginal lining by a protozoan pathogen called *Trichomonas*. It causes itching and vaginal discharge;

  (e) *AIDS* (acquired immune deficiency syndrome) is caused by the *HIV* virus which attacks the body's defence system, so that it becomes unable to fight off other diseases from which the person eventually dies. The virus can be present in semen, vaginal fluid, and in the blood, and may be passed on by intimate contact with any of these infected fluids.

The female menopause

The menopause marks the end of the reproductive phase of life, and occurs between the ages of 39 and 59, 47 being the average age. The ovaries cease to respond to the *gonadotropic* hormones at this age, and menstrual cycles become less frequent until they cease altogether. The *ovaries* shrink and no longer produce ova, and the production of oestrogen and progesterone is reduced. Other tissues of the body change in response to the reduced oestrogen level.

There is atrophy of the fallopian tubes, uterus, vagina and vulva. As the vaginal epithelium becomes thinner the secretion becomes less *acid*, so the protection against infection is reduced. The *breasts* shrink as the glands and ducts atrophy and the amount of adipose tissue is reduced. The mammary *blood vessels* narrow, so blood flow to the breast is reduced. The *nipples* become smaller and less erectile.

The bones become structurally weaker due to the loss of calcium, resulting in some degree of *osteoporosis*. The cholesterol level in the blood rises, and *atherosclerosis* results from fatty deposits in the arteries, which leads to the increased risk of coronary thrombosis in post-menopausal women. *Hair* in the axillae and pubic regions becomes sparse. Some women may suffer from *vascular disorders* such as hot flushes and excessive sweating. Headache and muscular pains and cramps are also common. There may be *emotional* disturbances severe enough in a few cases to cause clinical depression. In some cases *hormone replacement therapy* may be a possible treatment for the symptoms of reduced oestrogen levels in post-menopausal women.

The breasts

The two breasts or **mammary glands** are involved in milk secretion or *lactation,* and are modified *apocrine sweat* glands. They occur on the anterior surface of the thorax over the pectoralis major muscles to which they are attached by a layer of connective tissue. Each breast extends from the second to the sixth rib, and from the edge of the sternum to the axilla.

External structure

Just below the mid-line of the hemispherical breast is a small projection, or **nipple**, onto which about 15 milk ducts open. A circular pigmented area of skin called the **areola** surrounds the nipple. The surface of the areola appears rough because it contains modified sebaceous glands, which secrete a fatty material to protect the skin of the nipple. The skin of the areola and nipple is hairless and very thin.

Internal structure

The mammary glands are *branched tubuloacinar* glands, and the layer of connective tissue which attaches them to the underlying muscle is the *deep fascia*. Each mammary gland consists of 15 to 20 **lobes**, arranged radially round the nipple, and separated by an amount of adipose tissue which determines the size of the

Figure 14.4
Vertical section through a mammary gland (breast)

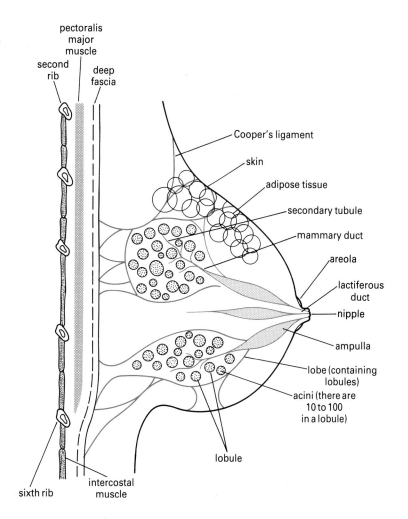

pectoralis
major
muscle

second
rib

deep
fascia

Cooper's ligament

skin

adipose tissue

secondary tubule

mammary duct

areola

lactiferous
duct

nipple

ampulla

lobe (containing
lobules)

acini (there are
10 to 100
in a lobule)

lobule

sixth rib

intercostal
muscle

breast. Thus the amount of milk secreted by a mammary gland is not related to the size of the breast. Excessive milk production is known as *Galactorrhoea.*

In each lobe are many smaller **lobules** 1 to 8 mm in diameter and composed of connective tissue in which the milk-secreting cells occur. Between the lobules are strands of fibrous connective tissue called **Cooper's ligaments.** These suspensory ligaments run between the skin and the deep fascia, and support the breasts. They are better developed over the upper part of the breast. The tubuloacinar glands form grape-like clusters in the lobules. The milk they secrete passes into **secondary tubules** which drain into larger **mammary ducts.** Where these ducts converge on the nipple, each widens to form an **ampulla** where the milk may be stored. From each ampulla a **lactiferous duct** continues, and opens on the nipple.

The blood supply to the breast

The *subclavian* and *axillary arteries* supply blood to the breast. The subclavian artery has an *internal mammary* branch which passes downwards alongside the sternum, and supplies the medial half of the breast. The axillary artery is a continuation of the subclavian artery, and has *lateral thoracic* and *subscapular* branches which supply the lateral half of the breast. From the arteries the blood passes into an extensive *capillary network*, and is collected from the breast by veins. Surrounding the nipple is a network of small veins called the *circulus venosus*, which drain into an *internal mammary vein*. This opens into a large *innominate* vein at the base of the neck.

Figure 14.5
Arterial blood supply to mammary gland (breast)

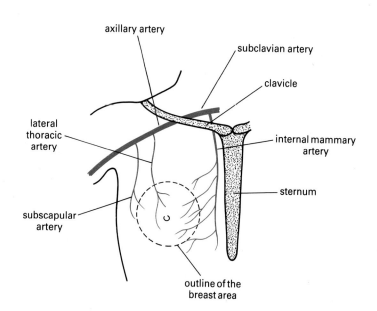

Lymphatic drainage of the breast

The *axillary lymph* nodes receive 75% of the lymph draining from the breast, and the *internal mammary* (parasternal) nodes receive the rest. The axillary nodes include four groups, the *subclavicular, central, subscapular* and *pectoral* nodes. The internal mammary nodes are a linear group following the edge of the sternum. The extensive lymph drainage allows *metastasis* (spread) of cancerous cells to other parts of the body if breast cancer develops.

Changes taking place in the breast

At **birth** the mammary glands in both male and female babies appear as slight elevations on the anterior chest wall.

At **puberty** in the female the breasts begin to develop, stimulated by the female sex hormones. The mammary glands enlarge and the ducts elongate. Additional adipose tissue is laid down, and the areola and nipple grow.

Figure 14.6
Lymph drainage of mammary gland
(breast)

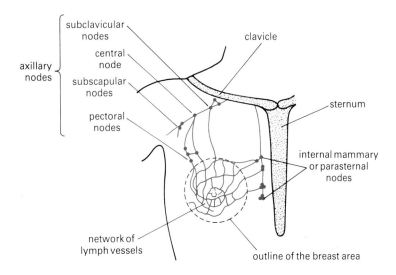

In **adolescence** sexual maturity is attained, and continues until the menopause. As the menstrual cycle becomes established and ovulation occurs, the increased production of *oestrogen* causes the ducts of the mammary glands to lengthen and branch. More adipose tissue is laid down in the breast as sexual maturity is reached. During this phase the volume of the breast is at its minimum between the fifth and seventh day of the menstrual cycle. The hormone *progesterone* which causes increased blood flow through the mammary vessels, and retention of tissue fluid, will increase breast size in the second half of the menstrual cycle, and may cause discomfort. Progesterone also stimulates the acini of the mammary glands to develop.

In **pregnancy** the increased production of the hormones oestrogen and progesterone stimulate further growth of the mammary glands, and the blood vessels dilate to increase blood flow. The areola and nipple enlarge and become darker in colour. The breasts enlarge further during the second month of pregnancy, and their upper surface becomes more rounded. In late pregnancy the milk ducts contain *colostrum*, a yellowish milk-like fluid rich in antibody proteins.

After **childbirth** when the levels of oestrogen and progesterone fall, the anterior pituitary lobe releases extra prolactin hormone which stimulates the glandular acini to secrete true milk. The constitutents of the milk are obtained from the blood flowing through the mammary glands. When the baby *suckles*, nerve impulses to the posterior pituitary lobe cause it to release the hormone *oxytocin*. This is carried in the blood to

Table 14.1
Summary of the effects of the
reproductive hormones on the body

Hormone	Origin	Effects on the body
Oestrogen	Ovarian follicles	Regulates the development of the sex organs and secondary sexual characters; stimulates LH and inhibits FSH production in the control of the menstrual cycle; initiates the thickening of the uterine wall; causes growth of the ducts in the mammary glands
Progesterone	Corpus luteum in the ovary	Inhibits LH and FSH production in the control of the menstrual cycle; causes further thickening of the uterine wall; causes tissues to retain fluid; stimulates acini of the mammary glands to develop
FSH	Anterior lobe of the pituitary gland	Stimulates follicle development in the ovary; causes the ovary to secrete oestrogen; interacts with ovarian hormones to control the menstrual cycle
LH	Anterior lobe of the pituitary gland	Causes ovulation; stimulates the development of a corpus luteum in the ovary; causes the ovary to secrete progesterone; interacts with ovarian hormones to control the menstrual cycle
Prolactin	Anterior lobe of the pituitary gland	Causes the mammary glands to secrete milk after childbirth
Oxytocin	Posterior lobe of the pituitary gland	Causes contraction of the uterus during childbirth; causes the release of milk from the breast

the breast where it stimulates milk flow to the baby. Suckling is also the principle stimulus in releasing *prolactin* which stimulates milk secretion. This is an example of *positive feedback*, since the harder the baby sucks, the greater the volume of milk produced.

Lactation often prevents menstrual cycles for the first few months after childbirth by inhibiting FSH and LH release. When the menstrual cycle becomes re-established, oestrogen and progesterone are again produced and prolactin secretion is suppressed. When lactation stops the ducts and glandular tissue of the breast are reduced, but the breast still remains slightly larger than it was before pregnancy. The lower surface of the breast is more pendant, and the nipple appears to be placed at a lower level.

At the **menopause** there is a shrinkage of breast tissue as the acini and ducts atrophy, and are replaced by connective tissue.

The lobular structure of the mammary glands therefore disappears. The amount of adipose tissue in the breast also decreases and the blood vessels become narrow, reducing blood flow. With the decrease in size the breasts become more pendant. The nipples become smaller and less erectile.

Figure 14.7
Successive changes in the shape of the breast

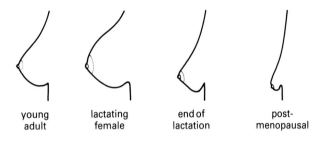

| young adult | lactating female | end of lactation | post-menopausal |

Abnormalities of the breast

Breast size

The size of the breast in different individuals can vary considerably mainly due to variations in the amount of fat present. Its size is determined by two genetic factors (a) the level of ovarian hormones in the blood, and (b) the sensitivity of breast tissue to these hormones.

- *Small breasts* can be enlarged by plastic surgery in which *breast augmentation* by implants is carried out. An incision is made around the areola, and sacs filled with *silicone rubber* or *saline* are inserted into the breast.

- *Atrophy* of the breast due to loss of adipose and glandular tissue occurs in all post-menopausal women. It may also be associated with general weight loss.

- *Hypertrophy* of the breast is its excessive enlargement, which can be counteracted by cosmetic surgery to remove some of the surplus tissue. In *breast reduction* an incision is made round the areola and down the front underside of the breast. Skin, fat and glandular tissue are then removed. Some hypertrophy of the breast is normal during *pregnancy* and *lactation* due to the enlargement of the mammary lobules.

Tumours of the breast

The female breast is highly susceptible to the development of tumours, which are often visible externally or can be felt under the skin.

- A *cyst* is a hollow tumour containing fluid or soft material, which forms a rounded lump in the breast. It may appear at any age, and though it is *benign* and does not invade the tissue it is usually removed by minor surgery. *Retention* cysts are due to blockage in milk ducts caused by inflammation.

- A *fibroadenoma* is a *benign* tumour composed of glandular and fibrous tissue which feels firm and rubbery, and is easily moved about under the skin. It occurs most frequently in young women taking the oral-contraceptive pill, and in childless menopausal women. It is usually removed by minor surgery.

- *Breast cancer* is due to *malignant* tumours which are not enclosed in a capsule and which invade and destroy the breast tissues. The symptoms of breast cancer are the presence of lumps, discharges from the nipple, or a nipple which becomes pulled in on one side. Puckering of the skin of the breast may also occur, but the tumour is seldom painful. Breast cancer is more likely to develop in post-menopausal women. It can be treated effectively if it is noticed in the early stages, and the beauty therapist may detect its presence in a client, who should then seek immediate medical advice.

Self-assessment questions

1 Where in the body could you expect to find:

(a) a newly fertilized ovum;
(b) a corpus luteum;
(c) a Cooper's ligament?

2 Name **two** gonadotropins, and state where they are produced in the body.

3 List **three** changes in the female breast which occur at puberty.

4 Explain the roles of prolactin and oxytocin in lactation.

5 Distinguish between galactorrhoea and dysmenorrhoea.

6 Give the causal agents of the following diseases:

(a) Gonorrhoea;   (b) AIDS;
(c) genital herpes.

7 Define the position of a mammary gland on the body surface.

8 List the ducts that a milk drop will pass through on its way from acini gland cell to a baby's mouth.

9 List the groups of nodes involved in lymph drainage from the breast.

10 What are the effects of progesterone on the body?

CHAPTER 15

Electrical Equipment

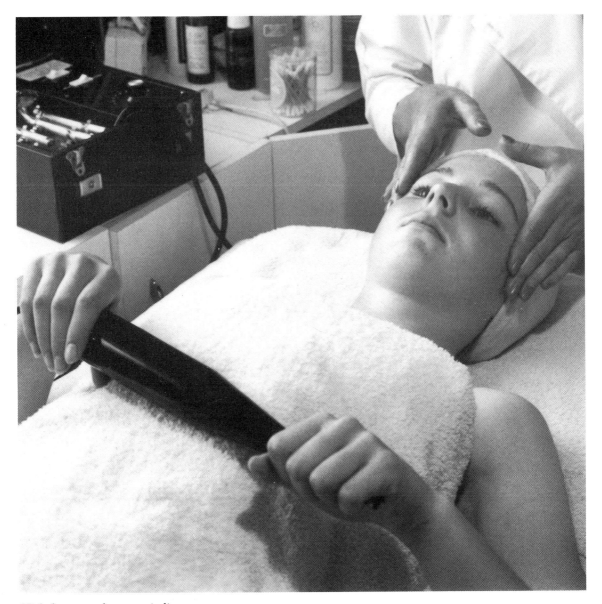

High frequency therapy – indirect method

The electrical equipment used in beauty therapy treatments contains a number of electrical devices whose actions are described below.

Electrical devices

Electromagnet

When an electric current flows through a copper wire coil, known as a *solenoid*, it acts as a *magnet*. The magnetic field is stronger when the coil is wound round a soft iron *core*. The *south* pole of the electromagnet is at the end of the wire coil where the current flows *clockwise*, and the *north* pole is at the other end where it flows *anticlockwise*. An electromagnet loses its magnetic effect when the electric current is switched off.

Figure 15.1
Simple electromagnet

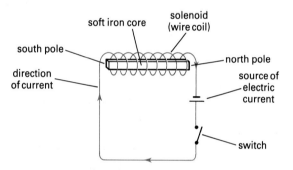

Electric motor

An electric motor is a device to convert electrical energy into *mechanical* energy. It contains a solenoid, the *rotor*, through which an electric current passes to produce an electromagnet. The rotor is placed between the two opposite poles of a *permanent* magnet. When the north pole of the electromagnet is close to the north pole of the permanent magnet it is *repelled*, causing the rotor to rotate. To keep turning always in the same direction, the electric current passing through it must change direction every half-turn of the rotor. A *split-ring commutator* is used for this purpose. The two free ends of the wire in the rotor are connected to one of the semi-circular plates of the split ring. These plates rotate with the coil and while doing so press against *carbon brushes*, which pass the electric current to them. Every half-turn the commutator halves interchange brushes, and the current flows through the rotor in the opposite direction. The rotor is attached to a *shaft* which is made to rotate continuously in the same direction as long as the motor is in operation.

Figure 15.2
Electric motor

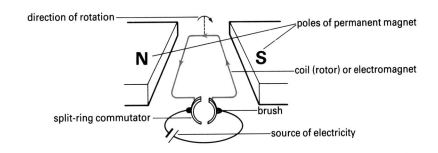

Changing the mains supply electric current

Many of the machines used in beauty therapy treatments require a different type of electric current to that supplied by the salon mains power circuit. *Mains* current has certain properties. It is an *alternating current* (AC), with a frequency of 50 cycles/second or 50 *hertz* (Hz). Mains current has a particular electrical pressure, or *voltage*, usually 240 volts.

There are a number of devices which will alter one or more of these properties of the mains current.

Transformer

A transformer is a device to change the *voltage* of an alternating current without changing its frequency. A changing magnetic field *induces* an alternating electric current in a copper wire coil. A changing magnetic field can be obtained by passing the mains alternating current through the coil of an *electromagnet*. The coil of the electromagnet carrying the mains current is called the *primary* coil. The coil from which the induced current of altered voltage is obtained is the *secondary* coil. The two coils are wound round a soft iron *core*, and insulated from one another.

A transformer which converts the mains voltage of 240 V to higher values is a *step-up* transformer. If the conversion is to a lower voltage it is a *step-down* transformer. In a step-up transformer the secondary coil has more turns than the primary coil. In a step-down transformer the secondary coil has the smaller number of turns.

Rectifier

A rectifier changes the mains alternating current into a *direct current* (DC) by acting as a 'valve', allowing electrons to pass through it in one direction only.

Electric heating and lighting are unaffected by the direction of flow of a current, but galvanism and electrical muscle stimulation (faradism) require direct current or the effect on the body would be counteracted each time an alternating current changed direction.

Although a rectified mains current only flows in one direction, the rate of flow still varies continuously. This variation is smoothed out to a *steady* value by the use of a capacitor.

Capacitor

A capacitor is a device which *stores* electric charge. It consists of two conducting metal plates with a thin layer of insulating material sandwiched between them. There is a build-up of charge on the two plates as electricity cannot readily pass through the insulating layer. A capacitor can *smooth out* a rectified mains current by storing charge when the current passing is high, thereby reducing it. By releasing charge when the current passing is low, the capacitor boosts it. The direct current then becomes an almost constant flow of electrons.

High frequency devices

In addition to requiring an alternating current of high voltage, beauty therapy equipment may need to produce a current of very *high frequency*, eg 20 000 Hz or higher. This must be generated from the mains current which has a frequency of only 50 Hz.

The basic principle of generating a current that changes direction at a frequency of very high value is to use an electronic switch called an *oscillator,* which can switch on and off several million times a second. Unfortunately, the rapid switching also generates *harmonics* of the required frequency. These harmonics must be filtered out by a circuit like that used to select a programme on a radio, ie a *tuning circuit.* A tuning circuit is usually made up of an *inductor* (coil) and a capacitor. In this way it is possible to choose the frequency of the alternating current produced.

The repeated rapid switching on and off by the oscillator is commonly produced by using either a *spark gap* or a *transistor.* A spark gap is a break in the circuit where there are two pieces of metal placed close together, but separated by a small air gap. Once the voltage has built up sufficiently in the circuit, it can pass current in the form of a spark across the air gap, so the voltage is suddenly reduced. The voltage then starts to build up again. A transistor is an electronic device that is fast enough for this switching on and off operation.

Figure 15.3
Induction coil

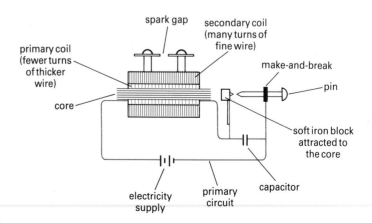

Figure 15.4
Oscillator and tuning circuit

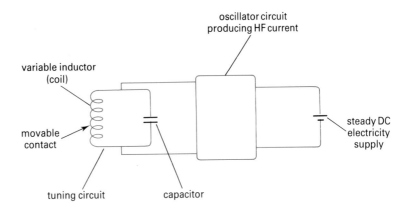

In the past, high frequency current of up to 20 000 Hz were produced from mains current by means of an *induction coil* containing a spark gap. An induction coil forms part of the traditional high frequency apparatus. Where very high frequencies of several million hertz are required, as in high frequency epilation equipment, an electronic oscillator must be used.

Potentiometer

A *potentiometer* is a variable *resistance* used as a volume control for radio, but in electrical stimulation machines it can be used to control the *size* (intensity) of the current. It consists of a *coil* acting as a resistance to the flow of current over which a *contact* is moved. The movable contact is attached via a *shaft* to the control knob.

Figure 15.5
Potentiometer intensity control

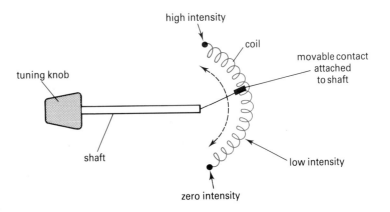

Electrical stimulation therapy

A number of different machines are available to increase the blood and lymph flow in the skin, and to stimulate motor nerves and muscles, causing muscle contractions.

Vacuum suction machine

- **Purpose**   It is used on the face to aid the movement of lymph through the superficial lymph vessels. It is used on the body for stubborn fat conditions, as it is thought to aid the softening of subcutaneous fat cells;
- **Effect**   The partial vacuum produced beneath the suction cup causes the skin to arch upwards into the cup. This stimulation brings an increased blood supply to the treated area of skin. Moving the suction cup along the path of a lymph vessel increases the rate of lymph flow;
- **Apparatus**   It consists of an *electric motor* which drives a *vacuum pump*. The pump sucks out some of the air from below the cup, and forces it through an outlet into the salon air;
- **Safety precautions**   The cup should be disinfected before use with an alcohol wipe. The skin should be previously lubricated with massage cream so that the suction cup will slide easily over the skin. Suction should not be applied over lymph glands, but only over lymph vessels;
- **Hazards**   If the machine dial is turned up too rapidly suction increases so strongly that bruising of the tissues due to capillary breakage may occur. It can also tear the skin.
  A photograph of the machine in use will be found on page 232.

Brush cleanser

- **Purpose**   It is used on the face and body for desquamation;
- **Effect**   Brushing loosens dead scales from the skin surface. It causes erythema due to the increased blood flow to the skin;
- **Apparatus**   It contains an electric motor driven by dry batteries which rotates the brush. The brush is moistened with a detergent solution;
- **Safety precautions**   The entire brush surface should be in contact with the skin to give uniform pressure. The brush size and texture should be suitable for the area of skin being treated. If too much liquid is applied to the brush spraying will occur. The brush should be disinfected with a 70% ethanol solution;
- **Hazards**   If the brush attachment is not firmly in place, the brush could fly off during use.
  A photograph of the machine in use will be found on page 155.

Belt massager (heavy vibrator)

- **Purpose**   It is used to stimulate the muscles of the thighs and hips;
- **Effect**   It improves the drainage of tissue fluid, reducing oedema which swells the tissues. It creates some erythema by increasing the blood flow due to frictional heating of the skin. The muscles are shaken and stimulated by the movements of the canvas belt;
- **Apparatus**   An electric motor rotates a disc, causing the end of the canvas belt attached to the disc to rotate also. This produces vibratory movements along the length of the belt;
- **Safety precautions**   The belt should be placed in a sterilizer before use to ensure that pathogens are not transferred from one client to the next;
- **Hazards**   It should not be used by clients with rheumatic conditions who are likely to bruise easily, or by anyone with a back problem.

  A photograph of the machine in use will be found on page 42.

Gyratory vibrator

- **Purpose**   It is used on the body to increase the rate of blood flow to the skin and muscles;
- **Effect**   The friction between the vibrator and the skin produces heat, resulting in erythema;
- **Apparatus**   It contains an electric motor which rotates a shaft to which the applicator is attached;
- **Safety precautions**   The applicator heads must be parallel with the skin surface during the treatment to give uniform pressure. A powder lubricant should be applied to the skin before starting the treatment. After use, applicators should be washed with hot water and detergent and dried with a paper towel. Alternatively an ethanol or ethanol/chlorhexidine wipe may be used for disinfection;
- **Hazards**   Bruising can occur if the treatment is prolonged, or an unsuitable applicator is used.

Percussion vibrator

- **Purpose**   It is used to massage localized areas of the body, using different types of applicator for different body regions. A sponge applicator is used for facial work, an ebonite one for the shoulders and back;
- **Effect**   The tapping movements of the applicators have their main effects on the skin surface. The frictional heat causes vasodilation in the skin blood vessels which increases the rate of blood flow and the activity of the sebaceous glands. Superficial dead skin scales are loosened and removed;
- **Apparatus**   An electric motor produces rotation which is then converted into an up-and-down tapping motion of the applicator;

- **Safety precautions**   The applicator heads must be parallel with the skin surface during the treatment. Powder should be used as a lubricant. All applicators should be disinfected after use. Some therapists believe that a percussion vibrator should not be used on the face;
- **Hazards**   Bruising can occur if the treatment is prolonged, or an unsuitable applicator is used.

Audiosonic vibrator

- **Purpose**   It is used on facial muscles to increase the rate of blood and lymph flow through the skin. It may be used to treat fibrositis nodules in the muscles of the neck and shoulders.
- **Effect**   The vibrations produced can penetrate the skin to reach the underlying muscles, where they produce heat for treating fibrositis and increasing blood flow. As there is no surface banging from the audiosonic vibrator, it can be used on the face and for mature sensitive skins.
- **Apparatus**   A coil is placed between the poles of a magnet, and an alternating current passes through the coil. The coil moves forward when the current is passing one way through the coil, and backwards when the direction of the current reverses. This is known as the electromotive effect, as a conductor moves in a magnetic field. The coil vibrates moving to-and-fro, and the movement of the coil is transferred to the applicator placed on the skin. The vibrations alternately compress and decompress (rarefy) the molecules in the surrounding air, as well as in the body tissues. The waves produced have particular frequencies, ie the number of compressions and decompressions produced per second, expressed in hertz. The frequencies to which the human ear responds are in the range of 20 Hz to 1500 Hz in the average person. Vibrations within this frequency range are described as audiosonic because they can be heard, and are produced by this type of vibrator.
- **Safety precautions**   Powder should be used as a lubricant when plastic applicators are used. Spongy applicators should be used where gentler stimulation is necessary, eg over bony areas of the face. Applicators should be disinfected before use.

Electrical muscle stimulation (faradic) machine

- **Purpose**   It is used on the *body* as a passive muscle exerciser for toning very specific areas, and on the *face* to improve facial contour. It is used in cases where taking active exercise may not be possible for medical reasons;
- **Effect**   The muscles which are stimulated contract and relax involuntarily, which improves muscle tone and prevents atrophy. The muscular movements increase the rate of flow of blood and lymph;

- **Apparatus**   The machine supplies an interrupted direct current, where the size (intensity) of the current rises and falls rapidly so that the current *pulsates*. The pulses last for such a short time that chemical effects will be too small to cause discomfort. Each brief pulse is followed by a longer interval when no current is flowing. The pulses of current pass through the body between two electrodes applied at different points on the skin over the muscle being treated. The interrupted direct current is produced by an electronic oscillator with a make-and-break circuit.

  The older type of faradic machine contained a *faradic coil* to reduce the frequency of the mains AC to around 30 Hz, which is low enough to stimulate muscle;
- **Safety precautions**   The current must not change in intensity too rapidly or the pain receptors of the skin may be stimulated in addition to the muscle;
- **Hazards**   The treatment is ineffective in the case of very obese clients as the electrical pulses cannot penetrate the thick layer of subcutaneous fat to reach the muscle.

A photograph of the machine in use will be found on page 100.

Galvanic machine

- **Purpose**   It is used on the face to introduce chemicals into the intact skin during *iontophoresis*, and for skin cleansing during *desincrustation*. It is used on the body to treat areas of hard fat;
- **Effect**   The direct (galvanic) current produces a chemical effect within the skin. Around the negative electrode (*cathode*) there will be an excess of *hydroxyl* ions resulting in increased pH. The effect of this increased *alkalinity* is to reduce the oiliness of the skin, and to break down the keratin of the dead skin scales. These effects are used in desincrustation.

  When used for iontophoresis, positive or negative ions thought to have therapeutic effects may be driven into the skin. This will occur if positive ions in solution are placed on the skin below the positive electrode (anode), while negative ions are placed below the cathode. The similarly charged electrode will repel the ions so that they are driven below the skin surface;
- **Apparatus**   The galvanic machine produces a direct current by means of a rectifier which converts the mains AC into DC. A smoothing capacitor produces a steady DC from the rectified current. Two metal electrodes connected by leads to the machine are placed on the skin. The current travels through the skin from one electrode to the other. The *active* electrode is placed over a pad soaked in electrolyte solution, and is the cathode when used for

desincrustation. When used for iontophoresis the active electrode may be either the anode or the cathode. The other electrode is wrapped in damp lint and held by the client. The damp pads improve the electrical contact between the electrodes and the skin;

- **Safety precautions**   The client's skin should be washed *immediately* after the treatment to dilute and remove the alkaline solution produced by electrolysis, which will soften the skin and cause redness. The size of the current should be changed gradually, and electrodes must not be suddenly lifted from the skin while the machine is operating. Sudden changes in current may cause muscles to contract violently. The pad should be evenly soaked with the electrolyte solution to prevent galvanic burns. The size of the current should be reduced where bony regions of the face are being treated. The absence of softer tissues causes reduced resistance to the current and galvanic burns may occurs;

- **Hazards**   If the current size is too great a galvanic burn may be produced in the skin due to high alkalinity. If the two electrodes are allowed to touch while the machine is operating, *short circuiting* may occur and damage the machine.

A photograph of the machine in use will be found on page 136.

Interferential machine

- **Purpose**   It is used on the body, but not on the face, to stimulate muscle contraction;
- **Effect**   It causes muscles to contract and speeds up the rate of blood and lymph flow. It causes little skin heating and affects motor nerves, but not sensory nerves, so there is little skin discomfort during treatment;
- **Apparatus**   The machine contains two oscillators which produce two high frequency alternating currents of slightly different frequencies. As these two currents flow through the same region of tissue, they mix to produce an interferential current whose frequency is the difference between the frequencies of the currents actually supplied. The difference between the frequencies of the two currents is usually between 0 and 100 Hz, so the interferential current is of low frequency. Interferential currents with frequencies at the lower end of the range (0 to 10 Hz) will cause muscle contraction. Currents with the higher frequencies (close to 100 Hz) do not cause muscle contraction, but increase the rate of blood and lymph flow and have an analgesic effect;

Safety precautions and hazards   The low current intensity makes interferential therapy a completely safe method of treatment.

A photograph of the machine in use will be found on page 240.

High frequency machine

- **Purpose**   On the face, the direct method is used to treat seborrhoea (greasy skin), while the indirect method increases the rate of blood and lymph flow through the skin and is beneficial for dry skins;
- **Effects**   It warms the skin, the high frequency current producing resistance heating which causes vasodilation. The ozone produced by the machine when using the direct method has an antiseptic action on the skin and may improve acne. These high frequency currents do not stimulate motor nerves to cause muscle contraction;
- **Apparatus**   The machine contains an oscillator which changes the frequency of the current from the 50 Hz of the mains supply to above 100 000 Hz. The voltage of the current is also increased to 2000 volts by a transformer, but the current is small and remains in the skin; it does not penetrate into the deeper tissues. A rectifier and capacitor convert the AC mains supply to the steady DC current required by the oscillator.
  In the direct method of treatment, frequent very short pulses of current flash across a spark gap inside the glass electrode which is placed on the skin. In the indirect method, the client holds the metal rod electrode (saturator) from which the current passes through the client's skin to the therapist who is carrying out manual massage on the face of the client. In both methods the current returns to the machine through the air and salon furniture to complete the circuit;
- **Safety precautions**   Metal objects such as jewellery should be removed as they can become hot enough through resistance heating to cause a burn. Electrodes should be disinfected with ethanol (surgical spirit) before and after use. The intensity should be reduced to zero and the current switched off before the electrode, or therapist's hand, is lifted from the skin. Sudden breaks in the circuit cause the client to feel discomfort. Shorter treatment times are required for dry mature skins;
- **Hazards**   The ozone produced during the sparking which occurs in the direct method is poisonous at high concentrations. The sparking itself may cause alarm in some clients.

A photograph of the machine in use applying the direct method will be found on page 254.

A photograph showing the indirect method will be found on page 267.

Epilation

Diathermy machine

- **Purpose**   It is used for the removal of unwanted facial hair;
- **Effect**   The hair root is destroyed by heat within the hair follicle. The hair can then be removed, and no further hairs will grow in the follicle;
- **Apparatus**   It resembles the high frequency machine described above. It produces an alternating current with a very high frequency of around 27 million hertz. This current is directed to the hair root from the tip of a needle electrode inserted down the hair follicle. Intense heat develops at the tip of the needle which destroys the matrix of the hair root.
- **Safety precautions**   It is essential when placing the needle that its tip should be in contact with the hair root. Regrowth of the hair will occur if the root is not destroyed;
- **Hazards**   Infection and scarring of the skin can occur if the upper part of the hair follicle is damaged by an incorrectly placed needle, or by moving the needle in or out of the follicle while the current is still flowing through it.

A photograph of the machine in use will be found on page 56.

Galvanic electrolysis

- **Purpose**   It is used for the removal of unwanted facial hairs, but is a slower method than diathermy;
- **Effect**   The region round the tip of the needle electrode inserted down the hair follicle becomes very alkaline. The hair root is therefore destroyed by a chemical (galvanic) burn, and can be removed from the follicle;
- **Apparatus**   A steady direct electric current is applied to the skin from a galvanic machine. It passes from an anode, consisting of a sponge pad soaked in salt solution, to a cathode which is the electrolysis needle inserted into the hair follicle. The tissue fluid acts as the electrolyte, conducting the current from anode to cathode;
- **Safety precautions**   The needle electrode must be placed correctly so that its tip is in contact with the hair root;
- **Hazards**   Galvanic burns may occur through over-treating a small area of skin. The positions of the sponge anode and needle cathode must not be too close together.

Blend machine

This method of epilation combines the galvanic method with diathermy, so that the hair root is destroyed by a combination of galvanic burn and resistance heating.

Contra-indications for electrical stimulation therapy

A number of disorders of the cardio-vascular system contra-indicate this type of treatment, eg heart disorders (angina), abnormal pulse rates, high or low blood pressure, varicose veins and highly vascular skin conditions. Skin lesions such as bruises, scar tissue, inflammation or pustules, and excessively loose, fragile, or hypersensitive skins also contra-indicate treatment.

Facial treatments are contra-indicated where the client suffers from asthma, migraine or sinus disorders. Neuritis, neuralgia, or the presence of much metalwork in teeth or dentures may also contra-indicate treatment.

Electrical stimulation treatments should not be applied to the abdomen during menstruation or pregnancy.

Inverse square law

All heat therapy and ultra-violet therapy treatments apply the principle of the inverse square law. This law states that the intensity of the radiation at the skin surface depends on the inverse square of its distance from the radiation source.

For example, if the distance of a radiant heat lamp from the skin is doubled, the intensity of the infra-red radiation on the skin is only one quarter ($\frac{1}{2}^2$) of the original intensity. Similarly, the intensity of the radiation on the skin 50 cm away from the radiant heat lamp is four times the radiation received when the lamp is placed 100 cm away.

The *duration* of a treatment is also determined by the inverse square law. To produce the same effect as exposure for one minute to an ultra-violet lamp placed 50 cm away from the skin, the client needs to be exposed for four minutes when the lamp is 100 cm away. The formula that can be used for calculating treatment duration is:-

$$\text{new time} = \text{original time} \times \left(\frac{\text{new distance}}{\text{original distance}}\right)^2$$

$$\text{eg new time} = 1 \text{ minute} \times \left(\frac{100 \text{ cm}}{50 \text{ cm}}\right)^2$$

$$= 1 \text{ minute} \times \left(\frac{2}{1}\right)^2$$

$$= 4 \text{ minutes}$$

Heat therapy

A number of appliances used in beauty therapy treatments involve the *heating effect* of an electric current as it flows through a *high resistance* wire which is present in the *heating element*. In some appliances the heating element produces steam by heating water.

Facial steamer

- **Purpose** It is used for preheating the skin, to aid the absorption of materials applied subsequently as masks or face packs. It is also used for deep cleansing of the skin of the face;
- **Effect** It has a *diaphoretic* effect, ie increases sweating. It causes vasodilation, increasing the rate of flow of blood and lymph. If the steamer also produces ozone its antiseptic action on the skin may improve acne;
- **Apparatus** An electric heating element, containing a *nichrome* high resistance wire, is present in a kettle in which distilled water is boiled. Distilled water is used to prevent scaling in the kettle. The steam produced passes into a pipe where it is mixed with air, and condenses forming a fine spray which is directed onto the client's face. The steamer may contain a high pressure mercury vapour lamp producing ultra-violet radiation which converts molecular oxygen in the air to ozone;
- **Safety precautions** The client's eyes can be protected by damp cotton wool pads;
- **Hazards** The steamer should be isolated from other electrical equipment as the presence of water makes the occurrence of electric shocks from faulty equipment more likely. The steam treatment may make the client's pulse rate rise and lower the blood pressure which could cause a client who already had abnormally low blood pressure to faint.

A photograph of the steamer in use will be found on page 181.

Steam bath

- **Purpose** For preheating the body prior to massage, and deep cleansing the skin;
- **Effect** The heat has a diaphoretic effect, and increases the rate of flow of blood and lymph due to vasodilation. Activity of the sebaceous glands increases, and muscular relaxation is promoted;
- **Apparatus** An electric heating element in a water tank heats water to 50–55 °C. The temperature is regulated by a thermostat and there is a thermal cut-out device in case the water level in the tank falls below the level of the heating element. The tank is contained in a thermally insulated cabinet from which the client's head will project. Warm air with a relative humidity of 95% surrounds the rest of the client's body;
- **Safety precautions** A towel soaked in cold water should be placed round the client's neck to keep steam away from the head. The slatted seat over the water tank should be covered with a towel to protect the skin of the buttocks. The therapist should make regular temperature and pulse checks throughout the treatment. There should be an internal door

handle to allow the client to come out of the cabinet immediately if she feels any discomfort during the treatment. A cooling down period of at least half-an-hour should elapse before a client is allowed to leave after treatment;

- **Hazards** Clients with low blood pressure, or who are on a low calorie slimming diet could faint during the treatment.

Sauna

- **Purpose**   To induce a feeling of relaxation followed by vigour;
- **Effect** The heat increases the rate of flow of blood and lymph due to vasodilation. There is a fall in blood pressure and the pulse rate rises. Sweating is increased;
- **Apparatus** The sauna is a heated wooden cabin where steam is made. The cabin walls are both thermally insulating and water absorbing. The cabin contains a stove inside which a thermostatically controlled electric element heats rocks. Water is poured onto the hot rocks to create steam. An air inlet is present just above floor level and there is an outlet near the top of the cabin. Warm air circulates by convection. The relative humidity of the air remains low at around 10%. An air temperature between 80 and 100 °C is usual for a ten minute treatment. Wooden benches on which the clients lie are provided in the cabin;
- **Safety precautions**   Clients should be watched for symptoms of faintness during the treatment. It should be followed by a cool shower, or a cooling down period of at least half an hour;
- **Hazards**   Heating elements can cause fires and burns and must be heavily guarded. Clients often over-estimate their ability to tolerate heat.

A photograph of a sauna will be found on page 201.

Far infra-red lamp

- **Purpose**   It can be used for preheating the skin;
- **Effect**   The heat rays produced do not penetrate below the epidermis of the skin, but the heat absorbed at the surface will spread downwards by conduction. The heat increases the rate of blood and lymph flow in the skin, and erythema results from vasodilation in the skin capillaries. Far infra-red rays are non-irritant and treatments of up to 30 minutes' duration can be tolerated;
- **Apparatus**   A coil of high resistance wire is embedded in fireclay to form the heating element. When an electric current passes through the wire it heats up and passes on the heat to the fireclay by conduction. The heating element produces only invisible *far infra-red* rays which have a wavelength of around 4000 nm (or 40 000 Angstrom units

(Å) where 10 Å = 1 nanometre). Far infra-red rays thus have a long wavelength. The rays are reflected and focused by a polished metal concave reflector behind the element. The front of the lamp is covered by a wire guard. The lamp takes between 5 and 15 minutes to heat up;

- **Safety precautions** The client's skin must be clean and free from greasy preparations. Goggles should be worn to protect the eyes when the lamp is used on the face. Treatment should never be continued for longer than 30 minutes or burning of the skin may occur;
- **Hazards** As the far infra-red radiation is invisible, it is impossible to tell by its appearance whether the lamp is switched on or off. There is thus the danger of burns due to touching the hot lamp. Too frequent use of these lamps can cause *cataract* by damaging the eye lens, and *mottling* of the skin with a network of dark brown lines.

These far-infra-red lamps have been largely replaced in beauty salons by radiant heat lamps which produce mainly near-infra-red radiation.

Radiant heat lamp

- **Purpose** To relieve muscle tension;
- **Effects** The heat rays produced penetrate more deeply into the body reaching the muscles. As the skin is warmed the rate of blood and lymph flow increases, and erythema occurs as a result of vasodilation. Sweating increases, and muscles relax relieving tension at the joints;
- **Apparatus** It consists of a glass bulb containing a tungsten filament which becomes hot when an electric current passes through it. The radiation emitted by the filament contains *near infra-red* of around 1000 nm (10 000 Å) wavelength, some white (visible) light, and a small amount of ultra-violet. The bulb has a red glass filter which allows only the infra-red and visible red light to pass through it. The ultra-violet rays and the other colours in the visible white light are stopped by the filter. The bulb is filled with an inert gas at low pressure, and the top half of the bulb is coated with polished metal to reflect the radiation downwards. The lamp has an electric power rating of 200 to 250 watts, and heats up immediately it is switched on;
- **Safety precautions** The client's skin must be clean and free from greasy preparations. The distance of the client from the lamp should be such that erythema does not occur until 10 minutes after the treatment starts. The application time should be short or the skin will burn. The lamp face should be parallel to the skin surface being irradiated so that a uniform heating effect is produced. The client's eyes should be protected by goggles to prevent cataract;

- **Hazards**   The glass bulb becomes very hot in use and will burn the skin if it is touched. The bulb must not be dropped, knocked, or splashed with water when hot or the glass will break. The bulb will then *implode* due to the partial vacuum inside it.

Figure 15.6
Infra-red bulb

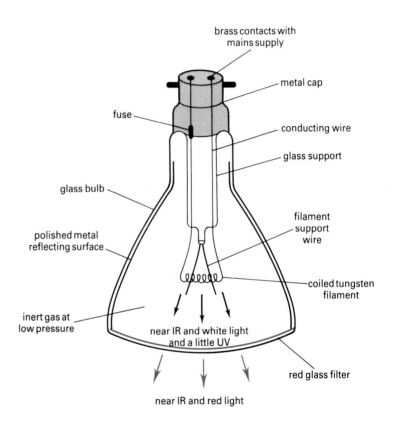

Contra-indications for heat therapy treatments

Cardio-vascular disorders (angina and high or low blood pressure), epilepsy, asthma and migraine are all contra-indicated. Diabetics, who have a reduced sensitivity to heat and could be unaware that skin burning was taking place, should not receive heat therapy. Other contra-indications are the recent consumption of alcohol or a heavy meal, being on a low calorie slimming diet, and menstruation or pregnancy.

Ultra-violet therapy

Ultra-violet (UV) is electromagnetic radiation used in beauty therapy for its property of producing a 'suntan'. It is invisible, with a wavelength range shorter than that of visible light. It is divided into three regions, UVA (wavelength 400–320 nm), UVB (wavelength 320–290 nm) and UVC (wavelength 290–100 nm). UVC radiation with a wavelength shorter than 250 nm will convert molecular oxygen into ozone.

The UVA radiation will pass through ordinary glass, but UVB and UVC will not. UVA and UVB both pass through Perspex (plastic). All three types of UV radiation will pass through quartz glass. UVA rays penetrate the skin most deeply, reaching to the lower levels of the dermis. UVB rays penetrate to the stratum basale of the epidermis, stimulating cell division. UVC rays only reach the outermost layers of the epidermis.

Some ultra-violet lamps produce UVC rays as well as UVA and UVB rays, while others produce mainly UVA radiation.

Low pressure mercury vapour (LPMV) tubes produce mainly UVA radiation, not more than 1% being UVB. The

Figure 15.7
Low pressure mercury vapour tube

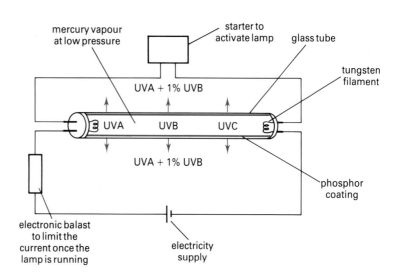

electric current passing through the mercury vapour inside these tubes produces some UVC, but this is absorbed by the special coating of *phosphors* on the inside of the tube and converted into UVA radiation which can pass out through the glass tube. *R-UVA* tubes have an internal reflector to boost the amount of UVA. The amount of UVB is reduced to 0.1%.

High pressure mercury vapour (HPMV or solarium) lamps

produce all three types of ultra-violet radiation. These lamps are often bulb-shaped and contain a quartz tube of mercury vapour at high pressure which produces the ultra-violet radiation when an electric current passes through it. The lamp is fitted with a filter to stop UVC rays, and to reduce the amount of UVB radiation to below 1% of the total.

Sunbeds and canopies

- **Purpose**   To produce a whole body tan;
- **Effects**   These are entirely cosmetic. The tanning effect is due to increased activity of the melanocytes in the epidermis of the skin. Slight erythema may preceed tanning. The skin is not protected against the UVB radiation in sunlight.
- **Apparatus**   The sunbed and canopy contain LPMV tubes so almost all the radiation emitted is UVA. The tubes in the sunbed are covered by a Perspex sheet over which the client lies. The canopy is supported from the ceiling at an adjustable height above the sunbed. A timer switch is incorporated, the safest type switching off the radiation automatically at the end of the selected treatment period.
- **Safety precautions**   The length of the treatment should be related to the amount of previous exposure to ultra-violet radiation, and to the client's skin type. The inverse square law applies, so the distance of the canopy from the client's body must be carefully controlled. Goggles should be worn by both the client and the therapist to protect the eyes. Cotton wool pads or sunglasses provide insufficient protection from reflected radiation. Creams or perfume, which can increase the skin's sensitivity to ultra-violet radiation, should not be applied to the skin before the treatment.
- **Hazards**   Sunburn and conjunctivitis will result from over-exposure to ultra-violet radiation. Premature ageing of the skin due to loss of elasticity, and the development of skin cancers, can result from over-exposure to UVB radiation. A photograph of the sunbed canopy in use will be found on page 194.

Individual tanning units

- **Purpose**   These units are used for tanning the face;
- **Apparatus**   They contain HPMV lamps which produce all three types of ultra-violet radiation;
- **Safety precautions**   Goggles must be worn to protect the eyes as UV rays cause conjunctivitis;
- **Effects and hazards**   As for sunbeds.

Contra-indications for ultra-violet therapy

Pregnancy, a hypersensitive skin prone to sunburn, and a susceptibility to cold sores (Herpes simplex) are all contra-indications for ultra-violet therapy. It is also inadvisable for clients taking drugs which cause photosensitivity, eg tetracycline.

Self-assessment questions

1   List **three** machines used in electrical stimulation therapy which contain an electric motor.

2   State the purpose of each of the following electrical devices:

(a) rectifier;
(b) electronic oscillator;
(c) step-up transformer;
(d) capacitor.

3   Distinguish between iontophoresis and desincrustation. Which type of machine is used in both of these processes?

4   In each case, name a machine used in beauty therapy which features the following:

(a) a partial vacuum;
(b) an electromagnet;
(c) an electromotive effect;
(d) resistance heating.

5   List **six** contra-indications for facial electrical stimulation therapy.

6   Describe the safety precautions you would carry out for a client having a sauna treatment:

(a) before starting the treatment;
(b) during the treatment;
(c) after the treatment.

7   List the beauty therapy treatments which necessitate protecting the client's eyes.

8   What are the effects of a radiant heat lamp on the skin?

9   Compare the type of radiation emitted from a low pressure mercury vapour tube and a high pressure mercury vapour lamp.

10   Explain the differences in the way a high frequency machine is used for the direct and indirect methods of treatment.

CHAPTER 16   *Cosmetic Preparations*

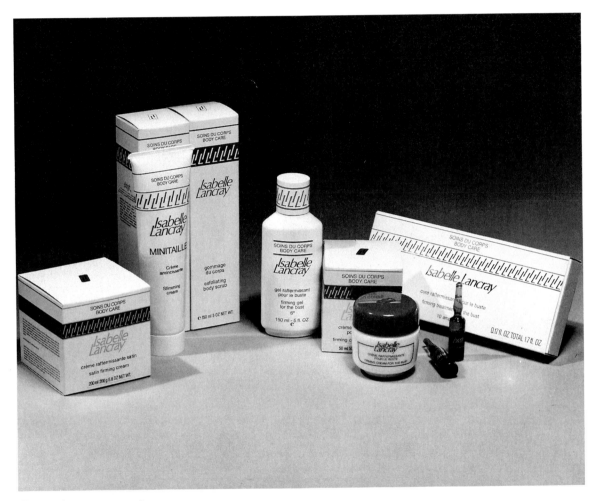

Beauty therapy preparations

Cosmetic preparations are intended to improve the appearance, or alter it to promote attractiveness. The main effects of cosmetics on the skin are to (a) **remove dirt;** (b) **alter the colouring;** (c) **retain water** in the epidermis and *delay* wrinkling; and (d) **protect** the skin from the harmful effects of *ultra-violet* radiation.

The wide variety of chemical substances used in cosmetic preparations have different effects on the skin, and in the past some of these substances have proved to be hazardous to the health of the users. There is now an *EEC directive* regulating the use of substances in cosmetics. The hormones oestrogen and progesterone, for example, may not be included in any cosmetic preparation. Certain other substances are only permitted in quantities below a specified maximum, eg hydroquinone must not exceed 2% of a skin bleaching cream, and para-dye must not exceed 1.7% in a hair tint.

Many of the chemicals used in cosmetics are listed in the *EEC Code*, and have *E numbers* like the food additives. The E numbers are given for just a few of the cosmetic ingredients listed in later sections of the chapter. In the case of *lipstick*, some of each application will inevitably reach the alimentary canal, being swallowed with food and drink. The same restrictions must therefore apply to its ingredients as apply to the food additives. As *eye cosmetics* come into contact with the delicate eye membrane (conjunctiva), stringent regulations apply here, particularly to the pigments permitted to colour the cosmetics.

A number of terms are used to describe the action of cosmetic preparations on the skin. These terms, with examples of the chemicals involved, are listed in the following section.

Descriptive terms applied to cosmetic ingredients

Emulsions

A cosmetic emulsion, or cream, is a suspension of droplets of one liquid in another (see Chapter 1) where the two liquid phases are *oil* and *water*. The chemicals used to form the oil phase are either esters (produced from organic acids neutralised by alcohols) or hydrocarbons (mineral oils and paraffin wax).

The **esters** employed are oils, fats and waxes of vegetable and animal origin:

- The non-volatile or *'fixed' vegetable oils* which are used include almond, olive, coconut and castor oils. Because they are unsaturated (see Chapter 7), they are liable to go rancid. They are insoluble in ethanol (alcohol) with the exception of castor oil;
- The *vegetable fat* cocoa butter from crushed cacao seeds is often included in cosmetic emulsions as it melts at body temperature and, being a saturated fat, does not go rancid;
- Carnauba *wax*, which is scraped from the leaf surfaces of the plant, makes cosmetic creams firmer in consistency;
- Waxes of *animal* origin such as beeswax, lanolin and spermaceti are also used. *Lanolin* comes from sheep's wool, and is a sensitiser, so it may cause dermatitis in some people. *Spermaceti* is obtained from the mixed oils of the sperm whale and consists mainly of cetyl palmitate and cetyl

myristate, which are esters formed from cetyl alcohol and fatty acids.

Hydrocarbons are not true oils and waxes, but are still used in the preparation of emulsions. The *mineral* oils and waxes used are obtained from petroleum. They are liquid paraffin, petroleum jelly and hard paraffin wax. *Synthetic* waxes (eg Lanette wax) derived from cetyl alcohol are also used as components of cosmetic creams.

The *emulsifying agents* (emulsifiers) used in making cosmetic creams include soaps, cetrimide (a cationic soapless detergent), lecithin (E322 from egg yolk and soya beans) and synthetic emulsifying waxes (Lanette). A soap may be made *in situ* from a mixture of a base and free fatty acids. Triethanolamine with stearic acid, and borax with beeswax (which contains some free fatty acids), produce such in situ soaps.

Emulsions can be *stabilised* (so that the oil and water phases do not separate out on storage) by adding gums, protein, starch or synthetic resin (eg PVP resin). When a cosmetic cream is applied to the skin, the two phases of the emulsion, which were homogeneously mixed, separate out. The water evaporates while the oil remains as a surface coating.

Humectants

A humectant is a substance which **attracts water vapour** from the atmosphere, ie it is *hygroscopic*. It will prevent a cream from drying out when exposed to air and thus becoming difficult to apply. *Glycerol* (E422), *sorbitol* and *propylene glycol* are added to creams as humectants. Glycerol must not be placed neat on dry skin or it removes water from the epidermis causing severe dehydration. It must always be applied with water.

Emollients

An emollient is a substance which **reduces water loss** from the dead stratum corneum forming the skin surface, thus preventing it from drying and cracking. By maintaining the water content of the epidermis it produces the emollient (ie *softening*) effect on the skin. *Fats, oils* and *waxes* are emollients as they form a waterproof film over the skin surface, and greatly reduce evaporation from it. The skin's natural emollient is the wax sebum.

Astringents

An astringent is a substance which has a **tightening** effect on the skin, making it look less flaccid. Some astringents (eg *ethanol*) are volatile liquids which cool the skin as they evaporate. *Fruit* and *vegetable* juices (lemon, carrot, cucumber) and *orange flower water* contain mild astringents. Stronger astringent effects are obtained from *witch-hazel, lactic acid, menthol* and *potassium aluminium sulphate* (alum). Stronger astringents should not be used on hypersensitive or dry mature skins as they are dehydrating.

Cleansers

A cleanser **removes** the skin's surface film of **sebum, sweat** and **scales,** together with soluble and particulate dirt and its associated bacteria and fungi. Water alone removes soluble dirt, but oily dirt must be emulsified by using a *detergent* with water. *Sodium stearate, potassium palmitate* (soft soap) and *lauryl sulphates* (soapless) are suitable detergents for use on skin. *Cream* cleansers consist of w/o emulsions where oily dirt on the skin mixes readily with the oily continuous phase, and particulate dirt adheres to the emulsion. Where the dirt to be removed is largely stale heavy make-up with a high wax content, the *mineral oil* liquid paraffin is an effective cleanser.

Natural clays or earths mixed into a paste and applied as a face mask can act as a cleanser. Surface dirt adheres to the inside of the paste mask, and is removed with the hardened mask at the end of the treatment. *Kaolin* (china clay from decayed granite), *bentonite* (a volcanic clay) and *fuller's earth* (aluminium silicate clay) used in these pastes must be *steam-sterilized* to destroy any spores of the *Bacillus tetani* bacterium which causes tetanus (lockjaw).

Desquamators (exfoliators)

A desquamator **removes** some of the outermost layers of the **stratum corneum** from the skin epidermis. *Comedones* (blackheads) and *milia* (whiteheads) are removed, and deeper cleansing occurs. *Soap* solutions applied with a facial brush, or skin massage with an abrasive (eg *oatmeal* granules or crushed *nuts*), are used for facial desquamation. *Pumice*, which is a stronger abrasive, can be used on the thick skin of the soles of the feet where callosities occur.

Lubricants

A lubricant allows other **surfaces to slide easily** over the skin, providing slip. Many of the machines used in beauty therapy treatments have applicators which are moved over the skin, and during manual massage the therapist's hands must slide freely and painlessly on the client's skin. There are two main types of lubricant: those based on powder, and those with a cream foundation.

- *Talc* (magnesium silicate), the *metallic soaps* (magnesium and zinc stearates) and *rice starch* are powder lubricants. These fine powders should not be shaken into the air as they damage the lungs when breathed in. Talc, like other minerals, must be *steam-sterilized* to destroy tetanus spores;
- Cream lubricants contain a high proportion of *petroleum jelly* in their oil phase, and silicones (derived from sand) are added for extra slip.
- Unscented *mineral oil* (liquid paraffin) is an excellent lubricant for massage.

Barriers

One type of barrier forms an impervious layer over the skin surface which **protects** the skin against dirt and some harmful chemicals, and is resistant to water. *Mineral oil* is the major component of *protective barrier creams*. An effective barrier cream should have a pH between 5.6 and 6.5, and should be non-sticky and stable to avoid the need for frequent re-application. Its protection against detergent solutions is short-lived however, as they will emulsify mineral oils as well as other oils and waxes in the cream.

Another type of barrier, called a *sunscreen,* is used on the skin to protect it against ultra-violet radiation. Talc, chalk, kaolin, magnesium oxide and zinc oxide, in a cream or lotion base, provide a mechanical barrier to prevent all types of ultra-violet radiation reaching the skin, so *tanning* cannot occur. Barriers are available which filter out the more damaging UVB radiation of shorter wavelength, but allow UVA radiation to reach the skin and cause tanning. *Para-aminobenzoic acid* acts as this type of barrier, but it can be a sensitiser and cause dermatitis in some people.

Opacifiers

An opacifier is a substance used to make a transparent or translucent cosmetic preparation *opaque,* so that visible light cannot pass through it and be reflected from the skin surface. Opacifiers are used in preparations formulated to **cover skin blemishes** such as scars, naevi or acne pustules. *Kaolin, titanium dioxide* (E171) and *zinc oxide* are all white mineral powders which are good opacifiers.

Colourants

Colourants are used in cosmetics to provide an overall skin-coloured **tint**, or to **highlight** particular features such as cheeks, eyes, lips and nails:

- *Soluble dyes* form coloured solutions with one of the liquids present in cosmetics, ie water, ethanol or oil;
- *Pigments* occur as solid coloured particles which are insoluble in any of these three liquids;
- *Lakes* are solid coloured particles obtained synthetically by adsorbing dyes onto the surface of insoluble metal oxides or hydroxides. For example, the dye cochineal adsorbed onto aluminium hydroxide forms the lake called *carmine.*

The insoluble pigments and lakes are usually used in cosmetic preparations as they neither 'run' by dissolving in sweat, tears or rain, nor permanently colour the skin by being adsorbed onto keratin molecules or dissolving in tissue fluid.

Natural pigments are inorganic materials and are non-sensitising, although lead- and mercury-containing pigments are highly *toxic* and not permitted in cosmetics. Examples of natural pigments that are used are *carbon black* (charcoal from burnt wood) and the mineral ores *chrome green, ultramarine* and yellow iron oxide (*ochre*).

Dyes used in cosmetics are mainly synthetic materials, although cochineal obtained from the Mexican cochinellid beetle is of animal origin. *Azo dyes* are synthetic dyes derived from the coal tar product aniline. Azo dyes are sensitisers and cross-sensitisers, but are commonly used to form lakes as they provide a wide colour range. Cochineal (E120) is also a sensitiser.

Diaphoretics

Diaphoretics are substances that **increase sweating** by providing a waterproof and thermally insulating layer over the skin. A layer of *wax*, *latex* (rubber) or *polyvinyl acetate* (PVA) resin applied as a face mask has this effect.

Antiperspirants

An antiperspirant **reduces** the flow of **sweat** to the skin surface from the sweat glands, so it has the opposite effect to a diaphoretic. Antiperspirants may function by increasing the permeability of the sweat duct wall, so that less of the sweat secreted reaches the surface pore. *Aluminium chlorhydrate* is the compound usually used as an antiperspirant, but it can cause contact dermatitis in some people, particularly if the skin has been damaged by removing unwanted hair.

Deodorants

A deodorant **removes unpleasant smells** (*body odour*) from the skin. The odour is caused by the breakdown of the sweat and sebum of the skin's 'acid mantle' and the fatty materials in stale make-up. When triglycerides are broken down by *bacteria*, free fatty acids are produced which are largely responsible for the unpleasant smell. Apocrine sweat produced in the axillae contains small amounts of protein and sugars which are also broken down by bacteria. Unpleasant ammonia-related compounds are produced from the proteins.

The bacterial activity on the skin can be reduced by *antiseptics* which prevent the bacteria multiplying. Hexachlorophene which used to be used as a deodorant is no longer thought to be non-toxic, and *hexamine* has replaced it. The amount of antiseptic allowed in a skin deodorant is controlled by EEC regulations.

Depilatories

A depilatory **removes unwanted hair** from the upper lip, chin, axillae and legs in women. The condition of terminal hair growth on the upper lip in women is *hirsuties*. The temporary removal of unwanted hair is known as *depilation*. It removes only the part of the hair shaft which projects from the skin, and does not destroy the hair root so the hair regrows.

Chemical depilatories break down the keratin forming the hair shaft by destroying its *peptide* and *disulphide* bonds. This weakens the hair sufficiently for it to break at skin surface level. Chemical depilatories contain *calcium thioglycollate* made alkaline by *calcium hydroxide* to give a pH between 10 and 12.5. Both these chemicals attack disulphide bonds, and the alkaline calcium hydroxide destroys the peptide bonds in the polypeptide chains of the keratin. Because of their action on keratin, chemical depilatories also damage the stratum corneum of the skin epidermis.

Depilatory waxes are used to remove hair from the legs. The melted paraffin wax applied to the skin solidifies and the hairs become embedded in it. When the solidified wax is stripped off the hairs break at skin surface level.

Perfumes

Perfumes add **fragrance** because they are absorbed by the outer layers of the skin. They are also used to cover the less pleasant smell of the oily components of skin cosmetics. A perfume consists of a blend of pleasantly smelling *volatile* plant products dissolved in *methanol*, to which *fixatives* are added to cause the scented molecules to evaporate at equal rates, so that the balance of the perfume does not change as it is used.

The volatile plant products used in perfumes are *essential oils* (bergamot, rose, citrus, lavender, jasmine etc), *resins* such as pine terpenes, and *balsams* such as myrrh which are mixtures of resins and essential oils. Unlike fixed plant oils, essential oils are *soluble* in the alcohols ethanol and methanol. The fixatives are usually *animal products* (ambergris, musk, civet and castor), but synthetic fixatives such as *benzyl benzoate* and *phthalates* may also be used. Some balsams and essential oils, particularly bergamot and citrus oils, are sensitisers and photosensitisers. Perfume should never be placed on the skin before sunbathing or ultra-violet treatment because of the photosensitisation risk.

Preservatives

A preservative is added to a cosmetic preparation to **prevent** large numbers of **micro-organisms** becoming established in it, and being transferred to the skin when it is applied. The vegetable oils, starches and proteins in cosmetics are a source of food for bacteria and fungal spores present in the air. Mineral oils cannot be used as a food source by micro-organisms and do not require preservatives. The preservatives added to cosmetic preparations include *para-* and *ethyl-hydroxybenzoates* (parabens and nipagin respectively) at a concentration of 0.2%, *benzoic acid* (E210), *cetrimide* and *essential oils*. All of these compounds may act as sensitisers causing dermatitis in some people. People with asthma may be particularly sensitive to benzoic acid.

Antioxidants

An antioxidant will **prevent** the **unsaturated oils** in a cosmetic preparation becoming **rancid**. This occurs when the double bonds ($C = C$) in their molecules are attacked by atmospheric oxygen to release unpleasant smelling fatty acids. *Ascorbic acid* (Vitamin C E300) and *lecithin* are used as antioxidants in most cosmetic creams. *Sodium sulphite* is used as an antioxidant in para dye base to prevent it darkening in the tube due to premature oxidation.

Bleaches

Hydroquinone is a skin bleach which acts by reducing the activity of the skin melanocytes so that less dark melanin pigment is produced. Hydroquinone is applied at a maximum strength of 2%, but it acts as a severe skin irritant on a number of people even at this low concentration, and these preparations may be a health hazard.

Cosmetic preparations for the face

Emollient cream (skin conditioner)

These creams are used on the face overnight and have a **softening effect** on the skin. They may be o/w or w/o emulsions containing spermaceti and lanolin, together with vegetable oils for their emollient action.

Moisturising cream

These creams are used on the face overnight or as a make-up base for dry mature skins. They are o/w emulsions containing a mixture of natural and synthetic waxes which will coat the skin to **reduce water loss** from the epidermis. Added silicone helps the cream to spread rapidly and evenly over the skin. The cream contains a preservative (paraben or nipagin), and a humectant to maintain its water content.

Moisturising creams are particularly valuable for all black skins and for ageing white skins. The older the skin becomes, the less efficient it is at retaining water. Moisturising creams *do not nourish* the skin as only the blood can supply nutrients. Adding collagen, elastin, lecithin or Vitamin E to the moisturising cream is ineffective as an anti-ageing aid.

Vanishing cream

This is an o/w emulsion used as a day cream and as a foundation for light make-up. Stearic acid and lanette wax or spermaceti are used for the disperse phase and are emulsified by an *in situ* soap formed from triethanolamine and stearic acid. A humectant such as glycerol may be included. A preservative (nipagin) and perfume are added.

A suitable formula for vanishing cream would be:-

Distilled water	73%
Lanette wax	15%
Glycerol	6%
Stearic acid	5%
Triethanolamine	1%
+ preservative and perfume	

Coloured foundation cream

A foundation cream must have good **holding properties** so that powder will cling to it. Adding lanolin to the blend of oils and waxes in the o/w emulsion achieves this. Pigments and lakes are added to give a uniform coloration to the skin of the face when the cream is applied. Titanium dioxide or zinc oxide are included to give opacity, and silicone to make the cream spread quickly and evenly. A preservative is required and perfume may be added.

Cold cream

This is a w/o emulsion which is used as a **skin cleanser**. When applied to the skin, the water in it quickly evaporates, and this has a cooling effect due to the removal of latent heat. Cold cream contains a high percentage of liquid paraffin which is effectively emulsified by an *in situ* soap produced from beeswax and sodium borate.

A suitable formula for a cold cream would be:-

Liquid paraffin	50.0%
Distilled water	32.0%
Beeswax	16.0%
Sodium borate	1.0%
Perfume	0.8%
Nipagin	0.2%

Figure 16.1
Stages of cleansing
Right: removing lipstick
Below left: removing eye make-up
Below centre: cleansing face
Below right: removing excess cleanser

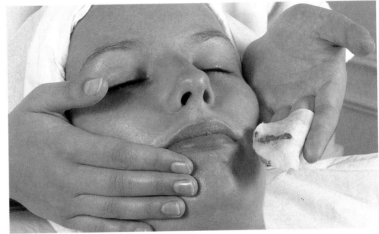

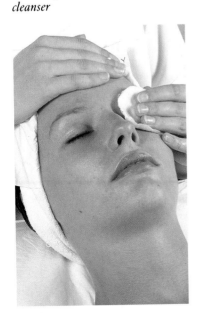
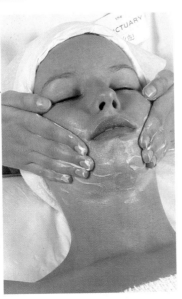
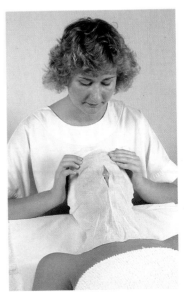

Acid cream (pH balanced cream)

These creams are used to counteract the effects of alkaline soap solutions on the skin by **maintaining a slightly acid pH** of 5.6 to 5.8. An acid cream is an o/w emulsion of the vanishing cream type which contains a weak acid, eg citric acid, and a buffer to maintain the slightly acid pH.

Face packs and masks

The effects on the skin produced by using the various types of face pack or mask may be cleansing, stimulating, astringent, diaphoretic or emollient:

A suitable formula for a clay based face pack would be:-

Distilled water	75%
Bentonite	15%
Glycerol	4%
Sulphonated castor oil	3%
Titanium dioxide	2%
Perfume and preservative	1%

- **Clay based face packs** are cleansing and stimulating in their action. They consist of a paste of clays and water which dries rapidly by evaporation of the water when it is applied to the face and neck. The pack is cleansing as surface dirt from the skin adheres to the clay. The warmth retained by the clay covering causes dilation of the skin blood capillaries, producing the stimulatory effect. The clay base is either *kaolin* or *bentonite*. By the addition of a humectant such as *glycerol* enough water is retained to keep the face pack flexible. *Titanium dioxide* is added to the clay base as a whitener to improve its colour. Perfume and a preservative (paraben) are added. These face packs are most suitable for naturally greasy skins.

- **Astringent masks** are clay based and contract as they dry producing the sensation of skin tightening. The clay base contains the more astringent *fuller's earth* and *kaolin* instead of bentonite. *Lactic acid, witch-hazel* or *orange flower water* are added to increase the astringent effect. These masks should not be used on mature or hypersensitive skins, but they may help in treating acne on a greasy skin;

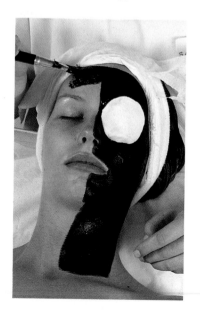

Figure 16.2
Clay base face pack application

- **Warm oil masks** are diaphoretic and emollient in their effect. A gauze mask is fitted over the face and neck leaving holes for the eyes, nostrils and lips. The gauze is then soaked in warm *almond oil*. An infra-red lamp is directed onto the mask, the additional warmth increasing the diaphoretic effect. This type of mask is very suitable for mature dry skins;

- **Wax masks** are diaphoretic and stimulating in their action. *Paraffin wax* blended with *petroleum jelly* or *cetyl alcohol* is melted and brushed onto the face and neck at a temperature very slightly above body temperature. It rapidly solidifies on the skin forming a waterproof layer which is thermally insulating. The blood capillaries of the skin therefore dilate and the sweat glands become more active;

- **Latex masks** are similarly diaphoretic and stimulating in their action. They are applied as an emulsion of *latex* and water. The water evaporates leaving a rubber film over the

Figure 16.3
Eyes must be protected during face pack application

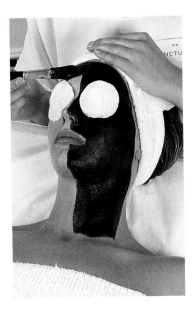

Figure 16.3
Eyes must be protected during face pack application

skin which is waterproof and thermally insulating. Emulsions of synthetic resins, eg *polyvinyl acetate*, can replace latex in this type of mask. Wax and latex or resin masks are all suitable for dry mature skins;

- **Hydrocolloid** (biological) **masks** consist of a sol or gel which is a colloidal suspension of *gums, starches,* or the proteins *gelatin* and *casein*. Polyvinyl synthetic resins may be used instead of the natural colloidal materials. Fruit or vegetable juices can be added to the colloids for particular effects, otherwise the masks are stimulating in their action.

  The sol or melted gel is applied over the face and dries quickly to form a plastic film which does not tighten. The fruit or vegetable juices can be selected to produce a slight astringency (eg cucumber), or to adjust the pH of the skin's surface film. Lemon juice will increase its acidity while carrot juice will reduce it. These hydrocolloid masks are suitable for mature, hypersensitive or dehydrated skins. They are useful for clients who dislike the greater tightening effect of other types of mask, or who prefer to have natural products used on their skin.

Certain *precautions* are necessary when applying face masks. The eyes must be protected by dampened cotton wool pads, and the preparation kept away from the nostrils, mouth and eyes. Clay based masks must always be made from *sterilized* materials because of the danger from tetanus spores.

Face powder

Figure 16.4
Application of face powder

A face powder is a mixture of inert white powders to which pigment is added to produce a flesh tint. Materials are included to give good opacity, lubrication, absorbency and skin adhesion, while providing a smooth matt finish of uniform colour to the

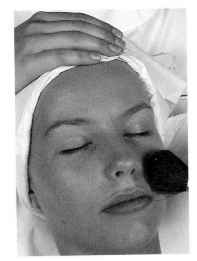

A suitable formula for a face powder would be:-

Sterilized talc	70%
Rice starch	10%
Precipitated chalk	10%
Magnesium stearate	5%
Titanium dioxide	5%
+ colour and perfume	

skin surface. *Titanium dioxide* and *zinc oxide* provide opacity while *talc* and *rice starch* give slip. The absorption of sweat and sebum is well-performed by *magnesium carbonate* and *precipitated chalk*, although chalk has a tendency to cake. *Silicon dioxide* (silica or sand) is anti-caking, but harmful to the lungs when breathed in. The *metallic soaps* (magnesium and zinc stearates) provide good skin adhesion, and *rice starch* gives a smooth matt surface. *Lakes* are the usual colourants. By the addition of a *gum* (karaya or tragacanth) to bind it, the powder can be marketed as a cake.

Rouge and blushers

Red lakes or pigments are added to a variety of bases and applied to the skin of the cheeks as rouge or blusher. The ingredients used in face powder form one type of base, but cream or wax bases may hold the colourants. *Silicone* is added to cream and wax bases to aid smooth application of the blusher.

Lipstick

The base for a lipstick consists of a blend of oils and waxes which allows easy application and good adhesion. *Castor oil* (to hold the colourant), *carnauba wax* (to harden the base), *beeswax*, *spermaceti*, *cetyl alcohol*, *petroleum jelly* and *lanolin* (emollient) are commonly included in lipsticks. *Silicone* increases their ease of application and gives improved staying power. *Pigments* and *lakes* are used as colorants, and adding *titanium dioxide* produces paler shades. Lanolin in lipstick may act as a sensitiser.

A suitable formula for a lipstick would be:-

Beeswax	30%
Petroleum jelly	25%
Carnauba wax	15%
Cetyl alcohol	15%
Castor oil	10%
Lanolin	5%

+ colourants, preservative and silicone

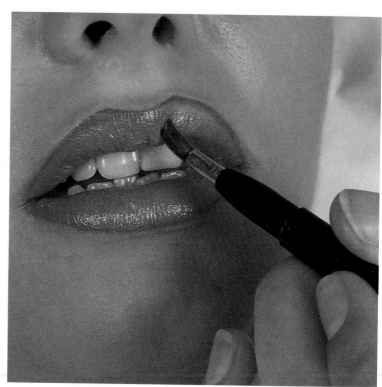

Figure 16.5
Application of lipstick

Mascara

Figure 16.6
Application of mascara

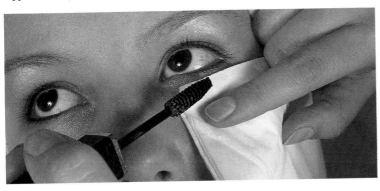

The base for mascara is either a blend of waxes similar to those used in lipsticks, or a w/o emulsion as cream mascara. Inorganic *pigments* which do not irritate the conjunctiva are used as colorants, eg carbon, ultramarine, chrome green and iron oxides. *Silicone* is added for easier application and improved staying power.

A suitable formula for mascara would be:-

Petroleum jelly	63%
Carbon black	20%
Cocoa butter	6%
Beeswax	4%
Spermaceti	4%
Cetyl alcohol	2%
Silicone + preservative	1%

Eye shadow and eye liner

The base for these preparations consists of an o/w emulsion similar to vanishing cream, or a mixture of waxes. Inorganic pigments are used as colorants.

Figure 16.7
Stages of eye make-up application
Right: highlighter
Below right: eye shadow
Below: eye liner

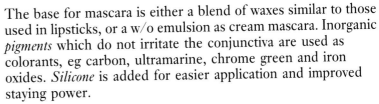

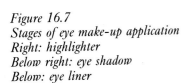

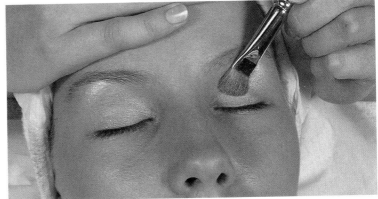

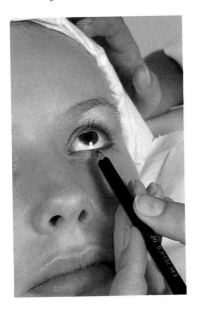

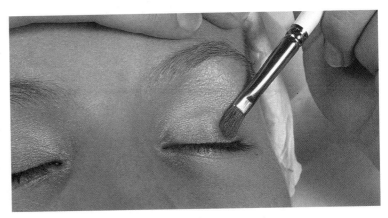

Eyebrow pencils

These pencils have a hard wax base which holds the inorganic pigments used as colorants.

Eyelash dye

Paratoluene diamine hair dyes oxidized by hydrogen peroxide are usually used to permanently colour eyelashes. As there is a high frequency of contact dermatitis due to these dyes, patch tests for sensitivity should be given 48 hours before the treatment, and great care exercised when applying the dye.

Cosmetic preparations for the nails

Nail cream

Like the rest of the skin keratin, nails lose water and become brittle, resulting in the disorder *Fragilitas unguium*. This is particularly likely to occur in older people, or where a person spends a lot of time with their hands in hot detergent solutions.

A cream for treating degreased dehydrated brittle nails is:

2% Salicyclic acid ointment	50%
Glycerin of starch	50%

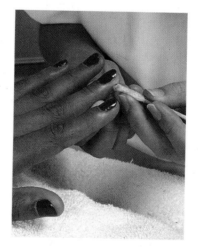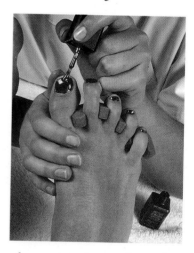

Figure 16.8
Application of nail lacquer
Right: to finger nails
Far right: to toe nails

Nail lacquer

Nail lacquer is a solution which, when painted onto the nails, leaves a film of *varnish* (enamel) when the solvent has evaporated. The film-former used in nail lacquer is *nitrocellulose* (produced from plant celluloses) which holds colorants well. As a nitrocellulose film does not adhere to the nail plate very firmly, and chips easily, an adhesive is added to the lacquer. *Formaldehyde resin* improves film adhesion and hardens the varnish, but can cause contact dermatitis in some people. Adding *silicone* will also toughen the varnish. *Phthalates* or *isopropyl myristate* are added as plasticisers to give the varnish elasticity and prevent flaking.

All these materials are dissolved in a mixture of volatile solvents which evaporate at slightly different rates. *Toluene* and ethyl, butyl and amyl *acetates* may be included in the solvent blend. These solvents are highly flammable so nail lacquer should be kept away from heat and flames, including lighted cigarettes. If inhaled, the solvents can damage the lungs. If the solvent evaporates too rapidly the lacquer will not flow well and brush marks will show in the varnish.

Coloured nail lacquer contains *inorganic pigments* or *lakes*, and *titanium dioxide* can be added to obtain paler shades. Adding *bentonite* helps to keep the pigments and lakes in suspension. Pearl nail lacquers commonly contain *Timicas* (mica flakes coated with titanium dioxide) or *bismuth oxychloride*. *Guanine* from fish scales may be used as an opaliser but is expensive.

Base coat

This is a clear lacquer which is applied to the nail and allowed to dry before brushing on coloured nail lacquer. Base coat contains a lower percentage of *nitrocellulose* and an increased percentage of *formaldehyde resin* to improve adhesion to the nail. It forms a harder varnish as less plasticiser is added. The coloured lacquer adheres more readily to this base coat of varnish than it does to the nail.

Cuticle remover

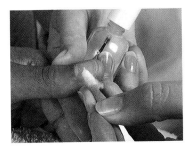

Figure 16.9
Application of cuticle remover

A 2% solution of the alkalis *sodium* or *potassium hydroxide* is caustic, and will soften the keratin of the cuticle by attacking its disulphide bonds. The cuticle can then be pushed back from the nail plate to expose the lunula of the nail more fully. Alkalis also remove sebum, so the skin round the base of the nail may become brittle and crack after using this preparation. A humectant such as *glycerol* is usually added to counteract its degreasing and dehydrating effect.

Less alkaline cuticle removers are available which contain *sodium phosphate* instead of sodium hydroxide. Sodium phosphate is the salt of a strong base and a weaker acid. It ionizes to form an alkaline solution, but the presence of the weak acid lowers the pH.

Liquid nail varnish remover

This preparation consists of a mixture of solvents which dissolve nail varnish readily, such as ethyl, butyl and amyl *acetates*. The mixture of solvents is not identical to that present in nail laquer, so the preparation cannot be used successfully to dilute thickened nail lacquer. These acetates are also fat solvents and remove sebum from the skin round the nail plate, so *lanolin* or *castor oil* are added to the preparation to counteract the degreasing effect. Nail varnish remover is flammable, and can damage the lungs if much is inhaled.

Nail hardener

This is a lacquer containing *formaldehyde resin* as the film-former so that the varnish adheres very firmly to the nail plate. This varnish helps to prevent soft nails chipping or peeling. Formaldehyde resin may cause contact dermatitis round the edges of the nail. It is therefore helpful if the cuticle and skin round the nails are protected by a film of *oil* before the nail hardener is applied.

Nail repairer

This preparation contains *nitrocellulose* and *formaldehyde resin* film-formers, together with fine suspended fibres of *rayon* or *nylon* which will reinforce the varnish. A *phthalate* plasticiser is added to keep the varnish flexible. The solvent is a blend of *toluene* and *ethyl acetate*. Several coats of this preparation are required to repair torn or damaged finger nails.

Nail white

Special pencils, containing a wax core in which *titanium dioxide* and *zinc oxide* are dispersed, are used to apply a film of white material below the translucent free edge of the nail.

Nail polish

To give shine to the nail and remove small irregularities, an abrasive powder or paste is applied and rubbed over the nail with a buffing pad. The frictional heat causes dilation of the blood capillaries below the nail. The best abrasive for this purpose is *stannic oxide*, which is mixed with *talc* to give slip. As stannic oxide is expensive, the cheaper precipitated *chalk* may be the abrasive ingredient.

Cosmetic preparations for black skin

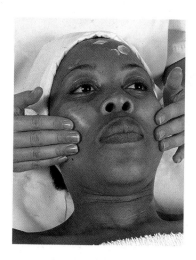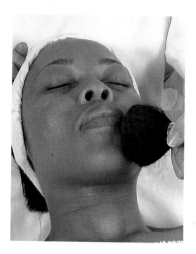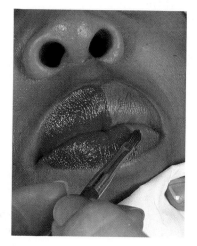

Skin bleach

Figure 16.10
Black skin
Above: moisturising
Above right: face powder application
Above far right: lipstick application

A skin bleach may be used by black women to lighten the complexion, so that its coloration is both paler and more even, and make-up has a greater impact. Skin bleaches containing *hydroquinone* are available, but only about 60% of treatments appear to give satisfactory results. A course of treatment requires two applications of the bleach daily for up to four months. The skin must not be exposed to sunlight over the treatment period.

Concentrations of hydroquinone above 2% are illegal in skin bleaches, but even at this low level hydroquinone can be a health hazard. It has been found to cause skin cancers or irreversible skin damage in some women. The permanent destruction of small groups of melanocytes commonly causes small white patches (vitiligo) on black skin.

Desquamators

These preparations are used on black skin to remove the outermost scaly layer of the stratum corneum, and leave a smoother less ashy surface for the application of make-up. The most suitable desquamators contain plant products, eg *oatmeal* granules.

Moisturising cream

As black skin though shiny is not oily, moisturising cream should be applied during the day as well as overnight, in preference to other types of cosmetic creams. The oil phase of the cream should consist of *plant* waxes and oils and fats such as cocoa butter, rather than mineral oils and glycerol which form a heavier film on the skin surface.

Cleansers

Highly degreasing cleansing lotions containing *ethanol* should not be used on black skins. Cleansing clay based face packs are effective and they also have a desquamating effect.

Foundation

White creams should not be used on black skins. A colourless *gel* base which will hold powder provides a suitable make-up foundation.

Face powder

Face powder should be composed of very fine particles of the usual inert powders with suitable colourants. Titanium dioxide or zinc oxide should not be present as these substances produce a greyish appearance on black skin.

Cosmetic preparations for the body

Massage cream

An emollient cream can be used to **lubricate** the skin during massage as an alternative to unscented mineral oil or talcum powder. The cream is usually a w/o emulsion with a high mineral oil content.

Talcum powder

This preparation is an **absorbent** powder which removes traces of water left on the skin after towel drying and absorbs sweat and sebum from the skin surface. Talcum powder also has **lubricating properties**, preventing skin surfaces from sticking together and allowing clothing to slide over the skin easily. It also provides lubrication for manual or electrical massage treatments.

For absorbency the powder contains precipitated *chalk, magnesium carbonate, silicon dioxide* or *kaolin. Talc* provides good lubrication, while *magnesium* and *zinc stearates* are necessary for skin adhesion. The talc used should be sterilized, and talcum powder should not be breathed in as it may cause lung damage.

A suitable formula for talcum powder would be:-

Sterilized talc	80%
Precipitated chalk	15%
Magnesium stearate	5%
+ perfume	

Foot powder

A foot powder has a *talcum powder* base containing *kaolin* for additional absorbency. Medicating agents may be added to protect against the fungal attack between the toes which causes athlete's foot, and bacterial breakdown of sweat causing hyperidrosis or bromidrosis. *Zinc undecenoate* is added as a fungicide, and *salicylic acid* reduces the bacterial activity which causes unpleasant foot odour.

Antiperspirant and deodorant preparations

Chemicals having these two effects on the skin are usually combined in a single preparation. It may be applied from an aerosol spray, a roll-on stick or as a cream, and is mainly used on the underarm area. In addition to *aluminium chlorhydrate* as the antiperspirant and *hexamine* as the deodorant, the preparation contains *silicone* to make it flow smoothly and dry quickly. Silicone also reduces any stinging sensation when the preparation is applied.

Artificial suntan lotion

Some of these lotions contain a brown *pigment* and when applied, their effect on the skin is entirely cosmetic as they give no protection against sunburn. They are difficult to apply sufficiently evenly to get uniform colouration, and the pigment is often unconvincing as a suntan.

Another type of artificial suntan lotion contains the colourless compound *dihydroxyacetone* as a 2.5% solution in an ethanol/water solvent. The dihydroxyacetone reacts with some of the keratin amino-acids to form a brown compound, so the tanning effect occurs gradually. This preparation can be used to disguise areas of skin where vitiligo occurs. Dihydroxyacetone may cause severe contact dermatitis in some people.

Suntanning pills

Suntanning pills containing *canthaxanthin* and *beta-carotein* have been available. They produce a tanning effect by colouring the subcutaneous fat. Although both the active ingredients of these pills are permitted food colourings, the pills have been found to cause eye damage and are being withdrawn. In no case should clients be persuaded to take suntanning pills containing canthaxanthin.

Sunburn lotion

Sunburn is treated by applying *calamine* lotion which is a suspension of *zinc carbonate* having a cooling effect on the skin. *Lacto-calamine* is a lotion containing 4% zinc carbonate, 5% witch-hazel and 0.2% phenol. The witch-hazel reduces skin inflammation, and the phenol acts as an anaesthetic to reduce the pain from sunburn, and prevents infection of the damaged skin. Soothing lotions of this type are known as palliatives.

Table 16.1
Summary of the characteristics of the major cosmetic ingredients

Name	Source or nature	Effect	Cosmetic use	Hazards
Acetone	Organic solvent	Degreaser	Nail varnish remover	Flammable
Almond oil	Fixed plant oil	Emollient	Warm oil mask	–
Aluminium chlorhydrate	Inorganic salt	Antiperspirant	Antiperspirant	Irritant
Amyl acetate	Organic solvent	–	Nail lacquer	Flammable
Ascorbic acid	Vitamin C	Antioxidant	Cosmetic creams	–
Azo dyes	From coal tar	Colourant	As lakes	Cross-sensitisers
Beeswax	Animal wax	Emollient	Creams; lipstick	–
Bentonite	Volcanic clay	Cleanser	Clay face pack	Tetanus spores
Calamine	Mineral salt	Coolant	Sunburn lotion	–
Calcium thioglycollate	Organic salt	Depilatory	Depilatories	Irritant
Carmine	Cochineal lake	Colourant	Rouge	Irritant
Carnauba wax	Plant wax	Emollient	Lipstick	–
Cetyl alcohol	Synthetic wax	Emollient	Emulsifier	–
Chalk	Mineral salt	Absorbent	Talcum powder	Dries the skin

Table 16.1 (cont)

Name	Source or nature	Effect	Cosmetic use	Hazards
Cocoa butter	Plant fat	Emollient	Creams	—
Dihydroxyacetone	Synthetic	Browns skin	Tanning lotion	Sensitiser
Essential oils	Volatile plant oil	Perfume	Perfumes	Sensitisers
Ethanol	Organic solvent	Astringent	Toners	Hardens skin
Formaldehyde resin	Synthetic resin	Hardens nail	Base coats	Irritant
Fuller's earth	Mineral clay	Cleanser	Astringent mask	Tetanus spores
Glycerol	From triglyceride	Humectant	Moisturisers	Dehydrating
Hexamine	Organic base	Antiseptic	Deodorants	—
Hydroquinone	Phenol derivative	Depigmentation	Skin bleach	Irritant; vitiligo
Inorganic pigments	Mineral ores	Colourant	Lipstick; mascara	—
Kaolin	Clay from quartz	Cleanser	Clay packs	Tetanus spores
Lactic acid	Sour milk	Astringent	Astringent mask	—
Lanolin	Sheep wool	Emollient	Hand cream	Sensitiser
Lauryl sulphates	Soapless detergent	Cleanser	Shampoo	Degreaser
Lecithin	Egg yolk lipid	Antioxidant	Creams	—
Liquid paraffin	Mineral oil	Emollient	Barrier cream	—
Magnesium stearate	Metallic soap	Lubricant	Talcum powder	—
Nitrocellulose	Plant celluloses	Varnish	Nail lacquer	—
Orange flower water	Essential oil	Astringent	Toners	—
Para-aminobenzoic acid	Organic acid	UVB filter	Sunscreens	Sensitiser
Paraffin wax	Mineral wax	Diaphoretic	Wax mask; depilatory	—
Paraben	Organic acid	Antiseptic	Preservative	Sensitiser

Table 16.1 (cont)

Name	Source or nature	Effect	Cosmetic use	Hazards
Phthalate	Ester	–	Plasticiser	Sensitiser
Polyvinyl acetate resin	Synthetic resin	Coating	Hydrocolloid mask	–
Propylene glycol	Organic alcohol	Humectant	Vanishing cream	–
Rice starch	From rice grains	Lubricant	Face powder	–
Salicylic acid	From willow bark	Desquamator	Desquamators	Irritant
Silicone	From sand	Lubricant	Lipstick; rouge	–
Sodium stearate	Hard soap	Cleanser	Toilet soap	–
Spermaceti	Animal wax	Emollient	Creams	–
Talc	Mineral	Lubricant	Skin powders	Tetanus spores
Titanium dioxide	Mineral	Opacifier	Powders; lipstick	–
Witch-hazel	Plant extract	Astringent	Toners	–
Zinc oxide	Mineral	Opacifier	Face powder; sunscreen	–
Zinc stearate	Metal soap	Lubricant	Talcum powder	–

Self-assessment questions

1 Distinguish between an emulsion and an emollient.

2 State the possible hazards associated with the following ingredients of cosmetic preparations:

(a) bentonite;
(b) lanolin;
(c) sodium hydroxide;
(d) amyl acetate.

3 Explain the reason for applying:

(a) base coat nail lacquer;
(b) talcum powder;
(c) a patch test.

4 List **four** components of nail lacquer, and explain the role of each component in the preparation.

5 In each case, state the effect on the skin of a cosmetic preparation containing:

(a) calcium thioglycollate;
(b) dihydroxyacetone;
(c) aluminium chlorhydrate;
(d) para-aminobenzoic acid.

6 State the source of the following components of cosmetic preparations:

(a) spermaceti;
(b) carbon black;
(c) talc;
(d) glycerol.

7 Distinguish between dyes, pigments and lakes. Which of these colourants would be most suitable for:

(a) mascara;   (b) blusher;
(c) lipstick?

8 For a mature dry skin, name a suitable type of:

(a) overnight cream;
(b) face mask;
(c) cleanser.

9 What is meant by:

(a) a diaphoretic;
(b) a humectant;
(c) a fixed oil;
(d) a perfume fixative?

10 Give the name of **one** ingredient in each case which gives the following properties to a face powder:

(a) skin adhesion;
(b) opacity;
(c) slip;
(d) sweat absorption.

APPENDIX I   *Anatomical terms*

Anterior or **Ventral**	Front side of the body. Palms of the hands are anterior
Posterior or **Dorsal**	Back or rear side of the body
Medial	Near the mid-line, ie a line running from the centre of the forehead to between the feet
Lateral	Further from the mid-line, ie at the sides
External	On the outside
Internal	On the inside
Superficial	Close to the external body surface but not actually on it
Deep	Further away from the surface lying underneath other structures
Proximal	Closest to the mid-line. In the case of the limbs, those parts nearest the trunk
Distal	Further from the mid-line. In the case of the limbs, those parts lying furthest away from the trunk
Superior	Closer to the head
Inferior	Further away from the head

APPENDIX II

Terms used in the description of bones

Condyle

A large projection, either convex or concave, at the end of a bone at the joint, eg the occipital condyles on the occipital bone at the base of the skull

Foramen

A round opening in a bone through which blood vessels, nerves, or ligaments can pass, eg a foramen occurs in each transverse process of a cervical vertebra for the vertebral artery and vein

Head

A rounded projection at the end of a bone, eg the head of the femur where it articulates with the pelvis

Process

A projection from a bone, eg the transverse processes project laterally from the centrum of a vertebra

Spine

A sharp slender process projecting from a bone, eg the neural spine is a posterior projection from the centrum of a vertebra, and the scapula has a ridge-like posterior spine

Sulcus

A groove along a bone in which a blood vessel, nerve, or tendon lies, eg the sulcus on the head of the humerus called the bicipital groove carries the tendon of the long head of the biceps muscle

Tubercle

A small rounded process, eg the tubercle on each rib which articulates with a transverse process of a vertebra

Tuberosity

A large rounded roughened area on a bone, eg the ischial tuberosity on the posterior region of the pelvis where the quadratus femoris muscle has its origin

BIBLIOGRAPHY

Bembridge, R.A., *Beauty Therapy Science*, Longman, 1985

Harvard, C.W.H. (ed.), *Black's Medical Dictionary*, 35th edn., A. & C. Black, 1987

Gersh, S. & Gersh, I.G., *The Biology of Women*, Junction Books, 1981

Gibney, M.J., *Nutrition, Diet and Health*, Cambridge University Press, 1986

Gray, H., *Gray's Anatomy*, 36th edn., R. Warwick & P.L. Williams (eds.), Churchill Livingstone, 1980

Hibbott, H.W., *Handbook of Cosmetic Science*, Pergamon Press, 1963

Hodgson, G., 'The hazards of beauty culture', *The Practitioner*, vol. 189, 1962. pp. 667–673 and pp. 778–787

Martindale, W., *The Extra Pharmacopoeia*, 28th edn., The Pharmaceutica Press, 1982

Pierantoni, H., 'Essential notions about black skin', *Les Nouvelles Esthetiques*, Paris, 1977

Rogers, A.W., *Cells and Tissues*, Academic Press, 1983

Rounce, J., *Science for the Beauty Therapist*, Stanley Thornes, 1983

Rowett, H.G.Q., *Basic Anatomy and Physiology*, 2nd edn., John Murray, 1973

Samman, P.D. & Fenton, D.A., *The Nails in Disease*, 4th edn., Heinemann, 1986

Simpkins, J. & Williams, J.I., *Biology of the Cell, Mammal, and Flowering Plant*, Mills & Boon, 1980

Stoppard, M., *Everywoman's Life Guide*, Macdonald & Co, 1982

Tortora, G.J. & Anagnostakos, N.P., *Principles of Anatomy and Physiology*, 3rd edn., Harper & Row, 1981

Thompson, C.W., *Manual of Structural Kinesiology*, 11th edn., C.V. Mosby Co., 1989

Young, A., *Practical Cosmetic Science*, Mills & Boon, 1972

Longer questions

1 (a) By means of a diagram **only**, describe a ring main circuit.
   (b) List **three** advantages of this type of circuit compared with older methods of wiring.
   (c) State where you would find the following structures in a ring main circuit:
       (i)   a conductor;
       (ii) a device to prevent electric shock;
       (iii) a 30 amp circuit breaker;
       (iv) a brown insulating cover.

2 (a) State the position, origin and insertion of the following muscles:
       (i)   Brachialis;
       (ii) Brachioradialis;
       (iii) Triceps brachii.
   (b) Give a labelled diagram of the joint where movement occurs due to the action of these three muscles.
   (c) Name the type of movement each muscle produces at the joint.

3 (i) Draw up a table to show the source, chemical nature and cosmetic use of the following cosmetic ingredients:
       (a) bentonite;
       (b) lanolin;
       (c) glycerol;
       (d) ethyl acetate;
       (e) para-aminobenzoic acid;
       (f) hydroquinone;
       (g) aluminium chlorhydrate.

   (ii) For each substance, explain the possible hazards of its use.

4 (a) Draw a simple labelled diagram of a section through the female breast.
   (b) Describe the influence of hormones on:
       (i) the development of the breast;
       (ii) lactation.

5 (a) Compare the chemical structure of starch and protein molecules.
   (b) Describe the digestion of starch and protein in the human alimentary canal, naming the region, digestive juices, enzymes and end products involved in each case.
   (c) What are the main uses of dietary starch and protein in the body's metabolism?

6 (a) Describe one appliance producing infra-red radiation and one producing ultra-violet radiation which are used in a beauty therapy salon.
   (b) Indicate any precautions which should be taken when using these appliances to treat a client.
   (c) Name any contra-indications associated with the use of these appliances.

7 (a) By means of a fully labelled diagram **only**, describe the blood supply to the liver.
   (b) Draw up a table to indicate the differences in structure and function of an artery and a vein.
   (c) List the functions of each of the following blood components:
       (i)   erythrocytes;
       (ii) leucocytes;
       (iii) thrombocytes;
       (iv) plasma proteins.

8 Give a diagram and explain the action of each of the following components of the nervous system:
   (a) a synapse;
   (b) a motor neuron
   (c) a reflex arc;
   (d) the fifth cranial nerve.

9 (a) Draw a simple labelled diagram of a longitudinal section through a finger nail.
   (b) Describe the effects on the nail of the following diseases or disorders:
       (i)   Pterygium unguium;
       (ii) Onycholysis;
       (iii) Agnail;
       (iv) Paronychia.
   (c) List the constituents of a nail lacquer and explain the function of each in this cosmetic preparation.

10 (a) Describe each of the following bones in terms of its type, position and main role in the body:
       (i)   femur;
       (ii) scapula;
       (iii) thoracic vertebra;
       (iv) patella;
       (v)   calcaneum.
   (b) Draw a clear labelled diagram of a thoracic vertebra.

INDEX